# Psychologically Informed Physiotherapy

## EMBEDDING PSYCHOSOCIAL PERSPECTIVES WITHIN CLINICAL MANAGEMENT

T0275469

For Elsevier

*Senior Content Strategist:* Rita Demetriou-Swanwick
*Content Development Specialist:* Nicola Lally
*Project Manager:* Janish Ashwin Paul
*Designer:* Christian Bilbow
*Illustration Manager:* Brett MacNaughton
*Illustrator:* Marie Dean

# Psychologically Informed Physiotherapy

## EMBEDDING PSYCHOSOCIAL PERSPECTIVES WITHIN CLINICAL MANAGEMENT

*Edited by*

**STUART PORTER, PhD, BSc(Hons), PGCAP, FHEA, Grad Dip Phys, MHS**
*Lecturer, University of Salford, UK*
*Visiting Lecturer, Corpus Christi Cambridge, UK*
*External Examiner, University of Liverpool, UK*

*Foreword by*

**MR ROBERTO MARTINEZ**
*Manager, Physiotherapist and Belgium National Football Team Manager*

**ELSEVIER**

Edinburgh  London  New York  Oxford  Philadelphia  St Louis  Sydney  Toronto  2017

# ELSEVIER

ISBN 978-0-7020-6817-1

**Notices**

Knowledge and best practice in this field are constantly changing. As new research and experience broaden our understanding, changes in research methods, professional practices, or medical treatment may become necessary.

Practitioners and researchers must always rely on their own experience and knowledge in evaluating and using any information, methods, compounds or experiments described herein. In using such information or methods they should be mindful of their own safety and the safety of others, including parties for whom they have a professional responsibility.

With respect to any drug or pharmaceutical products identified, readers are advised to check the most current information provided (i) on procedures featured or (ii) by the manufacturer of each product to be administered, to verify the recommended dose or formula, the method and duration of administration and contraindications. It is the responsibility of practitioners, relying on their own experience and knowledge of their patients, to make diagnoses, to determine dosages and the best treatment for each individual patient, and to take all appropriate safety precautions.

To the fullest extent of the law, neither the publisher nor the authors, contributors or editors assume any liability for any injury and/or damage to persons or property as a matter of products liability, negligence or otherwise, or from any use or operation of any methods, products, instructions or ideas contained in the material herein.

*The Publisher*

your source for books, journals and multimedia in the health sciences

**www.elsevierhealth.com**

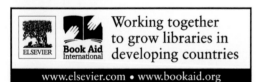

Working together to grow libraries in developing countries

www.elsevier.com • www.bookaid.org

The publisher's policy is to use paper manufactured from sustainable forests

Printed in Great Britain
Last digit is the print number: 10 9 8 7 6 5 4 3

# CONTENTS

# FOREWORD

It was back in 1994 that I got my full degree in Physiotherapy from the University of Zaragoza, Spain. At that point, I was almost obsessed with every possible injury or disease and the perfect treatment that I could find or develop to start helping and curing others. How wrong I was with that approach. It is now, after nearly 30 years of a professional career in football, that I understand that treating just the injury only delays future problems. It does not allow you as a medical practitioner to make a difference in people's health and lives. The true difference is made by treating the **human being** and not the **punctual injury or disease**.

Under Stuart Porter's editorship, this new book has accumulated different angles and experts giving a clear message in different ways. Treating the injury instead of treating the individual becomes a medical gamble. On the other hand, treating the individual will allow us to affect patient behaviour and ultimately improve his or her well-being and health state for the future. *Psychologically Informed Physiotherapy* will inspire any reader to consider a holistic care and approach where psychological strategies will become essential in any treatment.

Something that becomes apparent after working with elite footballers at Premier League or international level is that the main difference between good and exceptional players is in their brain and mental focus on their bodies. The power of the brain is clearly very much unknown as to the full influence that it can have upon our general condition and health or body in general, which makes a bigger need to treat the person and understand the person before you can have a total effect against a disease or injury. Understanding the mental state, character and mood of the patient will give clear clues for the successful outcome of medical care.

Stuart and his team have found a powerful way to focus and question the **psychological perspectives** in every area of medical care; from **holistic treatment** to relating to the patient and understanding the person and social influences.

This book will inspire every reader to search for a holistic approach in medical care and consider using different ways to manage the patient depending on the patient's personality, mind set and moment in their lives in order to cure and make the treatment totally effective for the needs of the patient.

This book will allow any medical care practitioner to master their own method of work towards the patient.

Inspiring work.

*Roberto Martinez*
Belgium Head Coach

# PREFACE

I have always liked quotes, and producing a new textbook has given me the opportunity to find some great ones. I therefore begin and end this preface with a quote. I trust that you will see its relevance to this book on psychologically informed physiotherapy.

*'It is far more important to know what person the disease has than what disease the person has.'*

*-Hippocrates*

As this book was nearing its final stages, so was the life of my father Brian who passed away on 20th October 2015. In an ironic turn of fate my father was cared for on the ward on which I worked for many years as a senior orthopaedic physiotherapist. I take no pride in saying that I had begun to view health care rather cynically, as a production line with little time to acknowledge the importance of the whole patient. A plethora of recent health care scandals in the UK merely fuelled my beliefs and as scandals and other stories flooded the media with worrying regularity they always seemed to have their genesis in failures to acknowledge the patient's psychological needs and the need to treat people holistically. Furthermore, as a lecturer, although I always tagged holistic care on to every essay or book chapter that I have ever written and every lecture that I delivered, in reality I do not think that I ever gave it the attention that it truly deserved.

As I sat with my father and watched the staff care for him, many of whom I had taught as students it quickly became apparent that my cynicism had been massively misplaced and that the quality of his care was largely as a result of the physiotherapists' acknowledgement of my father as a human being and not a patient with cancer, similarly viewing his family as integral parts of the process. What made the physiotherapists outstanding was not their knowledge of anatomy, rather it was their understanding of my father as a man that truly made the difference to his care. As a positivist with a passion for science, astronomy, biology and other 'hard data' it is now time for me to cast the net wider to acknowledge the role of psychology within physiotherapy practice.

To this end a group of international experts and clinicians have come together to provide a thorough and innovative text on the importance of psychology within physiotherapy. I am truly grateful to all of my colleagues for their efforts on what has been a new challenge for us all.

> *'If the only tool you have is a hammer, you tend to see every problem as a nail.'*
>
> *Abraham Maslow 1908–1970*

If this book gives the physiotherapist one more tool that they can use for the good of their patients then we have succeeded.

**Stuart Porter,** February 2016

# DEDICATION

I dedicate this book to Angela Kay (1966–2015) who always saw the good in everyone and who I was proud to call my friend.

# ACKNOWLEDGEMENTS

With thanks to Livie Orchard, Rachel Wilkinson, Mehrdad Shamali, Sana Asghar, Rachel Amelot, Rachael Kenny and Dr Robert Morris for posing for the photographs in the book.

This is the eighth book to bear my name and once again I thank Elsevier publishers for their faith in me and the Authors who give their time and immense knowledge so kindly when they have immense pressures of their own.

# CONTRIBUTORS

HELEN CARRUTHERS, MSc, BSc(Hons), PGCert, HECert
Lecturer in Physiotherapy, School of Health Sciences, University of Salford, UK

ALAN CHAMBERLAIN, MA, PgDPE, MCSP, RGN, HCPC, FHEA
Senior Lecturer in Physiotherapy, Department of Health, Psychology and Social Studies, University of Cumbria, UK

GRAHAM COPNELL, PhD, MSc, BSc(Hons), PGCert Ed
Senior Lecturer in Professional Health Sciences, Physiotherapy and Podiatry, School of Health, Sport and Bioscience, University of East London, UK

KATHERINE E CROOK, MA, BA(Hons), PGCE, BSc(Hons)
Assistant Lecturer, University of Coventry, UK

ANDREW EVANS, PhD, MSc, BSc(Hons), CSci, FHEA
Lecturer in Sport Psychology, Directorate of Sport, Exercise and Physiotherapy, Department of Health Sciences, Salford University, Salford, UK

SUSAN GREENHALGH, PhD, MA, GradDipPhys, FCSP
Consultant Physiotherapist, Royal Bolton Hospital, UK

JENNIFER E GREEN-WILSON, PT, MBA, EdD
Principal/Consultant, Institute for Business Literacy & Leadership, Rochester, New York, USA
Affiliate Faculty
University of Alabama at Birmingham (UAB), Birmingham, Alabama, USA
University of Vermont (UVM), Burlington, Vermont, USA

LOUISE HENSTOCK, MSc, BSc(Hons), BSc(Hons), PGCert, FHEA
Lecturer in Physiotherapy, School of Health Sciences, University of Salford, UK

ANTHONY HICKEY, PhD
Lecturer in Counselling/Psychotherapy/Research Methods, School of Health Sciences, University of Salford, UK

Lester E JONES, MScMed(PM)
Physiotherapist, Pain Educator empoweREHAB Victoria Pain Specialists
PhD Candidate, La Trobe University, Melbourne, Australia

ANDREW MITCHELL, MSc, BSc(Hons)
Sports Physiotherapist, Abu Dhabi Knee and Sports Medicine Centre, Health Point Hospital, Abu Dhabi, United Arab Emirates

CHRISTINF PARKER, MSc, PGCHEPR, FHEA

Senior Lecturer, School of Health Sciences, University of Salford, UK

ALEC RICKARD, MSc, BSc(Hons), FHEA

Programme Leader, BSc(Hons) Physiotherapy, School of Health Professions, Plymouth University, Plymouth, UK

JAMES SELFE, DSc, PhD, MA, GradDipPhys, FCSP

Professor of Physiotherapy, Department of Health Professions, Faculty of Health, Psychology and Social Care, Manchester Metropolitan University, UK

# PROFESSIONALISM AND THE PSYCHOLOGY OF PROFESSIONAL IDENTITY IN HEALTH CARE

GRAHAM COPNELL

## CHAPTER CONTENTS

One cannot produce a book on psychologically informed physiotherapy without first exploring what it means to actually be a professional and how this affects our client contact. The aim of this chapter is to provide a critical overview of the theoretical and empirical literature charting contemporary interpretations of the work of health care professions. This chapter is divided into two sections. Section one introduces key themes and debates regarding the sociology of the professions, included professional identity and power. Building upon this, section two considers the effect of marketization on health care professionals' roles and boundaries and considers future challenges with regards to professionalism, professional identity and autonomy.

Researchers and public sector professionals are interested in and concerned about how changes in health care policy affect the working practices, roles and identities of public sector professionals. Changes in how professionals involved in the delivery of health care are trained and regulated, and how they structure their practice have contributed to these concerns (Department of Health, 2000b; 2000c).

An expansion of the concept of governance within the public sector has created a plurality of actors and organizations involved in the development, regulation and control of

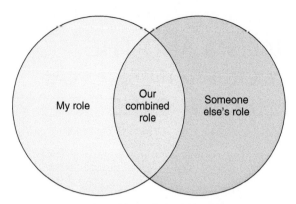

FIGURE 1.1 ■ Blurred boundaries in health care.

professional practice (Newman, 2006). Referring specifically to health care, there have also been changes to where health professionals deliver services with a move away from the traditional hospital provision to services being provided in a number of contexts. In addition to this, there has been an increase in the provision of NHS services by the voluntary and private sectors.

The view that changes in what professionals do, how they are regulated and how they are trained somehow affects their professional identity, roles and boundaries has been put forward by Hanlon (2000). What it means to be and act like a member of a specific profession is closely linked to the day-to-day activities an individual is involved in (Davis, 2002; Freidson, 1970; Hafferty and Light, 1995; Wenger, 1998), the language they use (Apker and Eggly, 2004; Lingard et al., 2002; Niemi and Paasivaara, 2007), their education and where they work (Baxter and Brumfitt, 2008). This final point is of particular interest when one considers the emphasis on services being delivered outside of the 'traditional' hospital setting, as this raises the question of context and its relationship to professional identity roles and boundaries.

There is a growing body of literature focusing on how public sector professionals are responding to changes in their work and working practices. Considerable attention has been paid to teaching and social work. With regards to health care professionals, current research addressing the changes outlined – and more specifically the relationship of context to roles and boundaries – has almost exclusively focused on doctors and nurses. Although forming a significant proportion of the health workforce, there has been very little attention given to how the changes outlined are affecting allied health professionals with regards to their roles and boundaries and professional identities. Although sparse, research from the UK and Canada has generally focused on roles, boundaries and power relationships, whereas research originating from the United States has focused on organizational factors affecting professions (Adams, 2014).

## KEY THEMES AND DEBATES REGARDING THE SOCIOLOGY OF THE PROFESSIONS

### Professions as a Distinct Group

Sociologists interested in the study of professions as a distinct aspect of the division of labour have focused on those occupations claiming to be professions, or those occupations perceived by researchers and academics to be professions (Bourdieu and Wacquant, 1992; Freidson, 1994). In contrast, the branch of sociology concerned with work and occupations focuses on the division of labour in the more general sense, for example incorporating concepts of social class and inequality (White, 2006). This is not to suggest that

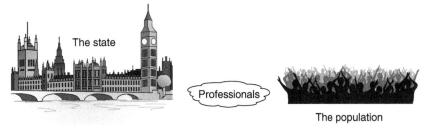

FIGURE 1.2 ■ Durkheims view of the role of a professional.

these concepts have not been addressed within the study of the professions, however, the literature exploring the role of professions as a distinct subset of occupations has adopted more varied and eclectic lines of enquiry. Analysis focusing on the relatively small subset of these occupations, the professions, has generated a far greater number of often conflicting interpretations, reflecting a number of different sociological paradigms. Professions have attracted a great deal of attention from sociologists mainly because of the higher rewards they receive and their apparent homogeneity with regards to empirical investigation (Bourdieu and Wacquant, 1992). However, viewing professions as a specific subset of occupational groups has tended to lead sociologists to either define the boundaries or factors indicative of that subset or outline the processes occupations move through in order to be classified within the subset (MacDonald, 1995). In addition to this, a focus on more macro theories of professions has contributed to the creation of a concept which is highly abstract, not easily lending itself to empirical research (Larson, 1990). The delineation of professions as an analytical subset of occupations can be extended when one considers the division between public sector and private sector

professions (Buelens and Van den Broeck, 2007). Contrasts have been made between professionals working in the public and private sector leading to the suggestion that a difference in values and beliefs exists between the two. Professionals working in the public sector are less committed to their organization, displaying more allegiance to their profession (Anderson 2009; Franco et al., 2002). This final point is of importance when we consider the role of health care professionals within contemporary health care (Adams, 2014).

## Classifying Occupations as Professions

Classifying occupations as professions has generated a great deal of literature for both its support and its criticism. Often referred to as the trait model of professions, this line of enquiry has focused on identifying those qualities which mark out an occupational group as a profession (Carr-Saunders and Wilson, 1933). There has, and continues to be, a great deal of literature highlighting, but also questioning, the key attributes which occupations identified as professions possess (Davis, 2002). There also appears to be little agreement on exactly which traits should be included to account for all professions (Moloney, 1986).

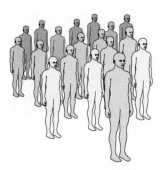

FIGURE 1.3 ■ Are physiotherapists and other professionals emotionally detached, neutral and somehow apart from 'ordinary people'? – discuss ...

The medical profession is often regarded as one of the prototypical professions possessing all of the desired attributes (Sullivan, 2000). Core characteristics such as practice autonomy, altruism, a defined body of knowledge and skills, control over how these are created (normally through prolonged education and eventual certification), defined ethics and scope of practice and control over access are often used to distinguish occupations as professions (Hoyle and John, 1995). Those professions allied, or seen as subsidiary to medicine (for example, physiotherapy), have been labelled as 'semi-professional' (Boyce, 1993; 2006; Etzioni, 1969), in that they fall short of the ideal (Burrage and Torstendahl, 1990). This has led a number of professions involved in the delivery of health care to attempt to emulate the professional ideal of medicine, often creating a tension between what they actually do when compared to what they (the profession) feel they should be doing (Mazhindu, 2003; Scholes, 2008).

Through its control of hospitals, the medical profession was, until relatively recently, able to structure and control the division of labour in health care. This meant in some cases controlling the knowledge base and activities of other professions (Ackroyd, 1996; Larkin, 1988; Miles-Tapping, 1985). The greater emphasis placed on primary as opposed to secondary care, in addition to challenges to medicine's control over how health services are delivered in the hospital setting, have led some authors to suggest that this once archetypal profession is also failing to live up to the ideal (Thistlethwaite and Spencer, 2008). As discussed in the second section of this chapter, changes in the delivery of health care have provided opportunities for the 'semi-professions' to expand and diversify their roles and provide services often only associated with medicine (Daker-White et al 1999; Dawson and Ghazi, 2004).

One of the key criticisms of the trait model as a means of structuring enquiry into the sociology of the professions is that the attributes identified and listed above are often seen as a given (MacDonald, 1995). To suggest that those occupations, either self-labelled or externally labelled as professions do not exhibit shared characteristics would be naïve. However, to suggest that such characteristics are the defining attributes of a profession would be to play into the hands of one social group to the detriment of another (Larson, 1990). This argument is supported by Larkin (1988), suggesting that medicine was (is) able to dominate paramedical professions, by the virtue of its position within society, a status reinforced to some degree by sociologists in the way they define medicine as the ideal profession. Taking this stance, a criticism of the trait model of professions is the potential for members of professions to use such explanations in order to justify, as opposed to explain, their role in society. Another criticism

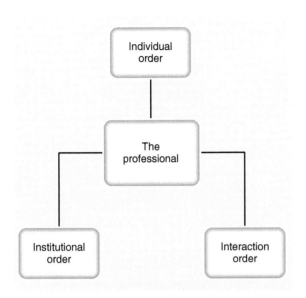

FIGURE 1.4 ■ Jenkins (2004) and identity.

is that there seems to be very little agreement on exactly which traits should be present (Moloney, 1986). The latter unfortunately still appears to be the case within the literature concerning professions, with a number of authors listing a variety of traits which they feel applies to the professions they are investigating (Chaska, 1990; Moloney, 1986; Sparkes, 2002). With regards to the first criticism a defence can be found in the functionalist origins of the trait model. Johnson (1972, p. 23) has stated that within functionalist classifications of occupations as professions:

> 'There is no attempt to present an exhaustive list of "traits"; rather the components of the model are limited to those elements which are said to have functional relevance for society as a whole or to the professional-client relationship.'

Durkheim (2002) viewed professions as a 'buffer', between the state and the general population.

The development of professions from a functionalist perspective therefore is regarded as an essential element in the development of industrialized societies. Professions serve society by acting as a medium between the laissez-faire ideologies of individualism and state collectivism (Johnson, 1972, p. 12). The traits associated with professions such as altruism and ethics give a sense of neutrality, setting professions apart from other occupations. Based on this, the status and perceived privileges associated with profession are justified. This explanation as to why industrial society needs professions and the roles they play within society has been criticized heavily over the past 40 years. Recently, Lunt (2008) has argued that the development of a litigation and blame orientated society has brought into question the neutrality of the professions, this being fuelled by a number of cases where professionals have been shown to be misusing their positions (Bolsin, 1998). Traits which were seen to be of importance to professional practice at the start of the twentieth century are being re-interpreted and restructured in order to fit within institutional and organizational expectations (Baxter, 2011). Empirically this is demonstrated in the work of Goode and Greatbatch (2005) who, when investigating nurses and call-centre workers in NHS direct, found that nurses no longer performed the role of buffer between the client and state, this role being adopted by the call-centre workers. Nurses, it appeared, had adopted the discourse of management and governance. This change in roles could be contributing to what Scholes (2008) has described as a crisis in the professional identity of nurses and has in part stimulated the current interest in professional identities,

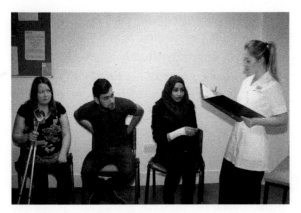

FIGURE 1.5 ■ Patient choice – here to stay and a driver for change in our profession?

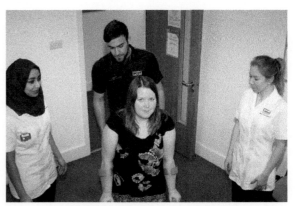

FIGURE 1.6 ■ Patient centred care – fact or fiction?

roles and boundaries discussed in the latter half of this chapter.

Although criticized by a number of authors (Evetts, 2011; Freidson, 1994; Hugman, 1991; MacDonald, 1995; Saks, 1996), functionalist theory still persists in the writings concerning professional development and the relationship between professions and external bodies such as the state or client (Foster and Wilding, 2000; Sparkes, 2002). Functionalist theory and trait classifications do offer useful explanations as to the relationship between professions and the state and provide insight into explaining how individual professionals may see themselves (Adams, 2014; Carmel, 2006; Evetts, 2011; Freidson, 1994; Mazhindu, 2003).

As indicated, the use of such models as a guide to empirical research has been questioned. Of major concern is the fact that both the trait model of occupational classification and the functionalist explanations of the role of professionals within society fail to recognize the temporal and contextual nature of the concepts of professional and profession/s (Freidson, 1994).

## Professions as Processes

Taking a more interactionist perspective and mainly drawing on the work of the social theorist Max Weber (Turner, 2006), a number of authors have proposed models suggesting that the attributes described by the trait approach and rationalized through functionalist writings, act primarily as a means of maintaining and legitimising the work of professionals. The characteristics often associated with professions serve only to protect their roles and maintain monopolies over certain areas of the labour market. Concepts such as the professional project (Larson, 1977), jurisdiction and conflict (Abbott, 1988) and social/market closure (Witz, 2003) have been used to describe how professionals seek first to establish themselves in the labour market and then maintain their privileged position. These more critical approaches to the sociology of the professions introduce the concept of competition and rivalry between professions as they strive to maintain and control their work (Abbott, 1988). As indicated, these models of professionalization (a term emphasizing processes as opposed to functions) draw largely from an interactionist perspective and demonstrate a shift from what professions are to what they do; this is significant in that it introduces the concept of social action (Burrage et al., 1990). From an empirical perspective, viewing professions as professionalization, where emphasis is given to social processes, moves the focus of investigation towards a more exploratory as opposed to descriptive enterprise. In the professional project, Larson (1977), focusing on the medical profession, extended the early work of Freidson (1970) by suggesting that through the development of specialist knowledge professions are able to justify and control their position within society. Larson's proposition, drawing on the work of Weber, is that through the development of specialized knowledge and collective action, professions place themselves in a position in which they can control access to this knowledge or at least be in a position which allows them to bargain with their patrons (eg, the state, employer or client) regarding access. Larson on the whole comments from a macro perspective generally omitting the content of professional activities over their form. Taking this into consideration, however, a number of authors have used Larson's work as a means of structuring empirical research (Edmunds and Calnan, 2001; MacDonald, 1984; 1995).

MacDonald (1995) champions Larson's work suggesting that it offers 'considerable analytical power' (MacDonald 1995, p. 34). Adapting the work of Larson, MacDonald (1995) suggested an analytical framework incorporating the notions of the professional project, but placed more emphasis on the role of the state, or more precisely the political culture, a key point raised by Johnson (1972).

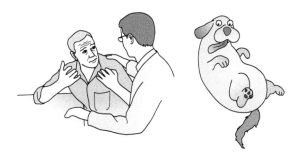

FIGURE 1.7 ■ Patient centred care – have we gone too far? Is the tail now wagging the dog?

The battle for, and maintenance (Witz, 2003) of, jurisdiction (Abbott, 1988) are also acknowledged by MacDonald. Finally, and of significance from both a theoretical and empirical view, is the importance placed on how individual professions see their roles. Extending Halliday's (1985) point that professions are not isolated groups with the sole aim of promoting their own agenda, consideration is given to the idea that professions and individual professionals have their client's interest at heart. It is made clear, however, that an emphasis on such traits as altruism and personal ethics is not a return to a trait model of identifying professional practice; rather such characteristics are essential in order for professions to persuade both their clients and their patrons of their unique place in society. MacDonald integrates the neo-Weberian perspectives developed by Larson and Abbott, but views them still as separate entities in his analysis; as a result he reinforces the concepts of closure, jurisdiction and the professional project without really advancing them. Again such a macro analytical perspective of professional work fails to acknowledge individuals and their often complex, contextually bound interrelationships. MacDonald clearly adds to the empirical foundations for

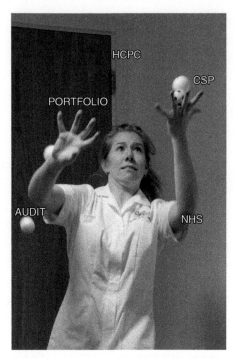

FIGURE 1.8 ■ Juggling our professional commitments.

investigating professionalization; however, his focus on the macro elements distracts from the local negotiations individual professionals are involved in, in their day-to-day work (Wenger, 1998).

Although not acknowledging Larson's work, Abbott (1988) builds on her basic propositions with regards to the idea of professions positioning themselves in the market. A key aspect of Abbott's work is the importance he places on the exclusivity of professional work leading him to suggest that:

'The central phenomenon of professional life is the link between a profession and its work, a link I shall call jurisdiction. To analyse professional development is to analyse how this link is created in work, how it is anchored in formal and informal social structure and how the interplay of jurisdictional links

between the professions determines the history of the individual professions themselves.'

*Abbott, 1988, p. 20*

Empirically, Abbott attempted to move from a micro perspective of observing what professionals do in practice, to the formulation of theory in which he terms the system of the professions. In critiquing Abbott's work, MacDonald (1995) has argued that, although reflecting Weberian theory, Abbott fails to recognize this in his work. Although the move from micro to macro has been criticized (Freidson, 1994), this focus on individuals and their day-to-day actions has allowed researchers to move beyond the more dominant sociological theories and explore professional practice from a more ethnographic perspective.

With regards to allied health professions, the work of Richard Hugman (1991) offers some useful insight into the professionalization of the caring professions. Of importance in Hugman's analysis is the concept of care and its relationship to power. Due to the content of their work, Hugman distinguishes nursing, the allied health professions and social workers, as being fundamentally different from other professions, for example, the medical or legal professions. Hugman acknowledges that all professions care about their work and in doing so accepts, to a degree, elements of the functionalist interpretations of professions. Extending this, however, Hugman argues that in contrast to professionals in medicine, who are seen as defining their work through rational scientific impartiality, nursing, the allied health professions and social work define their work through their relationship to patients. In addition to caring about their work, nurses, allied health professions and social workers, care for their patients (Hugman, 1991, p. 11). In their work as caring professionals, nurses, allied health professionals and social workers adopt roles and carry out tasks which are more accessible to the general public and as a result are seen as less expert. The value placed on these tasks is thus diminished. In charting the professionalization of the semi-professions, Hugman argues that the development (or lack of) of nursing, the allied health professions and social work as professions is reflective of the power relations between professions and wider social processes of gender and race.

The notion of interprofessional competition and jurisdiction is one which has attracted considerable attention (Adams, 2004; 2014; Borthwick, 2000; Edmunds and Calnan, 2001). An example of this with regards to health care professionals can be found in the work of Adams (2004). Investigating the apparent conflict between dentists and dental hygienists in Canada, Adams (2004) draws on Larson's work in order to provide an empirical frame of reference for her analysis. Adams argues that, through aspects of governance and the ideology of marketization, professionals are losing their bargaining power with both the state and the public, an assertion which has been put forward by a number of authors (Ackroyd, 1996; Foster and Wilding, 2000; Scourfield, 2006). Focusing specifically on allied health professions (Podiatry) Borthwick (2000) utilized the concept of jurisdiction as a frame of reference in his research on the development of podiatric surgery in the UK. Adopting a qualitative methodology using primarily interviews, Borthwick describes the strategies

employed by podiatrists in their attempts to gain jurisdiction over surgery in the foot and ankle and those used by orthopaedic surgeons in their attempt to retain their jurisdiction. Interestingly, Borthwick suggests that changes in the way health services are being commissioned and provided, with more emphasis on primary care, allowed podiatrists to encroach on the work of orthopaedic surgeons. The interrelationship between professions and the influence of changes in health care policy has also been highlighted by Edmunds and Calnan (2001). Focusing on the interactions between pharmacists and general practitioners (GPs), Edmunds and Calnan (2001) investigated the possible reasons for pharmacists wanting to expand their jurisdiction with regards to dispensing medications and the resistance provided by GPs. Using a telephone interview based qualitative approach, the authors suggested that, although the majority of pharmacists wished to extend their practice, they struggled with the concepts of entrepreneurialism and altruism, often seeing themselves as business people by the fact that they 'ran a shop'. From this snapshot of the literature it seems apparent that the local negotiations regarding professional jurisdiction and boundaries vary according to the professions involved and the contexts in which they work, as well as the profession's perceived identity and status.

What seems apparent from the sociological literature reviewed so far is that a key concept of the professions is the immeasurability of, and personal involvement in, their work. The concept of immeasurability has led a number of writers to question the role of professions in contemporary society where greater value is placed on choice, transparency and the value of money (Hanlon 1998; Southon and Braithwaite, 1998).

## Power and Professions

One concept in particular, which has influenced sociological thinking around professional relationships, is power (Johnson, 1972; Scott, 2001). Attributes such as autonomy and a high level of education and control of knowledge place professions in a position within society of relative power. Abbott's (1988) notion of jurisdiction and interprofessional conflict, Witz's (2003) work looking at professions in relation to the concept of patriarchy and Hugman's (1991) analysis of the caring professions are clear examples of where power forms a central concept. As a concept power, has been interpreted in a number of ways. Writers who have adopted a mainly Weberian stance with regards to professional practice on the whole appear to view power as the ability of groups within a society to secure access to and control over critical social resources (Poggi, 2006). In the case of professionals, examples of these resources would be knowledge and jurisdiction over practice. Although influential, this perception of power does not fully address the individual and individual interactions; nor does it take into consideration the points identified above, with regards to identity formation as an element of professionalization. An alternative to the Weberian concept of power can be found in the writings of Michael Mann (1986) and his concept of ideological power. Mann suggests that individuals and social groups create cognitive and normative frameworks in order to structure and give meaning to their activities. More specifically, through these frameworks individuals are able to give

meaning to their emotions and create and sustain their identities. Ideological power, therefore, 'emerges to the extent that a distinctive group establishes privileged control over the social activities and the cultural artefacts relating to the satisfaction of these needs' ie, their emotions and identities (Poggi, 2006, p. 467). From this, perspective power is inherently linked to contemporary concepts of professions and professional work.

One of the earliest writers to address the issue of power and the professions was Terence Johnson. Johnson's work (1972) concerning professions and power focused primarily on the relationships of occupations, perceived to be professions, with the client. Key points of relevance stemming from Johnson's work are firstly the suggestion that through the development of a collegiate network, professionals are able to establish and control their power base. The more abstract professional knowledge the greater control a profession will have over their clients; and finally the role of the state in mediating between a profession and a client, the suggestion being that the greater the state mediation the less powerful the profession. This final point is interesting, with Johnson suggesting that where the state mediates professional activities to the degree that professions become employees of larger organizations (such as the case in the NHS), professional knowledge becomes diluted and absorbed into the bureaucratic system. One consequence of this is that individual professionals may take on more divergent roles, depending on the organization they are working for. As Johnson suggests 'differences in the structural or organisational location of practitioners are, then, likely to generate divergences of orientation; there will be varying degrees of self-identification with the occupational community' (1972, p. 81). Of interest here is the use of the term self-identification, one of Johnson's key propositions being that professional power in part stems from their collegiate action.

Of growing interest in relation to the concept of power in the study of professions are the works of Michel Foucault and his theory of the relationships between knowledge and power. From a Foucaultian perspective, power is seen as a having no 'substantive content', rather it is a 'technology' or technique employed by different groups or individuals within society (Lechte, 1994). Viewing power, as a set of systems or techniques for control, places the focus of enquiry on to the 'channels through which power flows and the methods by which it is exercised' (Cohen, 2006, p. 213). Closely linked to Foucault's conception of power is the concept of governmentality. Seen as an umbrella term for a set of practices, institutions and technologies, governmentality is a system through which political power can be exercised (Cohen, 2006). It is important to mention that, although the state is often regarded as the source of political power, the concept of governmentality is much broader, representing a capillary system through which powerful discourses can flow. Foucault's ideas are beginning to influence writers with regards to interprofessional relationships and professional identity (Bondi, 2004; Evetts, 2006; Mackey, 2007; Manias and Street, 2001). Of particular interest is Foucault's 1973 work entitled 'The Birth of the Clinic'. Here Foucault suggests that the medical profession, via its control of the discourse of

disease and through the creation of hospitals as arenas in which medicine is practised, has taken ownership and control of this most intimate aspect of human life. Through the control of knowledge and the creation of the hospital as an institution, medicine is able to employ the technology of power.

The work by Freidson (1970), although not directly referring to Foucault, reflects some of his arguments, in particular the suggestion that social groups exert power over others through the creation and control of a powerful discourse. The power interplay between professional groups has been highlighted by Manias and Street (2001) in their study looking at the interplay regarding decision making between doctors and nurses in an intensive care setting. Using an ethnographic approach, Manias and Street found that the discourse of nursing was dominated by the medical paradigm and concluded that medicine was able to, through the use of knowledge, maintain its position of relative power.

Larson (1990), in one of her later works, focuses on how professions through the use of powerful discourse maintain and justify their position within society. Larson's main focus is on the relationship between knowledge and power, leading her to suggest that 'all professional or professionalizing phenomena must be theoretically linked to the social production and certification of knowledge' (1990, p. 25). As a concept, knowledge is not new within the sociology of the professions; however, here Larson is placing the production of knowledge at centre stage and offering a paradigm from which it can be analysed empirically. Drawing on both the works of Foucault and Bourdieu, Larson argues that professional practice is controlled by institutional domains (for example, professional bodies, universities or hospitals), which create and disseminate authoritative practice. Larson suggests that there is a core from which authoritative discourses originate, this being researchers in the case of professions. This core is surrounded by those trusted with the training of those wishing to join the profession. Larson also acknowledges that employers of professionals will influence their discourse, as will the context in which they work. At the periphery are the individual practitioners who, dealing with the lay members of society, are having to adapt and interpret the authoritative discourses, and it is here that any focus on discourse should begin; for as Larson suggests it is at this point that and different discourses are brought to bear upon codes of practice for which practitioners tend to invite, as their foundation, the 'true' discourse produced at the core (1990, p. 38). An interpretation of Larson's model of the creation of discourse is that through the control of knowledge production and the physical link between those tasked with creating the core knowledge and those tasked with passing it on, professions are able to socialize their members into the adoption of truth. As Larson argues, 'the control of knowledge always ultimately depends on controlling the subjects who know' (1990, p. 32). When challenged, it is the truth produced at the core which is used to defend practice, as this is seen as the most powerful.

A number of the propositions put forward in Larson's later work have not been tested empirically and are therefore open to interpretation. The idea that knowledge is controlled by institutional domains fails to recognize the concepts of interprofessional negotiation and the importance of the client with regards to professional practice as outlined above. In addition to this, Larson's focus is on the source of authoritative discourse, neglecting somewhat the concept of governmentality and the flow of power. There has, however, been some empirical work which suggests that through the processes of professionalization, professionals are socialized to accept a particular version of the truth. Apker and Eggly (2004), adopting a qualitative methodology based on observations, focused on the discourse of medical staff during 'morning report'; a purely doctor to doctor interaction. Their findings suggest and support Larson's proposition that through discourse, doctors reinforce a particular ideology (in this case a scientific model of medical practice), and this in turn leads to the creation of a distinct professional identity.

As indicated, Larson draws heavily on the work of Foucault suggesting that any empirical analysis of professions should focus on the various discourses employed. From an empirical perspective Foucault's works offer an interesting alternative to the largely interactionist lines of enquiry which dominate the sociology of the professions. The conceptualization of power as a technique, as opposed to a substantive concept, shifts the focus of enquiry onto the activities and interconnections individuals and groups engage in in their everyday lives. In contrast to the Weberian perspective, where the focus is more inclined towards the asymmetry of power, Foucault's concept views power more neutrally. In addition to this, Foucault suggests that through the concept of governmentality, power flows across society and infuses social life to the degree that the most powerful discourse is accepted as the norm. Taking Mann's concept of ideological power, Foucault offers a means of investigating the processes through which an individual's or group's frame of reference is shaped.

Extending the focus on discourse and the analysis of power in relation to professions, Evetts (2006) has argued that the concept of professionalism is now being seen as a complex form of organising occupational roles which at the same time serve to promote and provide a civic responsibility away from the more rigid Weberian concepts of bureaucracy. Crucially in Evetts, analysis, is the notion that control emerges from within professions and is exerted upon professions, the former being evidenced by professions claims to knowledge and collegial authority, the latter in the emergence of systems of governance and managerial control. The merger of these two discourses being seen as a means of gaining legitimacy within organizations and social institutions.

## The Contextual and Temporal Nature of Professionalism

Alongside the functionalist and postWeberian theories of professional work, there has and continues to be a view that the terms 'profession' and 'professionalism' are socially constructed, contextually and temporally bound, and as such they are open to negotiation. A number of authors such as Larson, in her later work (1990), Freidson (1994) and Wenger (1998) have placed individual professionals as the focus of their enquires into professions and professionalism. A focus on what professionals do at a micro interactive

level is significant in that it has prompted a line of investigation which has placed the day-to-day actions of individuals at the heart of empirical investigation (Allen, 2000). The adoption of more constructionist or phenomenological perspectives to the study of professions has allowed researchers to move beyond the macro theories of professions, which Friedson has argued have as their focus occupations and the division of labour, as opposed to professionals themselves. The adoption of a broader analysis of professions, which draws on a number of sociological frames of reference, not just the division of labour or occupations, has allowed sociologists to develop theories addressing professional practice which take account of the micro, individual elements of professionalism.

A focus on individual professionals and their work has prompted Freidson (1994) to suggest that any study of professions should primarily adopt a phenomenological approach. The term profession is viewed as a socially constructed concept and as a result, is used by a number of different social groups in different contexts and at different times, to mean different things. To view the term as being fixed is therefore inappropriate. Taking a more constructionist perspective, Freidson (1994) views the concept of profession as something which is contextually and temporally bound, in addition to this it is a concept which is continually negotiated. Any empirical enquiry moving beyond this negotiation moves beyond the concept of profession to the broader field of occupations. Friedson places more emphasis on the concept of professionalization than profession, stating that the process of professionalization: produces distinctive occupational identities and exclusionary market shelters which set each occupation apart from (and often in opposition to) the others (Freidson, 1994, pp. 16–17).

The formation of professional identities is of interest, with Freidson noting that this appears to be a particular idiosyncrasy of professions in the UK and the United States (when compared to Europe). Freidson draws attention to the socialization processes through which members of professions pass, giving particular attention to the long periods of formal education normally associated with professions and the ways professional work is organized. It is through these processes individuals develop particular professional identities, which as Freidson suggests bring individuals within a particular profession to identify more with their profession than their employer:

*'Organised specialised occupational identities get constructed. Knowledge gets institutionalised as expertise. The structure of meanings and commitments can override organisational goals and commitments.'*

**Freidson, 1994, p. 90**

Freidson echoes the work of Witz (2003) (market shelters) and Abbott (1988) (jurisdiction); however, from an empirical point of view, he offers a direction which addresses one of the key criticisms of the more macro perspectives. Viewing the concept of profession as socially constructed allows one to move away from any overarching definition. Liberation from an ideal or fixed concept allows researchers to focus on the 'untidiness and inconsistency of the empirical phenomenon' (Freidson, 1994, p. 25). Any analysis, it is argued, should therefore focus on illumi-

nating how groups and individuals negotiate their identities within a particular organization. As Freidson suggests:

*'The strategy of analysis, therefore, is particular rather than general, studying occupations as individual empirical cases rather than as specimens of some more general fixed concept.'*

**Freidson, 1994, p. 26**

Freidson's arguments are convincing and have clearly influenced researchers working in the sociology of professions (Bligh, 2005; Carmel, 2006; Mackey, 2007; Øvretveit, 1985). Such a focus is not, however, without criticism, with MacDonald (1995) suggesting that by focusing on the micro perspectives of individuals, research fails to address the influence a particular group in society has over other groups at a more structural level. Analysis focusing solely on individuals without regards for the context in which they work (both physical and political), or reference to broader social theories of occupations would be very narrow. Friedson makes it clear that any investigation at a micro level needs to acknowledge the context and build this into the mode of enquiry. Over all, Freidson argues for a bottom up approach to the study of the professions. This approach is reflected in a number of studies focusing on professional processes and professional identities, the majority adopting an ethnographic approach.

An important turn in the study of the professions was the development of negotiated order theory (Strauss et al., 1963). Emerging primarily within the sociology of medicine and reflecting core elements of symbolic interactionism, negotiated order theory provides an empirical and theoretical basis for the study of individuals within organizations, recognizing both an individual's agency and the contexts or structures within which they operate. Social order is continually formed and reformed through the active negotiation of social actors. Focusing on social relations and the contexts in which these are formed, negotiated order theory has and continues to be utilized in the study of the relationships within and between health care professions (Allen, 2000; Germov, 2005; Nugus et al., 2010; Svensson, 1996). In saying this, however, it is not without its criticisms. Although conceived in part as a reaction by social interactionism to the acknowledgement of both contexts and structures, negotiated order theory fails to provide a basis for the influence these elements may have on social action. As Day and Day argue:

> 'There is an implied dialectical relationship in which the informal structure of the organisation acts upon the formal structure, producing change.'

**Day and Day, 1977, p. 26**

The relationships between social action and social structures therefore remains obscured.

Although not contributing to the sociology of professions directly, the work of Anthony Giddens (1984; 1993), in particular his theory of structuration, offers a useful, theoretical foundation from which to formulate an empirical approach, allowing the researcher to give equal attention to both macro (structural) and micro (agentic) elements in the construction of professions and professional work. Drawing on structuration theory and social identity theory, Hotho (2008) investigated the relationship between professions and individuals with regards to the formation of professional identities in the hospital context. Although only based on data from a pilot study, Hotho's work provides an example of the utility of structuration theory in the sociology of the professions and professional identity formation.

Reflecting on the literature reviewed in this section there appears to be three core elements with regards to the theoretical and empirical discussion of professionalism and professional practice; that any empirical investigation into the professions needs to take into consideration individuals, the processes in which individuals engage in order to enact their concept of professionalism and finally the micro and macro culture in which those individuals and processes are situated.

## Contemporary Issues in the Study of Professions

### Professional Identity

Developments in the thinking regarding professions and professionals over the past 30 years has led to an interest in professional identity in general and the individual's identity as a professional in particular. The focus on identity has taken two very broad approaches, although there are arguments which suggest that the two fields overlap considerably (Cote and Schwartz, 2002), these being a psychological perspective and a sociological perspective. Taking the concept of profession and interpreting it as an element of the broader concept of identity has allowed researchers to span the spectrum of individual to collective/institutional process and action in order to interpret professional action in contemporary society (Baxter, 2011).

Psychology has a long tradition of focusing on identity and identity formation

(Weinreich and Saunderson, 2002). At a very simplistic level, identity, from a psychological perspective, can be defined as 'the internal, subjective concept of oneself as an individual' (Reber, 1985, p. 341). In general, most psychological theories of identity focus on its formation, viewing it as a maturation process over the course of an individual's life (Cote, and Schwartz, 2002). One criticism of the psychological 'statuses'[1] of identity formation is that they fail to take into consideration the broader social-contextual elements which contribute to the development of one's identity (Côte and Levine, 1988). In response to this criticism the more psychostructural theories of identity, for example 'othering', suggest that we define our identities by indicating what we are not (Ashforth and Mael, 1989). Marking differences as opposed to similarities allows us to situate ourselves and our identities in a more fluid and open way (Barbour and Lammers, 2015; Shapiro, 2008).

Social identity theory (Tajfel, 1992) has been used by a number of researchers to interpret the processes via which individuals and groups form identities. Davis (2002) has suggested that the creation of a professional identity, through the process of othering[2] has created an identity that is emotionally detached, neutral and somehow apart from 'ordinary people'.

Taking binary thinking as a frame of reference, Davis argues that by setting themselves apart from others, professionals could be dismissing core elements of their identities, for example emotional involvement and doubt, which are equally as important in the delivery of health care services.

Utilising critical discursive psychology as an analytical frame of reference, Reynolds (2007) investigated how professionals use different discourses when working in the multiprofessional setting. In her analysis Reynolds comments on how, through the process of othering, individuals create barriers to interprofessional working. In addition to this, however, Reynold's suggests that the rigid binary divisions identified by Davis (2002), for example doctor and patient, qualified and unqualified, have been diluted by the introduction and emphasis on interprofessional working. One potential outcome of this is greater interprofessional collaboration. Although not indicated in her study, the work by Reynolds offers some theoretical explanation away from the more dominant post-Weberian perspectives, as to why interprofessional teams face difficulties. More recently Kreindler et al. (2012) used a social identity approach as a theoretical lens through which to analyse research papers focusing on professional identity. They concluded that through the creation of profession specific identities, professions create 'silos' which could be used to either block or facilitate changes in working patterns. Overall, Kreindler et al. (2012) argued that, although useful, research which focuses primarily on identity from a psychological perspective neglects broader social interactions.

As indicated, although psychological theories of identity can provide some explanations as to how and why professionals function,

---

[1] Referring to the identity status paradigm (Marcia, 1966) which proposes that identity formation occurs as a process of maturation. Four identifiable periods or statuses form a hierarchical typology of self-regulation and social functioning (Marcia, J. E. (1966) 'development and validation of ego identity status'. Journal of Personal and Social Psychology, 5, pp. 551–558

[2] Defining self through differentiation from others

they have been criticized heavily for being too deterministic and 'intrapsychic'[3], often neglecting the broader social and contextual factors which go into shaping one's identity (Baxter, 2011; Cote and Schwartz, 2002). In contrast, sociological theories of identity adopt the stance that identity and identity formation is an active process. 'Identifying ourselves or others is about meaning, and meaning always involves interaction: agreement and disagreement, convention and innovation, communication and negotiation' (Jenkins, 2004, p. 4). A sociological stance on identity places emphasis on the contextual and temporal elements of identity and identity formation. The concept of individualization, drawing on the work of Beck (1992), for example, suggests that individuals have greater flexibility in the formation of their identities, this formation being both contextual and temporal and crucially negotiated as opposed to fixed. As indicated, sociologists have tended to focus their attention on groups as opposed to individuals with regards to identity and, as such, identity as a concept is regarded as something which is created through interactions and institutions. Identity is a process as opposed to a thing. Jenkins (2004) pulled together some of the key themes concerning the sociological stance on identity and has suggested that identity can be best understood as three distinct orders: namely the individual, interaction and institutional order. The individual order of identity is, put simply, what goes on in an individual's head, the interaction order is concerned with the relationships between individuals and finally the institutional order is 'the human world of

pattern and organisation, of established ways of doing things' (Jenkins, 2004 p. 17). Of importance is the acknowledgement which Jenkins (p. 18) makes when he states that 'it is almost impossible to talk about one without at least implying the others'.

There is a clear overlap with Jenkins's taxonomy and the terms 'professionality' and 'professionalism', with professionality concerning itself with the internal representation of professional identity and professionalism corresponding with the interaction and institutional orders (ie, the culture of professional practice). Baxter (2011) in her review of the literature on public sector professions, has suggested that the term professionalism refers more to the external control mechanisms associated with professions, for example regulation, whereas in contrast professionality is more reflective of the agentic elements of a professional's work, this being more indicative of their 'salient professional identity' (p. 33).

Expanding on the final two elements of Jenkins taxonomy, namely the interactional and institutional orders, Jenkins argues that through our interactions with others, we construct our identities and they are to some degree constructed for us. The process is one of perpetual change and negotiation, for example through the processes of labelling (Goffman, 2009), group identification (Barth, 1969) and categorization (Tajfel, 1992). In addition, the institutional element of the identification process creates the notion of identity as something which exists externally to an embodied individual (in contrast to the arguments presented regarding professionality). Institutions, from a sociological perspective, can be regarded as either concrete social

---

[3]Referring to internal psychological processes

forms, for example the family or the Church (Turner, 2006), or more subtle 'patterns of behaviour that are regulated by norms and sanctions into which individuals are socialised. Institutions are an ensemble of social roles' (Turner, 2006, p. 301). Institutions give a normative reference point as to how things should be done (or not) and thus involve control (Jenkins, 2004, p. 135). Referring back to the work of Giddens (1984) and Sewell (1992), social structures, for example institutions and organizations, provide social actors with rules and resources through which they can give meaning to their actions and identities. Of importance however, is the recognition of the reciprocal relationship between agents and structures. This duality is captured with regards to identity in the interpretations offered by Barth (1969), Berger and Luckmann (1991), Wenger (1998) and Cohen (2002).

## THE MARKETIZATION OF HEALTH CARE

The introduction of market principles into health care has radically changed the operating culture of state based systems such as the NHS (Bach, 2000). The balance of power between managers and health care professionals and between providers and purchasers has been shifted in light of the 'quest for choice and value for money' (Fournier, 2000, p. 67).

With regards to health care professions generally, the concept of a health care economy has been interpreted as both positive and negative. Hanlon (1996) commenting on the UK has argued that the introduction of a market ethos into the NHS will ultimately erode the altruistic nature of professional practice. An alternative view is that through the marketization of health services and the resulting management and bureaucratic infrastructure, professional practice and knowledge will become more diffuse and thus available to consumers and employers; however, the same such bureaucratic structures will be utilized by professions in order to retain a sense of ownership and control over their work (Ackroyd, 1996). What both of these arguments acknowledge is that professionalism is not divorced from the context in which professionals practise. A change in the organizational ideologies and hierarchies of health care systems clearly affects professionals. Focusing specifically on allied health professions, although limited, there is literature suggesting that, although initially poorly prepared, the allied health professions have adapted their professional discourses to reflect central elements of policy reform.

### Market Orientation and Professionalism

The need for cost effectiveness has long been recognized within health service delivery (Bach et al., 2008; Page and Willey, 2007). The introduction of the internal market into the NHS in the UK and its subsequent continuation has led organizations responsible for the delivery of health services to adopt a 'market orientation'; this is reflected in their values or processes, the principal aim of which is the creation of high value and desirable services (Hampton and Hampton, 2004, p. 1042). Key elements of a market orientation such as patient centred practice, a flexible workforce and cost effectiveness are reflected throughout reforms seen in health care services in the UK, the United States and Australia (Adams, 2014). The adoption of a market orientation in health care has been shown to improve performance (Raju et al., 1995). There is an assumption that staff working in market-orientated organizations reflect to some degree the ethos and values of their employers, and there is evidence to suggest that this is the case in private sector organizations (Ruekert, 1992; Whitchurch, 2008). Professionals working in the public sector are seen, however, to be a different kind of worker, in that their values and beliefs are more fragmented reflecting a particular professional orientation as opposed to the central values of marketization (Southon and Braithwaite, 1998). The ethos of professionalism is seen by some as being fundamentally at odds with that of marketization (Doyle and Cameron, 2000; Hafferty and Light, 1995; Hanlon, 1998; Wallace, 1995). This has led Baxter (2011, p. 9) to suggest that marketization of the public sector is having an effect on individuals' 'professional values, sense of salience and professional identities'.

There is evidence to suggest that the introduction of market incentives into health care affects professionalism. Focusing on nurse midwives working in the United States, Hampton and Hampton (2004) attempted to measure the relationship between professionalism and market orientation. Adopting a quantitative methodology Hampton and Hampton utilized a variety of measurement scales to assess professionalism, perceived rewards, market orientation and job satisfaction. Acknowledging that the sample is representative of only one profession, Hampton and Hampton concluded that there is a strong relationship between professionalism

and market orientation, suggesting that the two concepts are closely related in that they are both concerned with the standard of service provided to clients. The relationship between professionalism and marketization has been questioned by Poses (2003) who, again commenting on the US health care system, identified the introduction of market incentives as distracting professionals (doctors in this case) from their core professional values ie, altruism and a core body of knowledge. The latter point is supported by Rastegar (2004), who argues that the introduction of evidence-based practice along with the industrialization of health care is moving knowledge away from professionals, placing it under the remit of managers and wider bureaucracies, a point echoed by Bach (2000). Both Poses and Rastegar offer critical commentary from the United States and are concerned with the plight, in the most part, of the medical profession.

Empirical research investigating the argument that the introduction of the market dilutes or alters professionalism has been provided by a number of authors. McDonald et al. (2007) conducted a UK based ethnographic study looking at the effect on GPs' motivation of recently introduced financial incentives for the quality of care provided. The findings of McDonald et al. demonstrated a change in practice for doctors and nurses with the former adopting a more managerial role, choosing to delegate the more technical aspects of their work to nursing staff. Interestingly McDonald et al. (2007) noted that the delegation of tasks previously undertaken by doctors to their nursing colleagues caused a degree of unease, with nurses feeling that their work was being scrutinized in more detail than before. Although changes in practice were noted, McDonald et al. concluded that internal motivation, or what could be regarded as professionalism, was not affected. Cohen and Musson (2000) used a qualitative case based approach to examine the discourse of GPs at a time when the new GP contracts were introduced in the UK. Cohen and Musson's findings indicate that the concepts of managerialism and marketization were strongly represented by doctors in their accounts of their work; however, such discourses did not precede or replace what they felt was their central identity, that of a GP. Elston and Holloway (2001) adopted a grounded theory approach to investigate the perspectives of doctors, nurses and managers regarding changes in the organization of primary care in the UK. Their findings suggest that on the whole, while the GPs were willing to take on and/or retain their role as leaders, they were hesitant in relinquishing power to either the nurses or managers. The nurses interviewed in this study were keen to be recognized and valued, and they were eager to take on the extra responsibilities and roles relinquished by the doctors. Elston and Holloway (2001) concluded that differences in interpretations of professionalism led to some conflict between professions in light of the introduction of service reforms. This final point was observed by Grant et al. (2009) who, based on data from an ethnographic study focusing on the work of four GP practices at the time of the introduction of the quality and outcomes framework (DoH, 2003), found that the extent of change in roles and identities was highly individual with 'both winners and losers being located within rather than between professions' (Grant et al.,

2009, p. 242). Based on the evidence reviewed it is clear that the relationship between marketization and professionalism is complex and is not restricted to either profession specific or individual factors, but should be seen to be a combination of the two.

Although limited in number, the empirical evidence seems to suggest that the introduction of market values into the delivery of health services has influenced the identity of health care professionals; this being primarily reflected in their discourse and day-to-day actions. It is important to note that the literature considered so far has almost exclusively addressed the identities of the medical profession and more specifically doctors working in primary care in the UK. Doctors working in this environment have traditionally been independent and entrepreneurial and it is not surprising to see that they have adopted managerial traits in light of the marketization of health care. Taking into consideration the recent changes in policy discussed it will be of interest to assess the extent of the effects these will have on GPs' professional roles and identities. Although not researched, a number of commentators have suggested that GPs will, on the whole, reject the additional managerialism now incorporated into their roles and simply hire ex primary care commissioners to fulfil this role (Asthana, 2011; Pollock and Price, 2011). The empirical data, however, seem to suggest more of a mixed picture (Checkland et al., 2012). Research focusing on members of the medical profession working in secondary care indicates more unease with, and often resistance to, marketization. Doolin (2002), again adopting a qualitative case based methodology, incorporating interviews, observations and documentation analysis, aimed to analyse the extent to which enterprise discourse was evident in hospital based doctors in New Zealand. He found that since the introduction of market values into health care delivery many doctors had changed their identity (as reflected through their discourse) to reflect market values. A point observed by Doolin was that doctors changed their discourse depending on the context in which they were working. Doolin stresses, however, that, although adapting to the introduction of the market into hospitals, doctors remained uncomfortable. This notion of dual identities has been demonstrated by Kitchener (2000), who again focusing on doctors working in hospitals, used a qualitative case based approach to investigate the impact of marketization and professional identity. As in the previous studies cited, Kitchener noted the adoption of managerial and market-orientated discourses by doctors and suggested that through this change in discourse, doctors were diluting their professional identity and subsuming it within that of management. He goes on to suggest that they were in effect being 'deprofessionalized'. This concern echoes that of Hafferty and Light (1995) and may contribute to the rationale for the current focus on professional identity within medical education (Monrouxe, 2010; Thistlethwaite and Spencer, 2008).

The importance of context is apparent and may be explained when one considers the organizational complexities and hierarchies within hospitals (Reed and Anthony, 1993). In addition to this, those studies which have investigated other professions alongside medicine appear to suggest that changes in how doctors work, and subsequently their identities, has an impact on the professional identities of those around them.

### Nurses and Allied Health Professionals

Nurses and allied health professionals have been the focus of recent UK NHS policies aimed at driving patient centred practice within health care services (Skills for Health, 2006). Of note are the continued calls for team work in the delivery of health care by these professions and the demand for greater flexibility from these professions in the type of services they provide. The impact of marketization on nurses and the allied health professionals appears more complex when compared to the medical profession. Larkin (1988) has suggested that greater management and supervision of professional work may affect the semiprofessions more than medicine. The empirical data, although limited in volume, appears to suggest that nurses and allied health professionals are struggling to incorporate aspects of marketization into their identities, the result being a degree of self-reflection by these professions regarding their professionalism. In addition, a number of changes in how and where these professions work appears to be reinforcing as opposed to reducing their individual professional identities and cultures (Brown and Greenwood, 1999; Herdman, 2001; Mackey, 2007; Mazhindu, 2003). A current focus of research in the UK is on the effect social enterprise schemes are having on this section of the health care workforce (Miller et al., 2013). A growing interest has emerged and is directed towards discussing if and how entrepreneurial skills should be developed by nurses and allied health professionals (Cook, 2006; Drennan, et al., 2007; Sankelo and

Akerbald, 2008). The introduction of social enterprise schemes across the NHS is a recent development; however, other elements of marketization have been in position for some time, for example patient centred practice, skill mix and competency frameworks.

## Professionalism and Team Work

The need for more patient centred services has reinforced the call for interprofessional team work (Lowe and O'Hara, 2000). The concept of team work as a means of providing more joined up services was introduced as long ago as the 1920s (Consultative Council on Medical and Allied Services, 1920). Although primarily seen as a way of structuring the work force in primary care, team work is now regarded as a core attribute of patient centred care in the delivery of almost all health services (DoH, 2008).

There is some evidence to suggest that team work improves patient outcome (McCallin, 2001); however, the empirical evidence supporting what makes a good team remains limited (Neumann, et al., 2010). From a theoretical perspective there appears to be some agreement on what elements are required for teams to be effective. Clear goals and operational policies need to be in place, in addition, members of a team need to adopt a culture of mutual trust and respect with a willingness to share knowledge (D'Amour et al., 2005; Neumann et al., 2010). The primary purpose of team work in the delivery of health services is the provision of a range of knowledge and skills from a number of highly skilled clinicians all focusing on one client. For teams to be effective they need to therefore be multidisciplinary. A number of authors (Finlay, 2000; Laidler, 1994; Øvretveit, 1997) have

defined multidisciplinary teams as different professions working with the same client towards the same goal. This joint working could primarily take two forms; the first is when professionals work together with little or no exchange of information or changes to their working practices. The second is characterized by the overlapping of roles; however, this often occurs in an unplanned way 'which may lead to duplication and possible fragmentation of roles and interprofessional conflict' (Pethybridge, 2004, p. 30). Taking into consideration the potential limitations of multidisciplinary team working, Laidler (1994) and Øvretveit (1997) have suggested the concept of interdisciplinary working as being more appropriate for patient centred care. Interdisciplinary team working can be described as when professionals from different professions work in an 'interwoven' and overlapping way, where knowledge and skills are openly shared and roles are actively blurred (Pethybridge, 2004, p. 30).

With regards to professional identity there is a growing body of research indicating that the traditional demarcations between professional groups impairs the development of effective team working (Axelsson and Axelsson, 2009; Easen et al., 2000; Freeman and Ross, 2000; Lingard et al., 2002; McCallin, 2001; Miller and Ahmad, 2000). Salhani and Coulter (2009), focusing on the micropolitical struggles within interprofessional health care teams, conducted an ethnographic study in a psychiatric hospital in the UK. Using Abbott's (1988) concepts of jurisdiction and interprofessional competition, Salhani and Coulter argued that the traditional hierarchies (the dominance of the medical profession) within the hospital setting prevented some professions (nurses) from fully developing their professionalism. Cohen (2003) writing from an occupational therapy perspective, has suggested that the traditional elements of professionalism, as conceptualized in the work of Abbott (1988) and Larson (1977), block the introduction of interdisciplinary team work as the changes in attitudes required by individual health professionals are at odds with the concepts of jurisdiction and market closure. Reflecting the work of Salhani and Coulter (2009), the importance of context and its interaction with team work has been highlighted by Baxter and Brumfitt (2008). They conducted a qualitative case based study focusing on interdisciplinary teams working with stroke patients. Three teams were investigated, one based on an in-patient ward, one in a specialized stroke unit and one based in the community. Their findings suggest that in the case of the stroke unit and the community based teams the traditional hierarchies between the professions were being eroded in favour of the more inter-disciplinary model described above. However, this was not the case with regards to the ward based team where the traditional demarcations between the various professions involved were still evident. Xyrichis and Lowton (2008) have conducted a literature review focusing on what factors facilitate or prevent interprofessional team work. Taking into consideration the review was descriptive as opposed to critical; their findings indicated the importance of clarity in both purpose and roles for effective team working. From the work outlined above it would appear that the 'rhetoric' of interprofessional team working fails to take into consideration the sociological theories of the professions. Although not necessarily providing an answer as to how interprofessional teams could work, the sociological perspectives of professional practice do provide some indication as to why interprofessional teams do not always work. What is interesting from Baxter and Brumfitt's (2008) research is that context seems to play a role in how teams of professionals work together.

## The Redistribution of Roles Across Professions

A key element of interdisciplinary working is the need for role overlap, an aspect, it has been argued, that is at odds with the very definition of a profession (Baxter, 2011). In addition to interdisciplinary working, the marketization of health care has led policy makers to review the current roles and activities individual health professions play in the delivery of health care services. The redistribution of roles across professions has in part been the result of changes in how doctors work. However, this redistribution of skills across the health care workforce is being facilitated by changes in policy which are directly impacting the way allied health professionals and nurses practice (Hoskins, 2012; Nancarrow and Borthwick, 2005). Predominantly stated, funded health care systems such as the NHS have been accused of not being designed around the needs of patients and of having outdated working practices, with the current demarcations among staff being unrepresentative of clients' needs. One of the main ways the NHS is addressing these apparent shortcomings is by looking at how the current workforce is employed. Based on the theory of business process reengineering (Hyde et al., 2005), workforce redesign, ie, a redistribution of skills across a range of staff within health care organizations, may create a more flexible and responsive workforce. The overall aim of this being an improvement in the quality of care and a more patient centred approach, in that services are designed around the needs of the consumer (Adams, et al., 2000; Bach, 1998).

Addressing the aims of value for money and productivity, there is some research to suggest that a focus on skills, for example, through staff development and training, has a positive impact on productivity and profit (Hyde et al., 2005; Nolan, 2004; West et al., 2002). Research carried out in the UK by Bach (1998) in the mid-1990s demonstrated that by altering the skill mix of the health workforce employers are able to save considerable amounts in terms of pay expenditure. Although blocked initially by trade unions and professional bodies, the move towards role reprofiling, skill mix and a more transparent pay structure for all health workers (with the exception of doctors and dentists) has now been introduced in England (DoH, 2004). The work of Goode and Greatbatch (2005) illuminates to some degree the relationship between professionalism and the redistribution of roles between professions. In a qualitative study involving interviews and participant observations, Goode and Greatbatch (2005), investigated the boundary work between nurses and call handlers working for NHS Direct. Their findings suggest that nurses reinforced their professionalism as a means of constructing a boundary between themselves and the call handlers. Hoskins (2012) provides a discursive as opposed to an evaluative summary of the literature concerning the effects of marketization and professional identities. Focusing specifically on the emergence of non-medical roles in emergency care, she argues that as a result of changes in policy there has emerged a spectrum of overlap between professions. At one end of the spectrum professionals are simply duplicating tasks, whereas at the other, professionals are substituting for each other's roles. Although concerned with just one aspect of medical care, Hoskins develops an academic argument to suggest that the effects of policy change are not uniform within or across professions.

## A Skills Based Workforce

Health care systems are adopting a predominantly skills based approach to workforce development, focusing more on the needs of patients (as opposed to the knowledge and skills of individual professions). The types of skills health professionals have should represent the needs of the clients they serve, and so a demand based system of professional education has been introduced (Page and Willey, 2007; Payne and Keep, 2003). The introduction of a competency based skills framework for health care practitioners is a fundamental shift in how the skills health professionals have are developed. In the past, skills were determined by diverse groups – higher education institutes, professional bodies and overly complex centralized organizations – all attempting to predict the needs of industry. The introduction of a demand-led system places the power to determine what skills should be taught in further and higher education institutions firmly in the hands of employers and the various external agencies determining health care services.

There are, however, concerns that the introduction of a skills based work force could have a significant influence on both professional practice and the overall existence of professions as they are currently recognized (Duckett, 2005). Doyle and Cameron (2000, p. 1023) have suggested that 'as the "core" skills and responsibilities of the different groups change, the organization of the NHS labour force will be increasingly out of line with the traditional map of the health care professions'. The characteristics of any profession are thought to be developed through a process of socialization, this occurring during preregistration education (Sparkes, 2002) and through shared experiences in the workplace (Hyde et al., 2005; Lingard et al., 2002). A system which potentially dilutes this socialization process may inevitably fragment both the knowledge and practice of currently distinct occupational groups. Such an outcome may enhance professional practice and deepen professional integration; on the other hand, it may lead to professional protectionism (Cohen, 2003) and greater demarcations between groups, as individual professions attempt to claim legitimacy over distinct areas of practice and reinforce their professional identities (Brown and Greenwood, 1999; Hall, 2005). In light of the empirical work concerned with interdisciplinary team working, there appears to be support for this latter argument. Using the professional project (Larson, 1977) as a means of conceptualising contemporary professional practice, gives support for the notion

put forward by Southon and Braithwaite (1998, p. 23) that the current restructuring of health care services are 'fundamentally affect(ing) the nature of professionalism'. As with the introduction of market forces into the types of services available, it may be that by focusing on who delivers services, recent NHS policies increase the already embedded competition between professional groups. A third outcome may be that the traditional characteristics supposedly associated with public sector professionals are lost altogether, being replaced by characteristics more akin to the private sector, namely individualism, organizational allegiance and a consumer orientation that privileges value for money over quality of care (Hanlon, 2000; McDonald et al., 2007; Stubbings and Scott, 2004).

## Professional Regulation and Autonomy

Consistency of practice is a key focus of debate regarding contemporary professional practice. There have been, and continue to be, highly publicized failures and inconsistencies in the services health professionals provide (Walshe and Benson, 2005). A consequence of this has not only been a focus on the knowledge and skills professionals have, but also on how professions are regulated (Allsop and Saks 2003; Chamberlain, 2010). Changes introduced in policy (DoH, 1997; 2000a) and legislation (1999 Health Act) have radically altered how health professions are regulated in the UK (DoH, 2000a). With regards to allied health professions, the Council for Professions Supplementary to Medicine has been replaced by the Health Professions Council (HPC) (DoH, 2000a). This new regulatory body has been given tougher powers to tackle poor conduct and performance, has a role in the quality assurance of professional education and for the first time introduced mandatory continued professional development linked to reregistration and the right to practise. The primary role of the HPC is to protect the public. This is accomplished by keeping a register and a record of all allied health professionals' education, performance, behaviour and health. At the time of the HPC's introduction the professional body for physiotherapists, the Chartered Society for Physiotherapists (CSP), reacted angrily to the proposed changes in regulation. Its concerns and recommendations, however, were not reflected in the final proposals for allied health professionals (Frontline, P 6. June 2000). Of significance is the development and implementation of common standards of practice for all professions which come under the regulative powers of the HPC. The HPC regulates 14 individual professions which now share common standards of performance and ethics. This commonality of standards of practice could be seen as another means of blurring the boundaries between professions. In addition to the change in how allied health professionals are regulated, there have been a number of initiatives concerned with the modernization of health care in the UK which could potentially impact professionalization. The introduction of external agencies tasked with monitoring and informing health care delivery, for example National Institute for Health and Clinical Excellence and the Care Quality Commission, in addition to the reinvigorated culture of audit at the local level could be seen as removing clinical decisions from the individual profes-

sional (Miles et al., 2001). The plurality of relationships between individual professionals, professional groups and external institutions has created a system of governance which is more open and complex and it could be suggested disadvantageous to the once powerful professional bodies whose primary role was to regulate their members (Newman, 2006). The introduction of external agencies with a responsibility for the content of professionals' education and practice could be seen as diluting the professionalization processes and professionalism of those professions involved. Although examples to illustrate the key points regarding professional autonomy and regulation have been drawn from the UK, they are by no means limited to this region. Adams (2014) in her narrative literature review of publications in the sociology of the professions, identified professional regulation as the second most published issue in the sociology of the professions in Australia and the third in the UK. Interestingly, Adams's review identified that beyond gender, immigration, ethnicity and professionalization, work satisfaction and practice experiences were the most discussed issues in the US literature. These international differences are in part a reflection of the contextual and highly politicized nature of professional work in contemporary societies.

## Summary

Reflecting wider global financial agendas, as opposed to individual state based party politics, policy agenda for the health care economy is one which promotes multi and interprofessional and multi and interagency collaboration, role overlap and, related to health care delivery, the development of entrepreneurial professionals.

Smith et al. (2000) view the removal of professional boundaries as a key in the development of the 'new' NHS. The traditional demarcations between professional groups have been highlighted in recent UK policy as one of the main obstacles to modernising services (DoH, 2000b; 2006). Although it is acknowledged that professionals have played an integral part in the development of the UK National Health Service (Baxter and Brumfitt, 2008; Rivett, 1998), there is growing concern that the current organization and allegiances of the various professions involved in the delivery of health care services prevents, as opposed to assists, change (Ackroyd, 1996; Baxter and Brumfitt, 2008).

## References

Abbott, A., 1988. The System of Professions. University of Chicago Press, Chicago.

Ackroyd, S., 1996. Organization contra organizations: professions and organizational change in the United Kingdom. Organization Studies 17 (4), 599–621.

Adams, A., Lugsden, E., Chase, J., Arber, S., Bond, S., 2000. Skill-mix changes and work intensification in nursing. Work Employ. Soc. 14 (3), 541–555.

Adams, T.L., 2004. Inter-professional conflict and professionalization: dentistry and dental hygiene in Ontario. Soc. Sci. Med. 58 (11), 2243–2252.

Adams, T., 2014. Sociology of professions: international divergences and research directions. Work Employ. Soc. 1–12.

Allen, D., 2000. Doing occupational demarcation: The "boundary-work" of nurse managers in a district general hospital. J. Contemp. Ethnogr. 29 (3), 326–356.

Allsop, J., Saks, M., 2003. Regulating the Health Professions. Sage, London.

Anderson, L.B., 2009. What determines the behaviour and performance of health professionals? Public service motivation, professional norms and/or economic incentives. Int. Rev. Adm. Sci. 75 (1), 79–97.

Apker, J., Eggly, S., 2004. Communicating professional identity in medical socialization: Considering the ideological discourse of morning report. Qual. Health Res. 14 (3), 411–429.

Ashforth, B.E., Mael, F., 1989. Social identity theory and the organization. Acad. Manage. Rev. 14 (1), 20–39.

Asthana, S., 2011. Liberating the NHS? A commentary on the Lansley White Paper, "equity and excellence". Soc. Sci. Med. 72 (6), 815–820.

Axelsson, S.B., Axelsson, R., 2009. From territoriality to altruism in interprofessional collaboration and leadership. J. Interprof. Care 23 (4), 320–330.

Bach, S., 1998. NHS pay determination and work re-organisation: employment relations reform in NHS trusts. Empl. Relats. 20 (6), 565–576.

Bach, S., 2000. Health sector reform and human resource management: Britain in comparative perspective. Int. J. Hum. Resour. Manag. 11 (5), 925–942.

Bach, S., Kessler, I., Heron, P., 2008. Role redesign in a modernised NHS: the case of health care assistants. Hum. Resour. Manag. J. 18 (2), 171–187.

Barbour, J.B., Lammers, J.C., 2015. Measuring professional identity: a review of the literature and a multilevel confirmatory factor analysis of professional identity constructs. J. Profes. Organ. 2 (1), 38–60.

Barth, F., 1969. Ethnic groups and boundaries: The social organization of cultural difference. Oslo Universitetsforlagent cited in Jenkins, R., 2004, Social Identity. Routledge, London.

Baxter, J., 2011. Public Sector Professional Identities: A Review of the Literature. The Open University, UK.

Baxter, S.K., Brumfitt, S.M., 2008. Professional differences in interprofessional working. J. Interprof. Care 22 (3), 239–251.

Beck, U., 1992. Risk Society: Towards a New Modernity, vol. 17. Sage, London.

Berger, P.L., Luckmann, T., 1991. The Social Construction of Reality: A Treatise in the Sociology of Knowledge, vol. 10. Penguin, London.

Bligh, J., 2005. Professionalism. Med. Educ. 39 (1), 4.

Bolsin, S.N., 1998. Professional misconduct: the Bristol case. Med. J. Aust. 169 (7), 369.

Bondi, L., 2004. A double-edged sword"? The professionalization of counselling in the United Kingdom. Health Place 10 (4), 319–328.

Borthwick, A.M., 2000. Challenging medicine: the case of podiatric surgery. Work Employ. Soc. 14 (2), 369–383.

Bourdieu, P., Wacquant, L.J. (Eds.), 1992. An Invitation to Reflexive Sociology. University of Chicago Press, Chicago.

Boyce, R.A., 1993. Internal market reforms of health care systems and the allied health professions: an international perspective. Int. J. Health Plann. Manage. 8, 201–217.

Boyce, R., 2006. Emerging from the shadow of medicine: allied health as a profession community subculture. Health Sociol. Rev. 15 (5), 520–534.

Brown, T.G., Greenwood, J., 1999. Occupational therapy and physiotherapy: Similar, but separate. Br. J. Occup. Ther. 62 (4), 163–170.

Buelens, M., Van den Broeck, H., 2007. An analysis of differences in work motivation between public and private sector organisations. Public Adm. 67 (1), 65–74.

Burrage, M., Jarausch, K., Siegrist, H., 1990. An actor-based framework for the study of the professions. In: Burrage, M., Torstendahl, R. (Eds.), Professions in Theory and History: Rethinking the Study of the Professions. Sage Publications, London, pp. 203–225.

Burrage, M., Torstendahl, R., 1990. Professions in Theory and History: Rethinking the Study of the Professions. Sage Publications, London.

Carmel, S., 2006. Health care practices, professions and perspectives: A case study in intensive care. Soc. Sci. Med. 62 (8), 2079–2090.

Carr-Saunders, A.M., Wilson, P.A., 1933. Professions cited in Eraut, M., 2002, Developing Professional Knowledge and Competence. Routledge, London.

Chamberlain, J.M., 2010. Portfolio-based performance appraisal for doctors: A case of paperwork compliance. Sociol. Res. Online 15 (1), 8.

Chaska, N.L., 1990. The Nursing Profession: Turning Points. CV Mosby, London.

Checkland, K., Coleman, A., Segar, J., McDermott, I., Miller, R., Wallace, A., et al., 2012. Exploring the Early Workings of Emerging Clinical Commissioning Groups: Final Report. Policy Research Unit in Commissioning and the Healthcare System (PRUComm), London.

Cohen, A.P., 2002. Symbolic Construction of Community. Psychology Press, London.

Cohen, E.F., 2006. Foucault, Michel. In: Turner, B.S. (Ed.), The Cambridge Dictionary of Sociology. Cambridge University Press, Cambridge, pp. 212–214.

Cohen, L., Musson, G., 2000. Entrepreneurial identities: reflections from two case studies. Organ. 7 (1), 31–48.

Cohen, Z.A., 2003. The single assessment process: an opportunity for collaboration or a threat to the profession of occupational therapy? Br. J. Occup. Ther. 66 (5), 201–208.

Consultative Council on Medical and Allied Services, 1920. Report on the future provision of medical and allied services (The Dawson report) HMSO, London. Cited in J. M. Griffiths and K.A. Lucker (1994) 'Intraprofessional teamwork in district nursing: in whose interest? J. Adv. Nurs. 20 (6), 1038–1045.

Cook, R., 2006. What does social enterprise mean for community nursing? Br. J. Community Nurs. 11 (11), 472–475.

Côte, J.E., Levine, C., 1988. A critical examination of the ego identity status paradigm. Dev. Rev. 8 (2), 147–184.

Cote, J.E., Schwartz, S.J., 2002. Comparing psychological and sociological approaches to identity status, identity capital, and the individualisation process. J. Adolesc. 25, 571–586.

Daker-White, G., Carr, A.J., Harvey, I., Woolhead, G., Bannister, G., Nelson, I., et al., 1999. A randomised controlled trial. Shifting boundaries of doctors and physiotherapists in orthopaedic outpatient departments. J. Epidemiol. Community Health 53 (10), 643–650.

D'Amour, D., Ferrada-Videla, M., San Martin Rodriguez, L., Beaulieu, M.D., 2005. The conceptual basis for interprofessional collaboration: Core concepts and theoretical frameworks. J. Interprof. Care 19 (1), 116–131.

Davis, C., 2002. Managing identities: workers, professions and identity. Nurs. Manage. 9 (5), 31–34.

Dawson, L.J., Ghazi, F., 2004. The experience of physiotherapy extended scope practitioners in orthopaedic outpatient clinics. Physiotherapy 90 (4), 210–216.

Day, R., Day, J.V., 1977. A review of the current state of negotiated order theory: An appreciation and a critique. Sociol. Q. 126–142.

Doolin, B., 2002. Enterprise discourse, professional identity and the organizational control of hospital clinicians. Organ. Stud. 23 (3), 369–390.

Doyle, L., Cameron, A., 2000. Reshaping the NHS workforce. Br. Med. J. 320, 1023–1024.

Drennan, V., Davis, K., Goodman, C., Humphrey, C., Locke, R., Mark, A., et al., 2007. Entrepreneurial nurses and midwives in the United Kingdom: an integrative review. J. Adv. Nurs. 60 (5), 459–469.

Duckett, S.J., 2005. Health workforce design for the 21st century. Aust. Health Rev. 29 (2), 201–210.

Durkheim, E., 2002. Professional Ethics and Civic Morals. Psychology Press, London.

Easen, P., Atkins, M., Dyson, A., 2000. Inter-professional collaboration and conceptualisations of practice. Child. Soc. 14 (5), 355–367.

Edmunds, J., Calnan, M.W., 2001. The reprofessionalisation of community pharmacy? An exploration of attitudes to extended roles for community pharmacists amongst pharmacists and GPs in the United Kingdom. Soc. Sci. Med. 53 (7), 943–955.

Elston, S., Holloway, I., 2001. The impact of recent primary care reforms in the UK on interprofessional working in primary care centres. J. Interprof. Care 15 (1), 19–27.

Etzioni, A., 1969. The Semi-Professions and Their Organization. Free Press, New York.

Evetts, J., 2011. A new professionalism? Challenges and opportunities. Curr. Sociol. 59 (4), 406–422.

Finlay, L., 2000. The challenge of working in teams. In: Brechin, A., Brown, H., Eby, M. (Eds.), Critical Practice in Health and Social Care. The Open university, London, pp. 164–187.

Foster, P., Wilding, P., 2000. Whither Welfare Professionalism? Soc. Policy Adm. 34 (2), 143–159.

Foucault, M., 1973. The Birth of the Clinic. Tavistock, London.

Fournier, V., 2000. Boundary work and the (un) making of the professions. In: Malin, N. (Ed.), Professionalism, Boundaries, and the Workplace. Routledge, London, pp. 67–87.

Franco, L.M., Bennett, S., Kanfer, R., 2002. Health sector reform and public sector health worker motivation: a conceptual model. Soc. Sci. Med. 54 (8), 1255–1266.

Freeman, C.M., Ross, N.M., 2000. The impact of individual philosophies of teamwork on multi-professional practice and the implications for education. J. Interprof. Care 14 (3), 237–247.

Freidson, E., 1970. Professional Dominance: The Social Structure of Medical Care. Transaction Books, London.

Freidson, E., 1994. Professionalism Reborn: Theory, Prophecy, and Policy. University of Chicago Press, Chicago.

Frontline, 2000, June, p. 6.

Germov, J., 2005. Managerialism in the Australian public health sector: towards the hyper-rationalisation of professional bureaucracies. Sociol. Health Ill. 27 (6), 738–758.

Giddens, A., 1984. The Constitution of Society: Introduction of the Theory of Structuration. University of California Press, California.

Giddens, A., 1993. New Rules of Sociological Method. Polity Press, Cambridge.

Goffman, E. (2009) Stigma: Notes on the management of spoiled identity. [Online] available at <SimonandSchuster.com> (accessed 30.04.12.).

Goode, J., Greatbatch, D., 2005. Boundary work. The production and consumption of health information and advice within service interactions between staff and callers to NHS Direct. J. Consum. Cult. 5 (3), 315–337.

Grant, S., Huby, G., Watkins, F., Checkland, K., McDonald, R., Davies, H., et al., 2009. The impact of pay-for-performance on professional boundaries in UK general practice: an ethnographic study. Sociol. Health Illn. 31 (2), 229–245.

Great Britain. Department of Health, 1997. The New NHS Modern and Dependable. Crown Copyright, London.

Great Britain. Department of Health, 2000a. The NHS Plan: A Plan for Investment, A Plan for Reform. Crown copyright, London.

Great Britain. Department of Health, 2000b. A Health Service of All the Talents: Developing the NHS Workforce. Consultation Document on the Review of Workforce Planning. The Stationary Office Ltd, London.

Great Britain. Department of Health, 2000c. Meeting the Challenge: A Strategy for the Allied Health Professions. The Stationary Office Ltd, London.

Great Britain. Department of Health, 2003. Investing in General Practice – the New General Medical Services Contract. The Stationary Office Ltd, London.

Great Britain. Department of Health, 2004. Agenda for Change Final Agreement. The Stationary Office Ltd, London.

Great Britain. Department of Health, 2006. Our Health, Our Care, Our Say: A New Direction for Community Services. The Stationary Office Ltd, London.

Great Britain. Department of Health, 2008. Quality for All, NHS Next Stage Review Final Report. The Stationary Office Ltd, London.

Hafferty, F.W., Light, D.W., 1995. Professional dynamics and the changing nature of medical work. J. Health Soc. Behav. 35, 132–153.

Hall, P., 2005. Interprofessional teamwork: Professional cultures as barriers. J. Interprof. Care 19 (1), 188–196.

Halliday, T.C., 1985. Knowledge mandates: collective influence by scientific, normative and syncretic professions. Br. J. Sociol. 36 (3), 421–447.

Hampton, G.M., Hampton, D.L., 2004. Relationship of professionalism, rewards, market orientation and job satisfaction among medical professionals: The case of certified nurse–midwives. J. Bus. Res. 57 (9), 1042–1053.

Hanlon, G., 1996. Casino Capitalism and the rise of the commercialised service class – an examination of the accountant. Crit. Pers. Acco. 7 (3), 339–363.

Hanlon, G., 1998. Professionalism as enterprise: service class politics and the redefinition of professionalism. Sociology 32 (1), 43–63.

Hanlon, G., 2000. Sacking the New Jerusalem? – The New Right, Social Democracy and Professional Identities. Sociol. Res. Online 5 (1), [Online] available at: <http://www.socresonline.org.uk/5/1/hanlon.html> (accessed 12.12.10.).

Herdman, E.A., 2001. The illusion of progress in nursing. Nurs. Philos. 2 (1), 4–13.

Hoskins, R., 2012. Interprofessional working or role substitution? A discussion of the emerging roles in emergency care. J. Adv. Nurs. 68 (8), 1894–1903.

Hotho, S., 2008. Professional identity–product of structure, product of choice: linking changing professional identity and changing professions. Journal of Organizational Change Management 21 (6), 721–742.

Hoyle, E., John, P.D., 1995. Professional Knowledge and Professional Practice. Cassell, London.

Hugman, R., 1991. Organization and professionalism: The social work agenda in the 1990s. Br. J. Soc. Work 21 (3), 199–216.

Hyde, P., McBride, A., Young, R., Walshe, K., 2005. Role redesign: new ways of working in the NHS. Pers. Rev. 34 (6), 697–712.

Jenkins, R., 2004. Social Identity. Routledge, London.

Johnson, T.J., 1972. Professions and Power. Macmillan, London.

Kitchener, M., 2000. The bureaucratization of professional roles: The case of clinical directors in UK hospitals. Organization 7 (1), 129–154.

Kreindler, S.A., Dowd, D.A., Dana Star, N.O.A.H., Gottschalk, T., 2012. Silos and social identity: the social identity approach as a framework for understanding and overcoming divisions in health care. Milbank Q. 90 (2), 347–374.

Laidler, P., 1994. Stroke Rehabilitations – Structure and Strategy. Chapman Hall, London.

Larkin, G., 1988. Occupational Monopoly and Modern Medicine. Tavistock Publications, London.

Larson, M.S., 1977. The Rise of Professionalism: A Sociological Analysis. University of California Press, Berkeley CA.

Larson, M.S., 1990. In the matter of experts and professionals, or how impossible it is to leave nothing unsaid. In: Torstendahl, R., Burrage, M. (Eds.), The Formation of Professions: Knowledge, State and Strategy. Sage, London, pp. 24–50.

Lechte, J., 1994. Fifty Key Contemporary Thinkers From Structuralism to Postmodernity. Routledge, London.

Lingard, L., Reznick, R., DeVito, I., Espin, S., 2002. Forming professional identities on the health care team: discursive constructions of the 'other' in the operating room. Med. Educ. 36 (8), 728–734.

Lowe, F., O'Hara, S., 2000. Multi-disciplinary team working in practice: managing the transition. J. Interprof. Care 14 (3), 269–279.

Lunt, I., 2008. Ethical issues in professional life. In: Cunningham, B. (Ed.), Exploring Professionalism. University of London, Institute of education.

MacDonald, K.M., 1984. Professional formation: the case of Scottish accountants. B. J. Socio. 35 (2), 174–189.

MacDonald, K.M., 1995. The Sociology of the Professions. Sage, London.

Mackey, H., 2007. Do not ask me to remain the same: Foucault and the professional identities of occupational therapists. Aust. Occup. Ther. J. 54 (2), 95–102.

Manias, E., Street, A., 2001. The interplay of knowledge and decision making between nurses and doctors in critical care. Int. J. Nurs. Stud. 38 (2), 129–140.

Mann, M., 1986. The Sources of Social Power, vol. I. Cambridge University, Cambridge.

Marcia, J.E., 1966. development and validation of ego identity status. PSP 5, 551–558.

Mazhindu, D.M., 2003. Ideal nurses: the social construction of emotional labour. Eur. J. Psych. Couns. Hea. 6 (3), 243–262.

McCallin, A., 2001. Interdisciplinary practice – a matter of teamwork: an integrated literature review. J. Clin. Nurs. 10 (4), 419–428.

McDonald, R., Harrison, S., Checkland, K., Campbell, S.M., Roland, M., 2007. Impact of financial incentives on clinical autonomy and internal motivation in primary care: ethnographic study. Br. Med. J. 334 (7608), 1357.

Miles, A., Hill, A.P., Hurwitz, B., 2001. Clinical Governance and the NHS Reforms: Enabling Excellence or Imposing Control. Aesculapius Medical Press, London.

Miles-Tapping, C., 1985. Physiotherapy and medicine: Dominance and control? Physio. Can. 37 (5), 289–293.

Miller, C., Ahmad, Y., 2000. Collaboration and partnership: an effective response to complexity and fragmentation or solution built on sand? Int. J. Sociol. Soc. Policy 20 (5), 1–38.

Miller, R., Hall, K., Miller, R., 2013. A story of strategic change: Becoming a social enterprise in English health and social care. J. Soc. Entrep. 4 (1), 4–22.

Moloney, M.M., 1986. Professionalization of Nursing: Current Issues and Trends. Lippincott, London.

Monrouxe, L.V., 2010. Identity, identification and medical education: why should we care? Med. Educ. 44 (1), 40–49.

Nancarrow, S.A., Borthwick, A.M., 2005. Dynamic professional boundaries in the healthcare workforce. Sociol. Health Illn. 27 (7), 897–919.

Neumann, V., Gutenbrunner, C., Fialka-Moser, V., Christodoulou, N., Varela, E., Giustini, A., et al., 2010. Interdisciplinary team working in physical and rehabilitation medicine. J. Rehabil. Med. 42 (1), 4–8.

Newman, J., 2006. Modernising Governance; New Labour, Policy and Society. Sage Publications, London.

Niemi, A., Paasivaara, L., 2007. Meaning contents of radiographers' professional identity as illustrated in a professional journal – A discourse analytical approach. Radiography 13 (4), 258–264.

Nolan, P., 2004. The changing world of work. J. Health Serv. Res. Policy 9 (1), 53–59.

Nugus, P., Greenfeild, D., Travaglia, J., Westbrook, J., Braithwaite, J., 2010. How and where clinicians exercise power: Inter-professional relations in health care. Soc. Sci. Med. 71, 898–909.

Øvretveit, J., 1985. Medical dominance and the development of professional autonomy in physiotherapy. Sociol. Health Illn. 7, 76–93.

Øvretveit, J., 1997. Interprofessional Working for Health and Social Care. Macmillan, London.

Page, S., Willey, K., 2007. Workforce development: planning what you need starts with knowing what you have. Aust. Health Rev. 31 (5), 98–105.

Payne, J., Keep, E., 2003. Re-visiting the Nordic approaches to work re-organization and job redesign: lessons for UK skills policy. Policy Studies 24 (4), 205–225.

Pethybridge, J., 2004. How team working influences discharge planning from hospital: a study of four multi-disciplinary teams in an acute hospital in England. J. Interprof. Care 18 (1), 29–41.

Poggi, G., 2006. Power. In: Turner, B.S. (Ed.), The Cambridge Dictionary of Sociology. Cambridge University Press, Cambridge, pp. 464–469.

Pollock, A., Price, D., 2011. How the secretary of state for health proposes to abolish the NHS in England. Br. Med. J. 342 (d1695), 800–803.

Poses, R.M., 2003. A cautionary tale: the dysfunction of American health care. Eur. J. Intern. Med. 14 (2), 123–130.

Raju, P.S., Lonial, S.C., Gupta, Y.P., 1995. Market orientation and performance in the hospital industry. J. Health Care Mark. 15 (4), 34.

Rastegar, D.A., 2004. Health care becomes an industry. Ann. Fam. Med. 2 (1), 79–83.

Reber, A.S., 1985. Dictionary of Psychology. Penguin, Harmondsworth.

Reed, M., Anthony, P., 1993. Between an ideological rock and an organizational hard place: NHS management in the 1980s and 1990s. In: Clarke, T., Pitelis, C. (Eds.), The Political Economy of Privatization. Routledge, London, pp. 185–202.

Reynolds, J., 2007. Discourses of inter-professionalism. Br. J. Soc. Work 37 (3), 441–457.

Rivett, G., 1998. From Cradle to Grave: Fifty Years of the NHS. King's Fund, London.

Ruekert, R.W., 1992. Developing a market orientation: an organizational strategy perspective. Int. J. Res. Mark. 9 (3), 225–245.

Saks, M., 1996. From Quackery to Complementary Medicine: The Shifting Boundaries Between Orthodox and Unorthodox Medical Knowledge. Complementary Medicine: Knowledge in Practice. Free Association Books, London.

Salhani, D., Coulter, I., 2009. The politics of interprofessional working and the struggle for professional autonomy in nursing. Soc. Sci. Med. 68 (7), 1221–1228.

Sankelo, M., Akerbald, L., 2008. Nurse entrepreneurs' attitudes to management, their adoption of the manager's role and management assertiveness. J. Nurs. Manag. 17 (7), 829–863.

Scholes, J., 2008. Coping with the professional identity crisis: Is building resilience the answer? Int. J. Nurs. Stud. 45 (7), 975–978.

Scott, J., 2001. Power. Blackwell Publishers, Cambridge.

Scourfield, P., 2006. What matters is what works? How discourses of modernization have both silenced and limited debate on domiciliary care for older people. Crit. Soc. Policy 26 (1), 5–30.

Svensson, R., 1996. The interplay between doctors and nurses—a negotiated order perspective. Sociol. Health Ill. 18 (3), 379–398.

Sewell, W.H., Jr., 1992. A theory of structure: Duality, agency, and transformation. Am. J. Sociol. 98 (1), 1–29.

Shapiro, J., 2008. Philosophy, Ethics, and Humanities in Medicine. Philos. Ethics Humanit. Med. 3, 10. [Online] Available at: <http://www.peh-med.com/content/3/1/10> (accessed 15.06.12.).

Skills for Health, 2006. Delivering a Flexible Workforce to Support Health and Health Services – The Case for Change. Skills for Health, Bristol.

Smith, S., Roberts, P., Balmer, S., 2000. Role overlap and Professional boundaries: Future implications for Physiotherapy and Occupational Therapy in the NHS. Physio. 86 (8), 397–400.

Southon, G., Braithwaite, J., 1998. The end of professionalism? Soc. Sci. Med. 46 (1), 23–28.

Sparkes, V.J., 2002. Profession', and professionalization: part 1: role and identity of undergraduate physiotherapy educators. Physiotherapy 88 (8), 481–492.

Strauss, A., Schatzman, L., Ehrlich, D., Bucher, R., Sabshin, M., 1963. The hospital and its negotiated order. The Hos. Mod. Soc. 147 (169), b52.

Stubbings, L., Scott, J.M., 2004. NHS workforce issues: implications for future practice. J. Health Organ. Manag. 18 (3), 179–194.

Sullivan, W.M., 2000. Medicine under threat: professionalism and professional identity. Can. Med. Assoc. J. 162 (7), 673–675.

Tajfel, H., 1992. Social Identity and Intergroup Relations. Cambridge University Press, Cambridge.

Thistlethwaite, J., Spencer, J., 2008. Professionalism in Medicine. Routledge, London.

Turner, B.S., 2006. Institutions. In: Turner, B.S. (Ed.), The Cambridge Dictionary of Sociology. Cambridge University Press, Cambridge, pp. 300–302.

Wallace, J.E., 1995. Organizational and professional commitment in professional and nonprofessional organizations. Adm. Sci. Q. 40 (6), 228–255.

Walshe, K., Benson, L., 2005. GMC and the future of revalidation: time for radical reform. Br. Med. J. 330 (7506), 1504.

Weinreich, P., Saunderson, W. (Eds.), 2002. Analysing Identity: Cross-Cultural, Societal and Clinical Contexts. Routledge, London.

Wenger, E., 1998. Communities of Practice: Learning, Meaning, and Identity. Cambridge University Press, Cambridge.

West, M.A., Borrill, C., Dawson, J., Scully, J., Carter, M., Anelay, S., et al., 2002. The link between the management of employees and patient mortality in acute hospitals. Int. J. Hum. Resour. Manag. 13, 1299–1310.

Whitchurch, C., 2008. Shifting identities and blurring boundaries: The emergence of third space professionals in UK higher education. High. Educ. Q. 62 (4), 377–396.

White, K., 2006. Occupations. In: Turner, B.S. (Ed.), The Cambridge Dictionary of Sociology. Cambridge University Press, Cambridge, pp. 421–422.

Witz, A., 2003. Professions and Patriarchy. Routledge, London.

Xyrichis, A., Lowton, K., 2008. What fosters or prevents interprofessional teamworking in primary and community care? A literature review. Int. J. Nurs. Stud. 45 (1), 140–153.

# 2

# THE BIOPSYCHOSOCIAL MODEL
## An Overview

ALEC RICKARD

## CHAPTER CONTENTS

## INTRODUCTION

Biological. Psychological. Sociological. Three words that should seem familiar, perfectly normal and 'every day' to us. Most health care professionals would have had, as part of their preregistration training, some form of specific education around these three domains. These may well have been taught (and learnt) in relation to each other at some point, but quite possibly also separately, particularly initially. Depending on how long ago you trained, there may well have been discrete sessions or modules on the individual subjects and then, maybe, later there were attempts to integrate them. Abbreviated together, the term 'biopsychosocial' should also be familiar to all physiotherapists, indeed every health care professional, ideally, whether indoctrinated during their initial training, or through subsequent continuing professional development via further education and just reading the literature. A recommendation of a biopsychosocial approach appears as a well-established tenet of clinical guidelines (Clinical Standards Advisory Group, 1994; Kendall et al., 1997; Mercer et al., 2006; National Institute for Clinical Excellence, 2004; Royal College of General Practitioners, 1999; Royal College of Physicians, 2004; Savigny et al., 2009).

Three words, three domains, not only abbreviated and conjoined together, but also, perhaps, conveying some further specific meaning. Although we may feel we know it, do we really *understand* it? Do we correctly utilize it, or even misue it perhaps through inadequate training (Gatchel and Turk, 2008)? Is it a case of, as Aristotle stated, the whole being more than the sum of its parts, and different from the sum of its parts (Upton et al., 2014)?

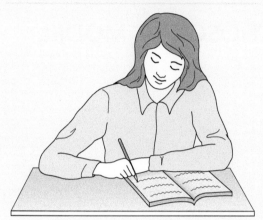

Before reading any further, try to write down brief answers to the following questions. You will be asked to review these again at the end.

■ What do you know/understand of the term 'biopsychosocial model' presently?
■ How do you utilize it in practice (if at all)?
■ Is there anything that prevents or hinders your use of it in practice?

## HISTORY OF THE BIOPSYCHOSOCIAL MODEL

The biopsychosocial model is largely attributed to Engel (1977), who sought to replace the traditional, predominant biomedical model, which fails to account for the social, psychological, and behavioural dimensions of illness. However, the concept is older, with the term 'biopsychosocial' itself first coined by Grinker some 20 years earlier (Ghaemi, 2009). Interestingly, although Engel wanted to ensure the psychosocial aspects were accounted for in medicine, and health care in general, it is thought Grinker's aim was to ensure the biological aspects were not forgotten within psychiatry, as a reaction to the profession's orthodoxy at the time.

Although undoubtedly playing a role in the assessment and treatment of disease (as opposed to *people,* perhaps?), particularly in the case of acute illness, the biomedical model is dualistic, reductionist and exclusionist by nature. This traditional disease model, also known more simply as the medical model, is dualistic, because it separates the mind from the body, in line with the Cartesian theory of pain, proposed by Rene Descartes in 1664 (Main et al., 2008). Thereby, a patient's signs and symptoms are conceptualized as either 'physical' (viewed positively and therefore *real* or *true*) or 'psychological' (usually viewed negatively and perceived as *fake* or *exaggerated*). It is also reductionist in that it assumes all disease is directly linked to specific physical pathology, which is confirmed by objective tests and that there is a linear relationship between the amount of damage and the pain experienced, as well as the severity of pain and the extent of disability (Asmundson et al., 2014; Main et al., 2008). Figure 2.1 illustrates the application of such reductionism. Finally, as Engel suggested, it is exclusionist because behavioural, psychological and social factors are not deemed important. Therefore Engel saw his model as a design for action in the real world of health care, because we must treat the whole person, in all their complexity (Waddell, 2004).

In terms of applying the biopsychosocial model to pain specifically, the gate control theory of pain cannot go without mention. Initially proposed by Melzack and Wall (1965) and subsequently modified (eg, Melzack and Casey, 1968 and others), it appears to be one of the first significant attempts to integrate biological and psychological mechanisms of pain within a single model (Asmundson et al., 2014). Although not displacing the

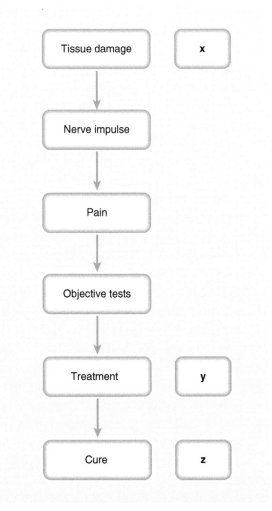

FIGURE 2.1 ■ A rather simplified view of physiotherapy – if only things were this straightforward ...

**BOX 2.2**
EDITED QUOTE FROM A LETTER TO THE
EDITOR OF *PHYSIOTHERAPY*

The Journal of the Chartered Society of Physiotherapy
'The great importance of psychological factors in rehabilitation has long been recognized by thoughtful and experienced physiotherapists. It is only recently, however, that articles in *Physiotherapy* have stressed this aspect of our work. Unfortunately many ... appear to be totally unaware ... and pursue their vocation oblivious to the psychotherapeutic effects ... successes may be attributed to this or that technique when in reality it is the knowledge and personality of the physiotherapist ...'

advancing pain science, has clearly not worked, with, for example, back pain being labelled a twenty-first century medical disaster (Waddell, 2004).

However, this does not suggest that physiotherapists, or other health professionals, have been solely operating under a strict biomedical model and not considering the psychological and social influences (Watson, 2000). Many would argue that physiotherapists have always been aware of these influences, it was just that this was less overt, not integrated, and, perhaps, deemed far less important. The prevalence in the literature of 'the biopsychosocial approach to health', 'the biopsychosocial model of pain' or variations thereof, including 'of disability' and 'wellbeing', suggests there has been a revolution in medical thinking (Smith, 2002). This revolution refers to a shift away from the biomedical model, which focused on physical pathology and physical damage and then fixing said damage (Asmundson et al., 2014), to one that, perhaps, focuses on the *person* and integrating all the different factors that contribute to their health and wellbeing state. However, have we really achieved this more *integrated* approach to health (Havelka et al., 2009)? Take a look at Box 2.2.

biomedical model, it challenged its primary assumptions by recognizing there was no longer a linear relationship between physical tissue damage and the actual experience of pain, utilizing a 'one-way' ascending-only system of nerve transmission. However, the prevailing chronicity of different disorders, spiralling health care costs and often limited, clear, efficacious management options, the biomedical model, even with the advent of

When do you think this was? A few years ago? Within the last couple of decades? This was actually from 1969 and the letter ended with:

> 'The few token psychology lectures are pitifully inadequate … Is it really more important to know about the inside of a short-wave machine?'

This last sentence of the quote does, perhaps, date it somewhat, but what if 'ultrasound' or 'TENS' replaced 'short-wave', would it seem more contemporaneous? With the apparent decreased popularity of electrotherapy generally at present, this may not be the best example, but could the sentiment equally apply to 'kinesiology tape', for example? More recently, Waddell (2004) similarly proclaimed that it is no longer sufficient for doctors and therapists to know about anatomy and physiology. Therefore the point is there has been a tendency to place greater emphasis on knowing about some*thing*, rather than some*one*. Waddell (2004) further emphasizes that health care demands we treat human beings, who suffer and are not simply neat packages of mechanics or pathology.

Over 40 years after the letter in Box 2.2, plus 50 from Melzack and Wall's seminal work on the gate control theory of pain and nearly 400 years from Descartes, we need to keep checking, evaluating, reflecting and asking the right questions, to see if we have truly moved forward.

## THE BIOPSYCHOSOCIAL MODEL IN PRACTICE

It must be stressed that the biopsychosocial model is not a panacea; it does not provide the specifics, the detail of what we should do with our patients. Waddell (2004) describes it more as a method or a set of tools, with the need for clinicians to also be counsellors, helping patients cope with their problem(s), but also suggesting that patients have to be less passive and more active in their role. Table 2.1 compares and contrasts the implications of the biomedical and biopsychosocial models. Perhaps the term biopsychosocial 'approach', often used interchangeably in the literature, is more apt than 'model'. It could be considered as ideally providing the fundamental, underlying approach to all health care, a framework for a problem-oriented approach (Waddell, 2004).

There have been a number of specific models and approaches that have been developed from this framework, such as the 'Mature Organism' model (Gifford, 1998) or the 'Fear-Avoidance' model (Vlaeyan and Linton, 2000). In fact, the late Louis Gifford wrote many articles and chapters on not only pain, but also patient experiences and management in general, managing to provide both philosophical, but pragmatic insight, grounded in clinical, real-world, experience and they are well worth reading. The World Health Organization's (WHO, 2000) International Classification of Functioning, Disability and Health (ICF) is based on the biopsychosocial model of illness and aligns well to it (Fig. 2.2).

If the dichotomous approach of the biomedical model is deemed unacceptable, we need to be careful this does not also happen with the biopsychosocial model. The 'bio', 'psycho' and 'social', by definition, underscores the important interactive contribution of the factors in each of these defining domains, and requires their individual assessments (Gatchel

| TABLE 2.1 | |
|---|---|
| **The Implications of the Medical (Biomedical) and Biopsychosocial Models** | |
| **The Medical Model** | **The Biopsychosocial Model** |
| Pain, disability, incapacity for work and sickness absence are more or less entirely a consequence of injury disease and impairment | Pain, disability, incapacity for work and sickness absence are *partly* a matter of the health condition, but *also* of how the individual thinks, feels and behaves |
| They are therefore out of the individual's control and he/she bears little or no responsibility | The individual must therefore share some responsibility |
| The health condition and recovery are a matter of health care | The health condition and recovery are *partly* a matter of health care, but *also* of the individual's own effort and behaviour |
| The patient is the passive recipient of health care | The individual must be an active participant in his or her own rehabilitation and recovery |
| Relief of pain will automatically cure disability | Management must both relieve pain, and at the same time, prevent disability |

*(Adapted from Waddell, 2004)*

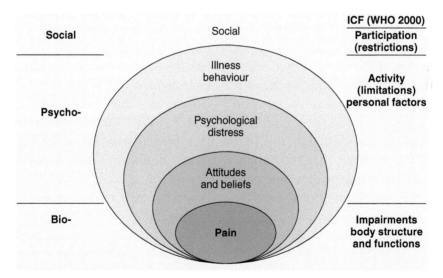

FIGURE 2.2 ■ The biopsychosocial 'onion' of low back pain and disability with mapping of the World Health Organization's (WHO) International Classification of Functioning, Disability and Health (ICF). *(Adapted from Waddell, 2004.)*

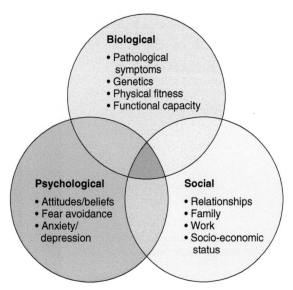

FIGURE 2.3 ■ Examples of the different domains and constructs of the biopsychosocial model traditionally represented in the literature.

and Turk, 2008). Figure 2.3 represents the biopsychosocial model as a Venn diagram, with the three core domains and then some examples of the constructs within each, with the potential overlap between them. The central area, overlapped by all three domains, could be viewed as the 'problem', be that illness or pain, for example, that the patient presents to us. Therefore their illness or pain is made up of the combination of the differing factors, to varying degrees.

Depending on the problem, or the severity, the prominence, influence and prioritization (the significance) of these individual factors will vary and may also vary at differing times during the course of the problem. Conversely, the central overlapping area could also represent being 'healthy/good health' or 'pain free', signifying absence of the influencing factors,

## *Case Study 1*

- 36-year-old male, right rotator cuff tear
- Difficulty elevating arm beyond 90 degrees
- Manager within local council's housing department – still in work
- Married with young family
- Runs local children's football club and has a strong social network with other parents

or at least balance or insignificance of the factors – the factors may still be there, they do not necessarily disappear, but are, possibly, below some preconceived threshold level of influence: nonthreatening. Although not receiving recognition for it, it appears the WHO did actually predate the biopsychosocial model by challenging the biomedical model as far back as the 1940s, when its inaugural constitution stated that, 'good health was not merely the absence of disease or infirmity' (WHO, 1948).

Consider the brief case study described in Box 2.3. What do you think are the primary factors that may influence his presentation, pain, disability and outcome? Although devoid of specific detail, can you allocate issues to each of the three domains as per Figure 2.3? Do that now before reading ahead. What if he is now off sick from work? What about if he did not have a social network or was single? Consider what influences this may now have on his presentation and, importantly, his management. Now look at the case study in Box 2.4 and see which domains apply as before and which may be a priority.

## Case Study 2

- 36-year-old male, right rotator cuff tear
- Difficulty elevating arm beyond 90 degrees
- Self-employed fisherman
- Single, lives with parents, but on waiting list for council house
- No specific social network, longstanding history of depression

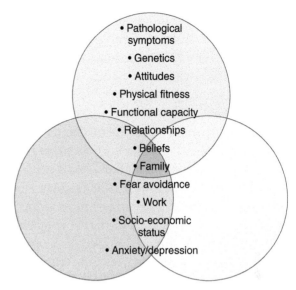

FIGURE 2.4 ■ Perhaps the reality (and messiness?) of the different domains and constructs of the biopsychosocial model.

The flag system (eg, Red Flags, Yellow Flags, etc.) provides a concise way of assessing the relative influence, dominance and potential urgency of these domains and their 'risk' factors (Greenhalgh and Selfe, 2006; Kendall et al., 1997; 2009; Main et al., 2008; Watson and Kendall, 2000). Do also read the chapters by Greenhalgh and Selfe (Chapter 2) and by Chamberlain (Chapter 7) in this book for further, interesting discussion on this. Watson (2000) additionally uses the term 'barriers to recovery' in relation to psychosocial Yellow Flags, which may help focus on the direct application to our own individual practice and can take into account individual competence to explore and manage these. However, there is a need to be cautious here, as it may be too easy to justify not exploring and managing these barriers ourselves, to pass the buck – 'I'm not a psychologist', 'it's not my role'. Unfortunately, this has been witnessed too often in practice with clinicians prejudging their patients – and sometimes writing them off from the first impression – proclaiming something along the lines of 'this one's covered in Yellow Flags', or 'don't think I can do much here, he's so yellow flaggy'. Yes,

we may not be psychologists and, yes, we need to be aware of our own scope of practice and competence, but we should also not underestimate what skills and ability we have and what may appear to be subtle, but actually significant, differences we can make by just taking the time to listen and attempt to rationalize with the patient their issues, worries and concerns. It is often not easy (although it is not always as difficult as perceived, but may be more time-consuming initially) – it would be simpler if we stuck to physical treatment of mechanical problems (Waddell, 2004), as per the biomedical model, but the reality is that many of the factors do so often overlap and are entangled, such that are they ever truly separate (see Fig. 2.4)? Borrell-Carrió et al. (2004) and others discuss 'complexity science' and causality as an attempt to understand these complex and changing factors that might be interrelated, but in different ways at different times. This can appear more linear, such as obesity leading to diabetes and arthritis; which may limit exercise capacity, adversely affecting blood pressure and cholesterol levels; which then may contribute to both stroke and coronary artery disease. Furthermore, some of the effects, such as depression after a heart attack or stroke, can then become causal resulting in a greater chance of a second similar event. This may also be circular, so that through a series of feedback loops, the specific behaviour patterns are sustained over time (Borrell-Carrió et al., 2004).

Each domain should be of equal importance, however there is, perhaps, a tendency for physiotherapists to still feel more comfortable with physical factors, such as the perceived – 'bio'— and have a preference for addressing this aspect (Bishop and Foster, 2005; Moffett and Mclean, 2006). The anecdote personally experienced being that 'we are "physio" – as in physical – therapists'. This may also be driven by the potential medical urgency needed with any identified signs of serious pathology, as part of the 'bio'; a sentiment quite rightly discussed in Selfe and Greenhalgh's chapter in this book (Chapter 2) about Red Flags ('Don't take the bio out of biopyschosocial'). The late Louis Gifford, in his foreword of Greenhalgh and Selfe's book on Red Flags (2006), similarly emphasized this, stating that, although assessing Red Flags (the 'bio') is an essential component of assessment, he also strongly conveyed (in his uniquely insightful way) the *person* at the centre of it. So, although distinct, the 'bio', 'psycho' and 'social' are not separate and it should not be about assessing or managing, for example, the 'bio' and then the 'psychosocial' (Jones and Edwards, 2006). Gifford further proclaims it is the patient's worry that drives their behaviour, to seek help, to be in front of you and Jones and Edwards (2006) highlight that this is from the interplay of the perceived threat balanced against the perceived ability to cope with it. So, without assessing the 'bio' (the pathology?), how can you reassure the 'psychosocial' (the person?)?

## REASSURED CONFIDENCE TO CONFIDENT REASSURANCE

Reassurance of the patient is needed to get them 'on board', convincing them we take their problem seriously as echoed by some other authors, in order that they will then listen to and actively engage in any management strategies. This is important, as all too often, from personal experience, any perception on the part of the patient that their health problem or pain is not deemed 'physical', results in them disengaging and feeling not believed or taken seriously. However, equally, reassurance about the 'bio' is needed for clinicians so that they are confident in appropriately managing the patient's problem and can have conviction in what they are telling the patient (eg, to deescalate patients' concerns about serious pathology and encourage, or to empower, even, to keep active – see discussion on Bishop and Foster's study in this chapter). Appropriate management may also include *not* treating them or *not* referring them for investigations unnecessarily. This is equally important as inappropriate investigations or treatments may not only be potentially physically harmful in their own right (eg, radiation exposure, adverse event from lumbar puncture), but can mislead treatment.

Many diagnostic tests demonstrate low specificity or sensitivity, resulting in false-negatives and positives with poor correlation between test results and symptoms and disability, especially between x-ray and pain (Waddell, 2004). Meta-analysis demonstrates clinical outcomes are not improved in lumbar spine imaging in the absence of clinical indication of serious pathology (Chou et al., 2009). In fact, Kendrick et al.'s randomized control trial (RCT) found that patients referred for x-rays reported greater pain and a poorer general health status (at 3 months) than those that did not. Even magnetic resonance imaging (MRI) does not appear to improve the situation, in fact it appears this more sensitive imaging technique produces even higher false-positive findings in asymptomatic 'normals' and that psychosocial factors are better at predicting functional disability as a result of disc herniation (Jarvick and Deyo, 2000; Maus, 2010). Really, this is not to be unexpected: if your car does not start in the morning, you would not take a photo of the engine and send it off to a mechanic, expecting them to diagnose and fix your problem? This is an analogy I have used in practice, along with sometimes likening their symptoms to the issue of software glitches in a computer, rather than hardware malfunction or failure, eg, if your computer crashes or freezes, you may not expect to find anything obvious from dismantling it, but a reboot seems to help (see Butler and Moseley's Explain Pain, 2003, however, apologies to the many more expert clinicians and academics, who I have probably heard describe similarly and may have absorbed this from,

via the likes of the Physiotherapy Pain Association's meetings, but am unable to specifically acknowledge!).

The use of flags and diagnostic triage (Waddell, 2004) can provide some assistance in beginning to broadly assign appropriate management strategies, usually by ruling out potential problems, rather than ruling in specific management. Psychosocial Yellow Flags do appear to have some prognostic value as risk factors for negative outcomes, if not consistently so, hence a combination of questionnaire and clinical interview is recommended for their evaluation (Nicholas et al., 2011). Furthermore, there are discrepancies in the literature as to the relative importance of each Yellow Flag/psychosocial factor, resulting in limited application for directing appropriate management. However, there is some evidence in low back pain patients that further subclassification, using the STarT Back Screening Tool, is possible such that we may allocate people in to low-, medium- and high-risk groups (Hill et al., 2008). This tool aims to categorize both physical and psychosocial aspects. There is some evidence that interventions targeting psychological risk factors result in better functional or return-to-work outcomes than those that did not and were more symptom-based (Nicholas et al., 2011).

## EDUCATION, EDUCATION, EDUCATION

Gatchel and Turk (2008) suggest that the failure of the biopsychosocial model in practice, or weakness in its application, may be as a result of the inappropriate training of health professionals. It has previously been suggested the assessment of psychosocial factors has not been a part of standard physiotherapy education and requires additional training (Hemmings and Povey, 2002; Watson, 2000). Bishop and Foster's (2005) large (n = 453) cross-sectional survey of experienced, musculoskeletal physiotherapists assessed their ability to identify psychosocial factors, via case scenario 'vignettes'. They demonstrated that, although most recognized when patients were at high risk of developing chronicity, contrary advice to restrict work and activity was common, therefore persistence of the biomedical model was suspected. It may be a problem of translation into practice, rather than lack of appropriate education and training, per se, although, perhaps a focus on the management of psychosocial factors is required, instead of assessment, in line with the previous discussion regarding confidence and reassurance. They did also cite that changing therapists' beliefs and practices requires exploration (Bishop and Foster, 2005). Audits of UK physiotherapy records have found significant numbers lacked evidence that psychosocial factors had been assessed (NHS QIS, 2009; Sparkes, 2005). Although this does not mean they were not assessed, it could suggest they were given lower priority, although further research is required to determine why.

Similarly, in Sweden it has been demonstrated that physiotherapists are aware of the importance of psychosocial risk factors, but struggle to specify which factors are important (Overmeer et al., 2004). Confidence and training issues may have been a factor in this survey, with only 43% (n = 102) feeling able to predict those that would develop chronic pain (the role of Yellow Flags). In addition, it

has also been found that a difference may exist between those that work in the UK's National Health Service (NHS) and in the private sector, as well as with experience. Although Pincus et al. (2007) found physiotherapists generally endorsed a psychosocial approach, this tended to be more so by those working in the NHS and there was a weak (but statistically significant) correlation between years in practice and tendency towards a biomedical approach.

Physiotherapists are not the only health professionals that do not seem to be fully implementing a recommended biopsychosocial-based approach. Although the majority of chiropractors appear to deem psychosocial factors important, less than half reported being able to assess them and only a third felt able to treat them (Walker et al., 2005). In the homeland of Yellow Flags (Kendall et al., 1997), Crawford et al. (2007) found that New Zealand General Practitioners' initial approach to acute low back was also influenced by biomedical factors, rather than published guidelines, with problems of time management, funding and lack of appropriate training identified.

Gatchel and Turk (2008) advocate not only appropriate biopsychosocial training of individual health professionals, but of teams, which, they suggest, should be integrated, under one roof and therefore all 'speaking the same language.' Multidisciplinary pain clinics may appear to be the pinnacle of an integrated biopsychosocial approach within most health care settings. Harding et al. (2010) found that all pain clinics in their study stated they subscribed to a biopsychosocial approach, but on further exploration that it was not as well integrated as first thought. Although clinicians focused on psychological approaches, in preference to physical approaches and readily embraced cognitive/behavioural strategies, there was relatively little consideration for the effect social factors played (Harding et al., 2010), of which work could be a major one. Harding et al. (2010) do admit that many of the social aspects, such as housing or financial issues, of chronic pain cannot be managed within a hospital clinic and may even lie outside the remit of health professionals, although they also suggest that some of these may have been implicitly considered within the psychological approaches.

## SUMMARY – A MODEL APPROACH NEEDED?

You may notice in this chapter that there has been little attempt to offer a specific, formal definition of the biopsychosocial model. That is very much deliberate. As Waddell (2004) stated, it is a framework and, although it may provide us with the tools we need, it should be seen as just that. It is established that biological considerations alone are not enough, but as it stands, is the biopsychosocial model also enough – is it at least the sum of its parts, if not greater? The biopsychosocial model has more than its share of detractors, but ones who also do not simply embrace the simpler life of biomedical model either (Borrell-Carrió et al., 2004; Gatchel and Turk, 2008; Ghaemi, 2009). Waddell (2004) himself, although a strong advocate for the biopsychosocial model, also warns that the literature may have swung too far towards psychosocial issues to neglect the physical. Although part of me laments that we still have a need to think in such linear, but potentially divisive

ways, perhaps it should be celebrated that most, if not all, of us, in wanting to do the best for our patients, strive to ensure that all components are considered. After all, this is the very essence of the original tenets of the biopsychosocial model and rather than being seen as a tidy, complete unifying theory, this would be far too rigid and inflexible to apply to individuals. Therefore it should simply be embraced as just the most obvious, common sense *approach* there is to how we should be dealing with people. Although we may refer to them as patients, clients or service users, at the end of the day we too are people; every bit as complex and potentially messed up.

Go back to Box 2.1 at the beginning of the chapter. Have any of your answers changed? This chapter is not about trying to provide answers, rather its aim is to get you to think and consider what you think you know. Therefore, more importantly, do you have any additional questions now? Yes, the factors influencing health and ill-health are complex, yes, people are complex and – guess what – society is (increasingly?) complex. It is only by questioning the status quo and striving for better that we may hope to achieve better.

## ACKNOWLEDGEMENTS

In addition to my ever supportive wife and children (despite my grumpiness), I would also like to thank many physiotherapy and pain clinic colleagues over the years, as well as my students, who I hope have got something out of me 'banging on about pain and those psychosocial issues'! However, a special acknowledgement goes to Linda Knott, dedicated and long-serving clinical specialist physiotherapist in pain management to South

Devon and active Physiotherapy Pain Association member, for the influence and support she gave me along the road to pain enlightenment (which, of course, is ongoing)!

## References

Asmundson, G.J.G., Gomez-Perez, L., Richter, A.A., Carleton, R.N., 2014. The psychology of pain: models and targets for comprehensive assessment. In: van Griensven, H., Strong, J., Unruh, A.M. (Eds.), Pain – a Textbook for Health Professionals, second ed. Churchill Livingstone, Edinburgh.

Bishop, A., Foster, N.E., 2005. Do physiotherapists in the United Kingdom recognize psychosocial factors in patients with acute low back pain? Spine 30 (11), 1316–1322.

Borrell-Carrió, F., Suchman, A.L., Epstein, R.M., 2004. The biopsychosocial model 25 years later: principles, practice, and scientific inquiry. Ann. Fam. Med. 2 (6), 576–582.

Butler, D.S., Moseley, G.L., 2003. Explain Pain. NOI Group publications, Adelaide.

Chou, R., Fu, R., Carrino, J.A., Deyo, R.A., 2009. Imaging strategies for low-back pain: systematic review and meta-analysis. Lancet 373 (9662), 463–472.

Clinical Standards Advisory Group, 1994. Back Pain: Report of a CSAG Committee on Back Pain. HMSO, London.

Crawford, C., Ryan, K., Shipton, E., 2007. Exploring general practitioner identification and management of psychosocial yellow flags in acute low back pain. N. Z. Med. J. 120 (1254), 27–39.

Engel, G.L., 1977. The need for a new medical model: a challenge for biomedicine. Science 196 (4286), 129–136.

Gatchel, R.J., Turk, D.C., 2008. Criticisms of the biopsychosocial model in spine care: creating and then attacking a straw person. Spine 33 (25), 2831–2836.

Ghaemi, S.N., 2009. The rise and fall of the biopsychosocial model. Br. J. Psychiatry 195 (1), 3–4.

Gifford, L.S., 1998. The mature organism model. In: Gifford, L.S. (Ed.), Physiotherapy Pain Association Yearbook 1998-1999. Topical Issues in Pain. Whiplash – Science and Management. Fear-Avoidance Beliefs and Behaviour. CNS Press, Falmouth.

Greenhalgh, S., Selfe, J., 2006. Red Flags: A Guide to Identifying Serious Pathology of the Spine. Churchill Livingstone, London.

Harding, G., Campbell, J., Parsons, S., Rahman, A., Underwood, M., 2010. British pain clinic practitioners' recognition and use of the bio-psychosocial pain management model for patients when physical interventions are ineffective or inappropriate: results of a qualitative study. BMC Musculoskelet. Disord. 11, 51.

Havelka, M., Lucanin, J.D., Lucanin, D., 2009. Biopsychosocial model – the integrated approach to health and disease. Coll. Antropol. 33 (1), 303–310.

Hemmings, B., Povey, L., 2002. Views of chartered physiotherapists on the psychological content of their practice: a preliminary study in the United Kingdom. Br. J. Sports Med. 36 (1), 61–64.

Hill, J.C., Dunn, K.M., Lewis, M., Mullis, R., Main, C.J., Foster, N.E., et al., 2008. A primary care back pain screening tool: identifying patient subgroups for initial treatment. Arthritis Rheum. 59 (5), 632–641.

Jarvick, J.G., Deyo, R.A., 2000. Imaging of lumbar intervertebral disk degeneration and ageing, excluding disk herniation. Radiol. Clin. North Am. 38 (6), 1255–1266.

Jones, M., Edwards, I., 2006. Learning to facilitate change in cognition and behaviour. In: Gifford, L. (Ed.), Topical Issues in Pain 5. CNS Press, Falmouth.

Kendall, N.A.S., Linton, S.J., Main, C.J., 1997. Guide to Assessing Psycho-Social Yellow Flags in Acute Low Back Pain: Risk Factors for Long-Term Disability and Work Loss. Accident Compensation Corporation and the New Zealand Guidelines Group, Wellington.

Kendall, N.A.S., Burton, A.K., Main, C.J., Watson, P.J., on behalf of the Flags Think-Tank, 2009. Tackling Musculoskeletal Problems: A Guide for the Clinic and Workplace – Identifying Obstacles Using the Psychosocial Flags Framework. TSO, London.

Kendrick, D., Fielding, K., Bentley, E., et al., 2001. Radiography of the lumbar spine in primary care patients with low back pain: randomised control trial. Br. Med. J. 322 (7283), 400–405.

Main, C.J., Sullivan, M.J.L., Watson, P.J., 2008. Pain Management: Practical Applications of the Biopsychosocial Perspective in Clinical and Occupational Settings, second ed. Churchill Livingstone, London.

Maus, T., 2010. Imaging the back pain patient. Phys. Med. Rehabil. Clin. N. Am. 21 (4), 725–766.

Melzack, R., Wall, P.D., 1965. Pain mechanisms: a new theory. Science 150, 971–979.

Melzack, R., Casey, K.L., 1968. Sensory motivational and central control determinants of p. A new conceptual model. In: Kenshalo, R. (Ed.), The Skin Senses. Thomas, Springfield.

Mercer, C., Jackson, A., Hettinga, D., et al., 2006. Clinical Guidelines for the Physiotherapy Management of Persistent Low Back Pain, Part 1: Exercise. Chartered Society of Physiotherapy, London.

Moffett, J., Maclean, S., 2006. The role of physiotherapy in the management of non-specific back pain and neck pain. Rheumatology 45, 371–378.

National Institute for Clinical Excellence, 2004. Management of Chronic Obstructive Pulmonary Disease in Adults in Primary and Secondary Care: NICE Clinical Guideline 12. National Institute for Clinical Excellence, London.

NHS Quality Improving Scotland, 2009. National Physiotherapy Low Back Pain Audit: Improving Back Care in Scotland. NHS QIS, Edinburgh.

Nicholas, M.K., Linton, S.J., Watson, P.J., Main, C.J., the 'Decade of the Flags' Working Group, 2011. Early Identification and Management of Psychological Risk Factors ('Yellow Flags') in Patients With Low Back Pain: A Reappraisal. Phys. Ther. 91 (5), 737–757.

Overmeer, T., Linton, S.J., Boersma, K., 2004. Do physical therapists recognise established risk factors? Swedish physical therapists' evaluation in comparison to guidelines. Physiotherapy 90, 35–41.

Pincus, T., Foster, N.E., Vogel, S., et al., 2007. Attitudes to back pain amongst musculoskeletal practitioners: A comparison of professional groups and practice settings using the ABS-mp. Man. Ther. 12 (2), 167–175.

Royal College of General Practitioners, 1999. Clinical Guidelines for the Management of Acute Low Back Pain, second ed. Royal College of General Practitioners, London.

Royal College of Physicians, 2004. National Clinical Guidelines for Stroke, second ed. RCP, London.

Savigny, P., Kuntze, S., Watson, P., et al., 2009. Low Back Pain: Early Management of Persistent Non-Specific Low Back Pain. NICE Guidelines. National Collaborating Centre for Primary Care and Royal College of General Practitioners, London.

Smith, R.C., 2002. The biopsychosocial revolution. J. Gen. Intern. Med. 17 (4), 309–310.

Sparkes, V., 2005. Treatment of low back pain: monitoring clinical practice through audit. Physiotherapy 91, 171–177.

Upton, J., Janeka, I., Ferraro, N., 2014. The whole is more than the sum of its parts: Aristotle, metaphysical. J. Craniofac. Surg. 25 (1), 59–63.

Vlaeyan, J.W.S., Linton, S.J., 2000. Fear avoidance and its consequences in chronic musculoskeletal pain: a state of the art. Pain 85 (3), 317–332.

Waddell, G., 2004. The Back Pain Revolution, second ed. Churchill Livingstone, Edinburgh.

Walker, S., Bablis, P., Pollard, H., McHardy, A., 2005. Practitioner perceptions of emotions associated with pain: a survey. J Chiropr Med. 1, 11–18.

Watson, P., 2000. Psychosocial predictors of outcome from low back pain. In: Gifford, L. (Ed.), Topical Issues in Pain 2. CNS Press, Falmouth.

Watson, P., Kendall, N., 2000. Assessing psychosocial yellow flags. In: Gifford, L. (Ed.), Topical Issues in Pain 2. CNS Press, Falmouth.

World Health Organization, 1948. Constitution of the World Health Organization. World Health Organization, Geneva.

World Health Organization, 2000. International Classification of Functioning, Dusability and Health (ICF). World Health Organization, Geneva.

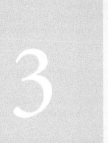

# SCREEN FOR RED FLAGS FIRST: DON'T TAKE THE 'BIO' OUT OF BIOPSYCHOSOCIAL

SUE GREENHALGH ▪ JAMES SELFE

## CHAPTER CONTENTS

The difficulty with diagnosing serious spinal conditions early and the catastrophic outcomes of delayed diagnosis are widely documented (Levack et al., 2002; Markham, 2004). Bin et al. (2009) identified how early symptoms of serious pathology are often fluctuating and vague, varying in intensity and evolution. Quinn and De Angelis (2000) concurred with these diagnostic difficulties, highlighting the fact that epidural spinal cord compression can imitate degenerative disc disease. Needless to say, with no previously existing back pain these symptoms can be difficult to spot. Consider a context of chronic low back pain and disability where new symptoms of serious pathology are now superimposed, ie, the chronic low back pain sufferer now has an additional cause for their pain, but this time serious; early diagnosis becomes considerably more challenging. This chapter discusses factors to consider and strategies to adopt to facilitate the diagnosis of serious spinal pathology in a patient with longstanding back pain.

## BACKGROUND

In the last decade musculoskeletal (MSK) disorders have increased and are now the greatest cause of disability among European Union (EU) member states and are the second greatest cause of disability worldwide. In terms of disability-adjusted life years (DALYs), low back pain (LBP) is listed in the top 10 causes worldwide. In Europe back pain ranks second to ischaemic heart disease as the largest cause of disability. People aged 45 to 54 are most commonly affected by these conditions, as musculoskeletal disorders have caused over 30 million years of disability combined in these age groups (The Global Burden of Disease, 2013).

It is estimated that up to 80% of the population will develop an episode of LBP at some

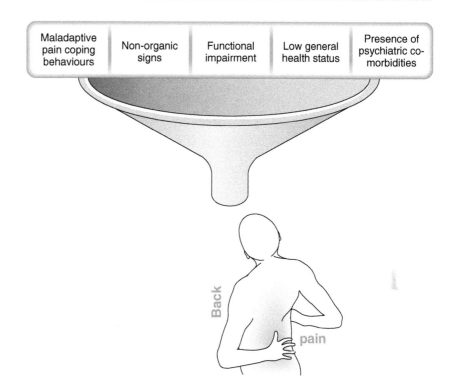

FIGURE 3.1 ■ Key baseline predictors of persistent disabling low back pain.

point in their life (Jones and Macfarlane, 2005) and in the UK approximately 14% of general practitioner consultations are related to LBP (Dunn et al., 2010). The prevalence of chronic LBP is about 23%, with 11% to 12% of the population being disabled by it (Airaksinen et al., 2006). States of chronic pain represent the greatest medical challenge, as they tend to be stable over time, can be resistant to intervention and consume most health care resources (Krismer and van Tulder, 2007). During a state of chronic pain psychosocial dimensions also become increasingly relevant and are important in explaining how people respond to back pain (Mannion et al., 1996). Low recovery expectations within the first 3 weeks of LBP onset can identify people at risk of poor functional outcome up to 6 months later (Iles et al., 2009).

The most helpful baseline predictors of persistently disabling LBP include the factors shown in Figure 3.1 below (Chou and Shekelle, 2010).

It is well recognized that the presence of Red and Yellow Flags are not mutually exclusive (Gifford, 2000) and 'although small, the prevalence of Red Flag conditions in patients with chronic back pain is not zero' (Bogduk and McGurk, 2002). Red Flags represent warning signs associated with serious spinal pathology, however serious spinal pathology is not a single condition; it is a group of highly heterogeneous conditions arising from different organ systems which are associated with a wide diversity of symptoms (Lyratzopoulos, 2014).

Red Flags are a list of prognostic variables for serious pathology. In relation to the spine this may include those listed in Table 3.1 below.

Over the last two decades the approach to the assessment and treatment of LBP has made an enormous leap forwards with regards to the holistic biopsychosocial approach, which no longer considers the sufferer from a reductionist biomedical perspective. During the initial consultation the identification of Red Flags is a clinical priority when

| TABLE 3.1 |
|---|
| **Common Examples of Red Flags** |

| | |
|---|---|
| Tumour: benign or malignant | 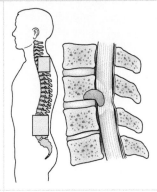 |
| Infection | 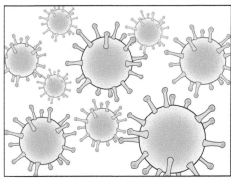 |
| Fracture | 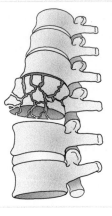 |

| TABLE 3.1 *cont* |
|:---:|
| **Common Examples of Red Flags** |

Cauda equina syndrome (CES)

The spinal cord per se ends at roughly the L1/L2 level, below this is the cauda equina; cauda equina (Latin for horse's tail) is a bundle of nerves located in the lumbar, sacral and coccygeal nerves and innervates the pelvic organs; the cauda equina extends to sensory innervation of the perineum and, partially, parasympathetic innervation of the bladder. Cauda equina syndrome may lead to permanent paralysis, impaired bladder and/or bowel control and loss of sexual sensation

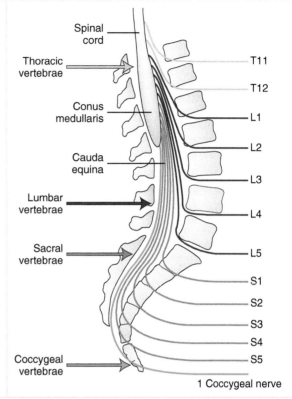

conducting diagnostic triage and the presence of Red Flags can represent a clear reason for further investigation or onward specialist referral, if identified, even in the presence of other important psychosocial factors. Red Flag questions routinely screen for serious underlying pathology often requiring urgent specific medical management. Fortunately serious pathology accounts for a very small percentage of patients, with the incidence estimated to be less than 1% (CSAG, 1994). However, although the incidence of patients presenting with metastatic bone disease to a spinal triage service is low, prevalence is likely to increase as a result of better treatment of

the primary cancer (Finucane, 2013) and increased life expectancy (NHS England, 2013). Osteoporotic fracture and malignant disease are the most common serious pathologies seen by musculoskeletal services, with osteoporotic fractures being by far the most common (Downie et al., 2013). Serious underlying disease must always be ruled out when 'osteoporotic' fracture is identified. If not diagnosed in a timely manner the outcome of delayed diagnosis for patients with underlying serious pathology could be catastrophic (Levack, 2002; Markham, 2004). Waddell (2004) clearly states that clinicians should 'always carry out diagnostic triage first. Exclude serious spinal pathology or a widespread neurological disorder before even thinking about "illness behaviour". So, although a very small percentage will have a serious pathology, every back pain sufferer must be screened for serious pathology, initially using Red Flags, to inform the clinical reasoning process.

The clinical guidelines for physiotherapy management of persistent LBP (Mercer et al., 2006) reported that there were 163 individual items that could be considered as Red Flags, with 119 items in the subjective history and 44 items in the objective examination. Clearly this presents a challenge in terms of the practical clinical utility of Red Flags. However, despite this, Gifford (2014) states,

'How can you be expected to be able to reassure patients that there's nothing seriously wrong and that it's safe to start loading and get moving if you don't know the major key signs of sinister pathology?'

This screening for serious pathology must be a continuing approach and reassessed at regular intervals to monitor important indicators, as the clinical landscape can change across time. Although chronic back pain sufferers do not have an increased risk of serious pathology, chronic LBP does not protect sufferers against the possibility of developing serious spinal pathology at a later date. Classic pain behaviours and poor coping strategies may, however, increase the risk of cancer developing through:

- Lack of exercise
- Obesity
- Smoking
- Excessive use of alcohol

thus highlighting the importance of life choices on our general health, see Figures 3.2 and 3.3 below.

It is important to realize that most Red Flags have a relatively weak evidence base and that LBP guidelines usually provide lists of individual Red Flags and leave their interpretation up to clinicians. However, a more effective screening tool could be recommended if data were available on how to use Red Flags in combination with each other. Ideally an effective series of Red Flag questions for spinal malignancy would highlight pertinent characteristics from the patient's

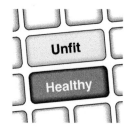

FIGURE 3.2 ■ We all face choices.

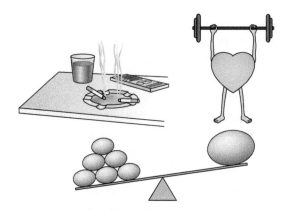

FIGURE 3.3 ■ Can we stack the deck in our favour by making the right choices?

| TABLE 3.2 | |
| :---: | :--- |
| **Sensitivity and Specificity** | |
| Sensitivity: true positives | Those patients who have a combination of Red Flags that do have serious spinal pathology |
| Specificity: true negatives | Those who do not have a combination of Red Flags that do not have serious spinal pathology |

*(Streiner and Norman, 2001)*

history and physical examination (Henschke et al., 2010). Waddell (2004) suggested that to arrive at an accurate and safe diagnosis key signs and symptoms need to be combined. The same is true for Red Flags; Klaber et al. (2006) state that 'clinicians should not uncritically accept any one Red Flag in isolation – the context is crucial.'

When trying to rule a diagnosis in or out, a diagnostic test must have a high sensitivity, ie, those who have a positive test should have the disease (Table 3.2). Unfortunately individual Red Flags have a low sensitivity in isolation. For example, Harding et al. (2005) conducted a prospective longitudinal study of 482 consecutive patients who were attending a back pain triage clinic of which 213 patients reported some night pain and 90 reported pain every night. On average patients had 5 hours of continuous sleep and awoke two and a half times per night, interestingly no serious pathology was identified in any patient. Although a significant and disruptive symptom for patients, these results challenge the sensitivity of night pain in isolation as a useful diagnostic indicator for serious spinal pathology in a back pain triage clinic. Southerst et al. (2012) also confirmed that other well-known Red Flags such as age over 50,

previous history of cancer, no relief with rest and constitutional symptoms such as unexpected weight loss, fever and fatigue individually have high specificity but low sensitivity. Combinations of Red Flags are therefore much more helpful; however, more work is needed to evaluate sensitivity and specificity of such combinations to evaluate their strength (Southerst et al., 2012). Currently Red Flags individually or in combination should be viewed as useful clinical sign posts to raise the index of suspicion as to the possibility of the presence of serious pathology; Red Flags would generally fail if they were used as binary classification tests within a classical diagnostic testing process.

For more than two decades a flag system has been used to assist in the diagnostic triage process. Both Red and Yellow Flags are considered to be key components of this process during the clinical examination of a LBP sufferer (Mercer et al., 2006). In addition there are Blue Flags (social and economic factors), Black Flags (occupational factors) and Orange Flags (psychiatric factors), although these will not be addressed in this chapter. A very useful mnemonic (ABCDEFW) has been posed by Waddell (2004) as an aide memoire to guide clinicians through the relevant themes related to the assessment of Yellow Flags, these are listed below and expanded upon at the end of the chapter in Table 3.5.

- Attitudes and beliefs about pain
- Behaviour
- Compensation issues
- Diagnosis and treatment
- Emotions
- Family
- Work

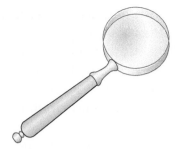

FIGURE 3.4 ■ Is it possible to look too hard for symptoms?

## Seek and Ye Shall Find – Is It Possible to Look Too Hard for Symptoms?

Judicious use of investigation has been highlighted as important within the biopsychosocial approach. Unnecessary investigation, such as magnetic resonance imaging (MRI) has been highlighted by Waddell (2004) as potentially detrimental in relation to the patient's psychological state see Figure 3.4. Commonly investigations reveal insignificant abnormalities, sometimes referred to as 'incidentalomas' which can unnecessarily raise anxiety for patients and their families. In the case of MRI, age related changes, reported as 'degenerative changes' can reinforce diagnostic 'labelling'. Littlewood et al. (2013) provide an important critique of the utility of diagnostic labelling and challenge its importance in clinical practice when considering the complex interplay between tissue damage, nociception, the central nervous system and the patient's pain experience. They describe pain as an output sensation, ie, a product of central nervous system processing, at the level of the spinal cord and brain, modulated by a host of other factors which may be intrinsic, such as the patient's beliefs about pain or extrinsic, such as societal, contexts. However, further clinical investigations may be appro-

priate and necessary if underlying pathology is suspected. Careful clinical reasoning when working in an extended scope arena will guide the clinician to order appropriate and timely investigations when the index of suspicion is raised. The clinician must always consider in advance what they suspect the investigation will show and how the results may influence the onward medical management. Ordering the correct investigation(s) at the correct point in the disease process will ensure that patient outcome is optimized. Whole spinal MRI in the case of suspected metastatic spinal cord compression (MSCC) is one example (NICE, 2008). If all test investigations are positive, the clinician's threshold prior to ordering the test is too high, therefore some serious cases will inevitably be missed in the early stages of the disease process. In this situation the decision to investigate is not being made until the clinician is almost certain that sinister pathology exists. If a large proportion of results are negative, the threshold is too low and a review of clinical reasoning may be required. The only exception to this general rule would be cauda equina syndrome (CES) as a result of the emergency surgical nature of the condition and the catastrophic outcomes if the surgical window is missed. Because of the large number of factors that can masquerade as CES symptoms (Woods et al., 2015) the 'gold standard' diagnostic tool, MRI, may be negative. Therefore in CES cases a positive 'hit rate' of 10% or less may be acceptable by MRI within your clinical environment. However, it is inappropriate to order an investigation such as an MRI simply because the clinician has no idea what is going on and is 'searching' for a diagnosis. Clinical reasoning should identify clear factors deeming further investigation necessary.

## RED FLAG COMPLEXITIES

Any new patient with multiple symptoms is very challenging as patients can have simultaneous combinations of benign musculoskeletal (MSK) problems, Yellow Flags and serious pathology as illustrated in Figure 3.5

During consultations with patients with complex conditions clinicians need to ask themselves:

- Is there a local lesion responsible for the condition?
- Is there one lesion producing a series of referred phenomena responsible for all of the symptoms, or is there a systemic pathology underlying the patient's problems?
- What is the balance between the physical symptomology and psychological/emotional health?

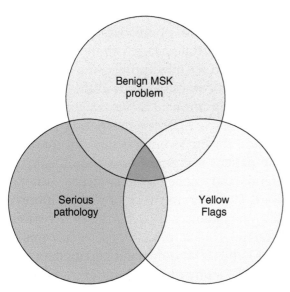

FIGURE 3.5 ■ Venn diagram illustrating the potential complexity and overlap of patients' conditions.

This is where the science and art of physiotherapy plays a major role. Instinct, clinical skill and experience are important when dealing with such complex patients (Mitchell, 2012), as Sackett et al. confirmed in (1996) when describing evidence based medicine.

*'The practice of evidence based medicine means integrating individual clinical expertise with the best available external clinical evidence from systematic research. By individual clinical expertise we mean the proficiency and judgment that individual clinicians acquire through clinical experience and clinical practice. Increased expertise is reflected in many ways, but especially in more effective and efficient diagnosis and in the more thoughtful identification and compassionate use of individual patients' predicaments, rights, and preferences in making clinical decisions about their care.'*

One of the consequences of multiple morbidities is that trying to unpick the complexity of the patient's condition can often lead to delays in diagnosis (Mitchell, 2012) (Table 3.3).

NB two case histories (Rose and Elizabeth) are presented later in this chapter but it is relevant to refer to them here in Table 3.3.

A delayed diagnosis is particularly important in cases of cancer (Levack, 2002) and CES (Gleave and Macfarlane, 2002) as the stage of the condition has a strong influence on clinical outcome. Up to 20% of all patients with newly diagnosed cancer in England have multiple consultations, ie, three or more visits to primary care prior to referral. This highlights the complexity associated with diagnosing cancer, in the absence of chronic pain states, rather than suggesting poor diagnostic

### TABLE 3.3
### Factors Influencing the Referral Pathway

| Complexity of Presentation | Patient |
|---|---|
| Coexisting morbidity | Rose and Elizabeth |
| Symptom suggests different initial diagnosis | Rose |
| Symptom suggests different malignancy | |
| *Patient – Mediated Factors* | Rose and Elizabeth |
| Time to re-present with ongoing symptoms | Rose |
| Time to re-present after initial treatment | |
| Declining investigation or examination | Elizabeth |
| Declining referral or admission | Elizabeth |
| Not attending follow-up | Elizabeth |
| *Diagnostic Process* | |
| Reassurance from negative investigation | Rose |
| Investigation suggests benign cause | Rose |

(Mitchell, 2012)

### TABLE 3.4
### Number of Consultations and Mean Time to Referral of Cancer Cases

| Number of Consultations | Median Time to Referral (Days) |
|---|---|
| 3 | 34 |
| 4 | 47 |
| 5 | 96 |

(Lyratzopoulos, 2014)

reasoning or suboptimal professional practice (Lyratzopoulos, 2014) (Table 3.4).

Cancer diagnosis in primary care can be particularly complex and challenging as it can be difficult to differentiate new potentially malignant symptoms and coexisting illness may readily mask the symptoms of a developing cancer (Mitchell et al., 2012). Southerst et al. (2012) highlight the findings of a retrospective case review involving patients suffering from primary sarcomas of the pelvis; delays in diagnosis included clinicians being deceived by the chronicity of the condition. In another specific example two-thirds of multiple myeloma patients initially present with back pain (Lyratzopoulos, 2014). In multiple myeloma, the multiplication of abnormal plasma cells within bone marrow causes a reduction in the number of normal blood cells and the resultant anaemia leads to constitutional illness symptoms such as tiredness, malaise and weakness (Southerst et al., 2012). According to NHS choices (2015) symptoms of clinical depression include, unexplained aches and pains, lack of energy and no motivation. In the case of a patient presenting to a musculoskeletal service with these symptoms it is easy to see how complex the clinical reasoning process can become in the presence of preexisting chronic LBP and ongoing depression (Fig. 3.5). Decisions relating to a new clinical diagnosis often benefit from observing patient symptoms over time to identify trends and changes, the so called 'watchful wait'. However, this type of clinical observation highlights a possible tension between effective clinical practice and policy makers and patients who demand speedy diagnosis. A recent study of significant event audits in the diagnosis of lung cancer showed several factors which contributed to multiple consultations, these included poor communication between primary and secondary care and patient preference for delayed referral (Lyratzopoulos, 2014) (Table 3.4).

The strongest predictor of multiple consultations is tumour site. Between 30% and 50% of patients subsequently diagnosed with multiple myeloma, pancreatic, stomach or lung cancer have multiple consultations, compared with <10% of patients subsequently diagnosed with breast cancer or melanoma. These differences reflect the challenges with identifying conditions associated with nonspecific symptoms, such as back or abdominal pain, compared to those with characteristic symptom signatures, such as palpable breast lump or visible skin lesion (Lyratzopoulos, 2014) (Box 3.1).

## HOW TO SPOT RED FLAGS IN A BUNDLE OF YELLOW FLAGS

Unfortunately serious pathology does not conform to a structured check list of items that present in a logical or tidy chronological order. A recent study investigating patients' experience with CES illustrated a clear variation in the order of symptom presentation (Greenhalgh et al., 2015). For instance some patients developed bladder dysfunction before any leg weakness was reported. Others reported significant leg symptoms before bladder function was affected.

> *'The first thing to go was my bladder function. I couldn't tell when I was going to go. I just felt like I always wanted to go and I didn't. I couldn't tell whether it was bladder or bowel.'*
>
> *Mr Blue*

> *'It was like you could not tell where your feet were in space. I was sort of losing control…my legs weren't working properly like they were made of rubber. It was as if I had been riding a horse for a week or something and obviously that was to do with the saddle numbness.'*
>
> *Mr Black*

In what initially seems to be a paradox, therapists reported that this was an important finding and actually found it useful to learn that there is no pattern in symptom presentation for CES (Greenhalgh et al., 2015). The clinician often needs to work through a maze of vague and ambiguous findings, cross-checking against recognized patterns before order is found and diagnostic hypotheses are formulated. There is a complex relationship between biomedical knowledge and clinical reasoning. A high level of biomedical knowledge is essential but does not necessarily translate into a high level of skill when considering clinical reasoning. What is known is that clinical reasoning should be an iterative continuous process, reinterpreting new emerging information in light of the hypothetical diagnosis in an ongoing cyclical loop, we have previously described this as 3D thinking (Greenhalgh and Selfe, 2006; 2010). In our model of 3D thinking we proposed that during patient consultations physiotherapists draw on their previous experience and knowledge and that each patient consultation simultaneously adds to the physiotherapists' knowledge and experience. Developing this model further, it is important to note that during a patient consultation each new piece of information gained by the therapist is assessed for diagnostic alternatives, each of which is simultaneously assigned with levels of certainty and plausibility by the therapist. Clinical reasoning is therefore not one single cognitive process based on certain biological difficulties. There needs to be an understanding over time, carefully establishing the patient's reaction to and their interpretation of the meaning of symptoms. This meaning – making over time is commonly known as narrative reasoning. Fleming and Mattingly (2000) describe narrative reasoning and active judgement as used collectively in the clinical setting to transport information from an ambiguous and chaotic situation towards reason and order. Gaining a good understanding of the patient's understanding of pain and illness enables this to be achieved more successfully; allowing patients to take a crucial role in the clinical reasoning process. Throughout the hypothetical deductive reasoning process, the clinician searches for diagnostic cues from the patient. Not just for severity of pain and location, but for behaviour such as changes in health seeking behaviour (Table 3.2).

The gate control theory developed by Melzack and Wall (1965) highlights that pain is not an unavoidable consequence of nociceptor stimulation but an experience significantly affected by cortical processes affecting attention and meaning. The biopsychosocial model of illness extrapolated these thoughts, initially described by George Engel in 1977 (Engel, 1977). Subsequent authors discussing the biopsychosocial model (CSAG, 1994; Gifford, 2014; Waddell, 2004) confirmed the link between psychological, social and physiological variables. The biopsychosocial model (Gifford, 2014) has thus become firmly established within physiotherapy, encouraging a holistic approach to clinical practice and is often depicted by the biopsychosocial onion (Fig. 3.6). Although extremely useful, it is important to consider the impact upon this model with the development of new nociceptor stimulation from a pathological cause. As discussed, it can be very difficult to differentiate new, possibly serious, symptoms

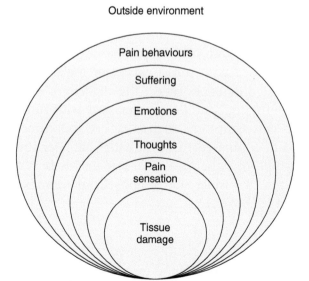

FIGURE 3.6 ■ The biopsychosocial onion. *(Gifford, 2014)*

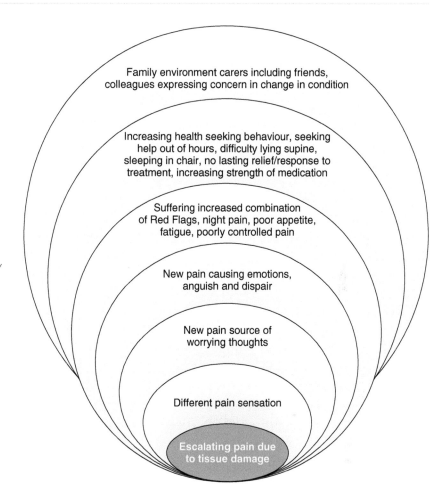

FIGURE 3.7 ■ A model of escalating Yellow Flags as serious pathology develops. *(http://www.paineurope.com/tools/who-analgesic-ladder)*

as a coexisting illness, especially if it is associated with a complex chronic pain state where it may initially mask the symptoms of serious spinal pathology (Mitchell, 2012). Figure 3.7 presents a model illustrating how as serious pathology develops increasing levels of new pain can also cause Yellow Flags to escalate. In patients with chronic pain new nociceptive pain can originate from the same wide variety of anatomical structures as patients without chronic pain and can also be as a result of benign nonserious and serious pathologies ranging from disc lesions to vertebral fractures. Importantly pain is the most common presenting symptom of spinal metastases or MSCC (Levack, 2002). Delays in diagnosis of chronic back pain sufferers complaining of new back pain only, in the absence of a known diagnosis of cancer, are therefore not unlikely. Also of great clinical relevance is that escalation of pain at the prodromal stage of serious disease can be intermittent; this in itself can be misleading, even in more straightforward cases where pain is often interpreted as improving in response to intervention rather than a waxing and waning phenomenon related to a serious cause. New pain which may be intermittent and/or even in the same site of long established chronic pain, is different with an altered quality. If previous clinical notes are available they are almost certainly worthy of investigation. It is vital to establish if the pain is new and never complained of before. This new escalating pain not surprisingly can lead to worrying thoughts, anguish and despair in chronic back pain sufferers. Further disease progression can then result in systemic illness: tiredness, lethargy and constipation, with symptoms from physiological conditions such as anaemia and hypercalcaemia. The presenting condition is now completely different from the established chronic pain situation, with patients suffering from an increasing number of Red Flags and pain affecting behaviours in new ways, eg, an inability to lie supine, sleeping in a chair and not going to bed. Quinn and DeAngelis (2000) highlight that epidural spinal cord compression, although mimicking degenerative disc disease, is worse at night while supine lying; in contrast, degenerative disc disease would normally be relieved by lying down and unloading the disc. Health seeking behaviour may change with increasing visits to a variety of health services, sometimes out of hours. Explore the recent history of health seeking even if the patient presents symptoms as being separate episodes, ie, fever and chills, tiredness, thoracolumbar pain. Always be vigilant in relation to Red Flags, even if these are brought up coincidentally when the patient attends for another reason or is discussing something else (Mitchell, 2012). It can be very helpful to get an overview of the patient's pattern of health seeking. How often

do they usually see their general practitioner? The following quote from Mr Orange in the context of his new pattern of daily health seeking should ring alarm bells.

> 'I was one of them people you know, up to being forty I'd never been in hospital in my life.'
>
> ### *Greenhalgh et al., 2015*

The therapist should be asking what has changed in this man's life (who, all his life has avoided the medical profession) that has triggered such a major alteration in his behaviour? He has clearly passed a 'personal' threshold that has caused a very significant change in his behaviour (World Health Organization (WHO), 2001). Mr Orange went on to develop CES and underwent emergency spinal surgery.

Friends, family and colleagues can often become increasingly concerned. The worried, anxious and complaining partner can actually be a very useful barometer for clinicians, rather than the sometimes perceived hindrance. Based on the experience of having lived with someone who has suffered for years with chronic pain, the partner is able to observe that this new pain experience is different to the underlying chronic condition and this often, correctly, causes a great deal of concern.

During the subjective examination it is important to establish if there is a change in medication use. The WHO has developed a three-step 'ladder' for cancer pain relief in adults (WHO, 2015) and this has been widely adapted as a core approach to the management of other pain states, including chronic pain. If pain occurs there should be prescription of drugs in the following order: nonopioids, such as aspirin and paracetamol, if necessary the prescription of mild opioids such as codeine is next on the ladder, and finally, strong opioids such as morphine should be prescribed. To maintain optimum pain relief, the WHO suggest drugs should be given 'by the clock', that is, every 3 to 6 hours rather than 'on demand.' This prevents large swings in analgesic levels in the blood stream and provides a relatively steady state for pain relief. If the patient is escalating up the analgesic ladder in a step by step progression, but still complaining of poorly controlled pain, this would be a worrying scenario indicative of a worsening condition see Figure 3.8. For a patient suffering from neuropathic pain, drugs such as amitriptyline or nortriptyline (off label), duloxetine, or gabapentin or pregabalin may also be added (NICE, 2015).

This is in contrast to the patient who presents with a haphazard, uncoordinated

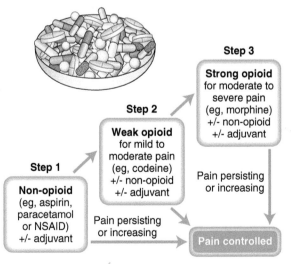

FIGURE 3.8 ■ The World Health Organization (WHO) analgesic ladder.

system of analgesia with no regulation of the dose or regime. Such patients often describe a reluctance to taking medication, a fear of becoming addicted and a dislike of swallowing medication; this chaotic regime would be a far less concerning situation.

Many of the issues previously discussed may not be identified by the clinician at one isolated consultation and so observation over time may be required. Consider other diagnoses in patients with a coexisting disease, rather than assuming the symptom is as a result of the primary chronic condition. Consider all possibilities and do not just go along with the patient's interpretation of the cause of the symptoms, it is all too easy to attribute ongoing symptoms to previous benign diagnoses (Mitchell, 2012).

### Safety Netting

We have established that serious pathology of the spine can often begin with vague, nonspecific symptoms. These can develop over time into well recognized Red Flags, or sometimes appear to resolve spontaneously, as in the case of some osteoporotic fractures. Because of the low sensitivity of Red Flags, their absence during the initial consultation does not necessarily rule out serious pathology. Frequent reevaluation over a period of time can identify unexpected deterioration in symptoms and a failure to receive a lasting benefit from a conservative management approach (Southerst et al., 2012). As a consequence, it is often appropriate to apply a period of 'watchful waiting' until the clinical picture becomes clear. This watchful wait is otherwise known as safety netting (National Collaborating Centre for Cancer, 2013). Clinicians have a responsibility to empower the patient to look out for significant changes in their condition and report them if and when they occur. Sufficient information should be given to patients at the start of such an observational process to give them some understanding of what to look out for and why in order to facilitate patients becoming active participants in the diagnostic process. When a patient presents with what appears to be a low risk for serious spinal pathology, but not no risk, the process of safety netting provides a structured and ordered approach to the observation of signs, symptoms and health seeking behaviour over time.

The following case illustrates how this type of observation over time can be very helpful. Rose (age 58) has a 42-year history of chronic LBP (Table 3.3). Over the last decade symptoms have been intermittently severe, but over the previous 12 months symptoms of back pain have very gradually progressed following a lifting injury at work. Five years previous, Rose had been treated for breast cancer. As a result the clinician's index of suspicion relating to the risk of serious spinal pathology was high at the time of receiving Rose's referral; however, the subjective and objective examination were unremarkable. At this first presentation Rose had only two Red Flags in her history:

▪ Age of 58
▪ Previous history of breast cancer

Rose presented as having mechanical back pain with no leg pain, no neurological signs or symptoms and with no worrying findings during the objective examination. Rose was insistent that this was 'her' chronic back pain. The clinician chose to observe her closely over time and treat with a gentle conservative

approach. Over the course of 4 weeks a significant improvement had been achieved and Rose was delighted with her substantial recovery. However, over the following 2 weeks Rose developed thoracic pain; the LBP, however, remained significantly better. At this stage a thoracic spinal x-ray was an appropriate investigation to request and this was reported as normal. The thoracic pain responded less well to a conservative approach, but 1 week later severe LBP returned suddenly. An urgent whole spinal MRI (NICE, 2008) revealed multiple spinal metastases from T5 caudally, affecting all but two vertebrae to the tip of the sacrum. Rose had been reviewed at the breast clinic 1 month before presenting to the orthopaedic service with back pain and was reassured that all was well. As a consequence, Rose would not have consented to being referred for a spinal opinion if she had not been 'encouraged' by her colleagues. Rose did not suspect that anything was serious until 2 days before the orthopaedic clinician saw her with the investigation results, 2 days after her MRI. The clinician's index of suspicion was high from the beginning, as according to Mitchell (2012), any patient with a history of cancer should be considered to have metastatic disease until proven otherwise, but initially Rose's presenting symptoms were vague and inconclusive. Over the course of 6 weeks the picture became much clearer to the clinician, yet to Rose her symptoms had been similar on and off for a decade. In hindsight Rose admitted at a later date that the quality of her pain had changed 10 months prior to diagnosis, but that this had caused her little concern as it was in the same site as the chronic pain which had been present for over 40 years. Importantly Rose had not previously been questioned about the quality of pain and whether this had in any way changed. The focus of clinical questioning had been exclusively on the nature, location and severity of her pain. In addition to a previous history of breast cancer, Rose reported that she would have valued more information about what sort of things to look out for in the future with respect to either the disease returning or spreading. A lifetime risk of developing invasive breast cancer is said to be 1:8. The median age of diagnosis is 61 with the most common age range for diagnosis being between 55 and 64 years of age. Only 6% to 10% of breast cancer cases have metastases present at initial diagnosis. It is estimated that breast cancer becomes metastatic in 30% of cases, ie, 60% do not develop metastases (Metastatic Breast Cancer Network, 2015). It is therefore neither appropriate nor cost effective to perform a whole spinal MRI on all patients with a history of breast cancer who develop back pain. However, a period of safety-netting in all of these patients is prudent.

It should also be noted that patients with mental health issues and those with multiple morbidities can also slip through safety nets relatively easily (Mitchell, 2012). In addition trying to gain an overview of patients with mental health issues, patterns of health seeking can also be very challenging. Mental capacity is an important concept in this context and relates to the ability of an individual to make a decision. The term 'a person who lacks capacity' means a person who lacks capacity to make a specific decision and at the time that decision needs to be made. Elizabeth was a 42-year-old lady who lived alone, her three children lived separately in a residential care facility. She was referred by accident and emergency (A&E) with a diagnosis of LBP. Elizabeth had initially attended A&E 1 month before with suspected CES. At her initial visit staff in A&E recorded a history of both bladder and bowel incontinence and a physical examination revealed lax anal tone but with no sensory loss, a consultant in A&E reported that CES was not present. Upon arrival to the orthopaedic clinical assessment and treatment support service (CATS) it was clear that Elizabeth was drowsy to the extent that she intermittently rested her head on the clinician's desk. She was slurring her words when questioned; she attributed this to her medication, Seroquel, prescribed for her paranoid schizophrenia which the clinician was unaware of until this point. The patient confirmed that she was under the care of a psychiatrist and thought that paranoid schizophrenia was her diagnosis, although she was not absolutely sure. Despite her unusual behaviour, inability to answer clearly many of the questions during the subjective examination and the diagnosis of paranoid schizophrenia the clinician at the time felt that Elizabeth's mental capacity was not impaired. During the subjective examination Elizabeth also disclosed that she had suffered from a significant and lengthy history of physical and mental abuse. Elizabeth described long standing back pain since childhood but she began with new leg pain the previous February whilst an inpatient in a psychiatric ward. The clinician suspected an L5/S1 disc irritating the S1 nerve root, but was also concerned about the integrity of the cauda equina. Consequently urgent MRI was organized in line with the locally agreed cauda equina pathway. MRI identified central disc prolapses at L4/L5 and L5/S1, more severely at L5/S1, with gross cauda equina compression and central spinal canal stenosis, particularly on the left, with exiting and transiting nerve root compression. Subsequent immediate contact with the patient confirmed that she was happy to be referred to the neurosurgeons at the Specialist Spinal Centre and onward emergency referral was organized. Surprisingly, however, Elizabeth did not attend her spinal appointments on four separate occasions. A case conference was organized with the patient, her designated community psychiatric nurse (CPN), a consultant orthopaedic surgeon from the CATS service and the safeguarding adults lead nurse from the Primary Care Trust (PCT). The central question addressed by this case conference was the mental capacity of the patient, ie, did Elizabeth have the capacity to make a specific decision about the urgency of spinal surgery. It was agreed that Elizabeth would be offered an appointment the next day with the consultant orthopaedic surgeon and the CPN to reassess her physical presentation of CES and her mental capacity to make a specific decision about the appropriate surgical treatment for her condition. At this meeting Elizabeth looked very well and appeared happy to attend. Elizabeth then revealed that she felt she was under severe pressure to comply with care suggested by medical professionals and she also revealed a strong aversion to hospitals and a real fear of surgery. She felt pressurized into agreeing to surgery and responded by retreating into social isolation, not answering the door, phone calls or written requests from any medical professional.

All health professionals have a legal duty to have a regard of The Mental Capacity Act (MCA, 2005) or its equivalent legislative framework across the British Isles when working with people over the age of 16 who lack capacity to make decisions for themselves.

An assessment of capacity can be made by anybody using the following two stage test:

1. Does the person have an impairment of, or a disturbance in the functioning of, their mind or brain?
2. Does the impairment or disturbance mean that the person is unable to make a specific decision when they need to?

A helpful way of applying this is to think, can the person understand, retain, reason and communicate the decision? Where a person lacks capacity to make a specific decision then a best interest decision can be made on their behalf. Consideration must be made if the person will regain capacity, as in some circumstances the decision could be delayed. In addition, the Code of Practice (2007) specifically states that the person must still be involved in the process by finding out their views, past experiences and by consulting others who know them. A decision made for someone who lacks capacity must always take the least restrictive option and be in the person's best interest.

It is interesting to reflect that the proposed criteria for intervention for medical treatment either in hospital or in the community are that:

■ The person has a mental disorder (Elizabeth had paranoid schizophrenia)
■ If medical treatment was not provided, there would be a significant risk to the health, safety or welfare of the person (CES has a very small window of opportunity for successful surgical decompression)

- Because of the mental disorder, the person has a significantly impaired decision-making ability in relation to treatment (Elizabeth's valid reasons for not attending her surgical appointments were not made clear to the medical team)

In Elizabeth's case it is this last criterion which was the deciding factor despite the other two still being present. The mental capacity assessment concluded that Elizabeth did have mental capacity to make a complex decision of this gravity. Elizabeth did not have surgery, at the time of writing her symptoms had returned to normal and she continued to be monitored and supported by her mental health team. This case is interesting as, although the initial assessment was challenging, a diagnosis of CES was arrived at swiftly and an appropriate management plan was initiated, however because of Elizabeth's complex psychosocial health status, the greater challenge arose in the subsequent management of the condition.

## COMMUNICATION

Good communication skills allow us to gain an understanding of the patient's world by achieving an understanding of what patients perceive is happening to them (Swain, 2004). Therapists therefore require excellent communication skills in order to establish the clinical causes underpinning the patients presenting Yellow Flag(s). Physiotherapists need to understand, in depth, key aspects of the patients' lived experiences of their own condition to truly be able to differentiate Yellow from Red Flags. Table 3.5 illustrates the sometimes subtle differences between Red and Yellow Flags that should be explored

during a consultation with a patient who has a chronic pain condition.

Good communication skills allow us to gain an understanding of the world around us by achieving a mutual understanding of what is really happening in the patient's life (Swain, 2004). One study by the authors of this chapter exploring patients' experience with CES identified that the language used by individual patients to describe their symptoms was frequently explicit, but often the language used by clinician's was ambiguous in nature. This appears to highlight the gap between what clinicians perceive they are asking and what patients perceive is being asked. Therefore the gravity of the clinical situation was not always recognized, resulting in delays to diagnosis. Clinicians should frame questions to patients in a way that highlights the gravity associated with their responses to increase the face value of the enquiry. Ensure that jargon is avoided and take care to listen to the patient's responses carefully. This study highlighted that in the context of severe pain concentration and the questions being asked, their relevance was often misinterpreted as illustrated by Mrs Red:

*'I don't think his questions weren't clear, I think that it was impossible to concentrate on anything other than pain management. That's the only way I can... it was impossible to do anything other than control what was going on inside and I think I sort of adopted strategies, ways of holding myself, ways of doing things and, but it was taking all my concentration to deal with the pain and my posture and whatever I needed to be myself. If somebody was asking me questions it was like look come back later, I can't deal with this and I think*

| TABLE 3.5 | | |
| --- | --- | --- |
| **Examples of Differentiation Between Yellow and Red Flags** | | |
| **Themes** | **Yellow Flags** | **Red Flags** |
| **Attitude and Beliefs** | Catastrophic thinking | Pain actually worse |
| | Fearing the worst | Pain has not been this bad |
| | Belief that pain is uncontrollable | This pain now is uncontrollable |
| | Worrying in case pain becomes progressively worse | Pain is becoming progressively worse |
| **Behaviours** | Consistent pattern of health seeking for back pain | Sudden increase in consultations with clinicians, GPs, physiotherapist, A&E, GP out of hours services, night consultations, NHS direct |
| | Use of extended rest, disproportionate down time | Change in functional ability, demonstrating difficulty/inability to lie flat, resting in chair, snoozing on and off |
| | Reporting escalating pain | Escalating medication; dosage and potency of medication |
| | Poor/reduced sleep quality | Significant increase in night pain; does not go to bed, sleeps in chair, pacing bedroom at night |
| | History of avoiding activity to avoid pain | Now not coping with pain at rest |
| **Compensation and Economic Issues** | Lack of financial incentive to return to work | Physically unable to return to work |
| **Diagnosis** | Worried about diagnosis and that something may have been missed | Developed symptoms warned about in previous episode |
| **Emotions** | Anxiety, depression, tearful, low mood, lack of motivation, anger | Increased anxiety causing anguish and despair (Turnpenney et al., 2013) Lethargy Feeling under stress at further change in physical ability, eg, poorly controlled pain, unable to go bed at night, change in sexual function 'Never assume that the screaming ab-dab patient has not got anything physically wrong with them!' (Gifford, 2014) |

| | **TABLE 3.5** *cont* | |
|---|---|---|
| | **Examples of Differentiation Between Yellow and Red Flags** | |
| **Themes** | **Yellow Flags** | **Red Flags** |
| **Family** | Solicitous/over protective family, friends and colleagues | Family, friends and care givers can become a barometer for change<br>Increased concern in relation to <u>change</u> in:<br>■ Appearance<br>■ Pain; night/day<br>■ Functional ability<br>■ Health seeking<br>■ Medication use |
| **Work** | Intermittent work loss episodes | Off work, unable to return despite financial loss<br>Work loss is a worry, but sometimes secondary to severity of symptoms |
| | Unsupportive employer and colleagues | Colleagues voice concern in relation to behaviour and appearance (another barometer) |

*(Adapted from Gifford, 2014)*

*that's why I started getting, well I was short with people.'*

### *Greenhalgh et al., 2015*

Finally, do not underestimate the value of case based discussion with trusted clinical colleagues, ensuring that aspects of confidentiality are respected. Expertise, pattern recognition and hypothesis generation are well known concepts in the diagnostic process. If in doubt, two or more heads can be better than one to optimize the patient's outcome (Kassirer, 2010).

## CONCLUSION

This chapter has highlighted the importance of always conducting diagnostic triage at initial assessment of all spinal patients presenting to musculoskeletal services, to first rule out serious pathology. It has then discussed the considerable challenge associated with identifying Red Flags in a bundle of Yellow Flags and the complexities of clinical reasoning that each clinician faces on a daily basis. One of the keys to success in this area is developing good two way communication to gain an insight into the lived experiences of patients. Clinicians should always be proactive in searching for information (Mitchell, 2012). It is often appropriate and can be very useful to observe the patient over time and evaluate Red Flags at each consultation. It is important to empower patients at risk of serious pathology of the spine, such as Rose, by giving them some control and explaining what Red Flags to look out for and what to do if they think these have developed. Collaborate with patients as partners in an attempt to achieve a timely diagnosis of serious pathology of the spine. In patients who have suffered benign chronic LBP for some time, this collaborative approach is likely to lead to better outcomes for the patient and greater clinical satisfaction for the therapist. Support your advice by giving patients appropriate literature or directing them to specific high quality electronic sources of information that you have vetted.

## KEY TAKE HOME MESSAGES

- Conduct diagnostic triage on all spinal patients to first rule out serious pathology
- Coexisting illness may mask the symptoms of serious pathology
- Reevaluate Red Flags at each consultation
- It can be very difficult to differentiate (new) symptoms of serious pathology
- Periods of watchful waiting can be valuable
- Be vigilant to Red Flags, even if these are brought up coincidentally
- Inform 'at risk' patients of key Red Flags to look out for and give advice about what to do if they occur
- If you are suspicious or puzzled about a clinical problem discuss with a colleague

## ACKNOWLEDGEMENTS

We would like to thank Dr Victoria Lyle, advanced orthopaedic practitioner, for her contribution and help in preparing the case study on 'Elizabeth' presented within this chapter.

## References

Airaksinen, O., Brox, J.I., Cedraschi, C., et al., 2006. Chapter 4. European guidelines for the management of chronic nonspecific low back pain. Eur. Spine J. 15, S192–S300.

Bin, M., Hong, W., Lian-shun, J., Wen, J., Guo-dong, S., Jian-gang, S., 2009. Cauda equina syndrome: A review of clinical progress. Chin. Med. J. 122, 1214–1222.

Bogduk, N., McGurk, B., 2002. Medical Management of Acute and Chronic Low Back Pain an Evidence Based Approach. Causes and sources of chronic low back pain. Elsevier, Chapter 14, p. 116.

Chou, R., Shekelle, P., 2010. Will this patient develop persistent disabling low back pain? JAMA 303, 1295–1302.

Code of Practice, 2007. HMSO, London.

CSAG, 1994, Report of a Clinical Standards Advisory Group on Back Pain. HMSO, London.

Department of Health, 2005. The Mental Capacity Act: England and Wales, HMSO, London.

Downie, A., Williams, C., Henschke, N., Hancock, M., Ostelo, R., Henrica, V., et al., 2013. Red flags to screen for malignancy and fracture in patients with low back pain: systematic review. BMJ 347, f7095.

Dunn, K.M., Jordan, K.P., Croft, P.R., 2010. Recall of medication use, self-care activities and pain intensity: A comparison of daily diaries and self-report questionnaires among low back pain patients. Prim. Health Care Res. Dev. 11, 93–102.

Engel, G., 1977. The need for a new medical model: A challenge for biomedicine. Science 196, 129–136.

Finucane, L., 2013. Metastatic disease masquerading as mechanical low back pain; atypical symptoms which may raise suspicion. Man. Ther. 18, 624–627.

Fleming, M., Mattingly, C., 2000. Action and narrative: two dynamics of clinical reasoning. In: Higgs, J., Jones, M. (Eds.), Clinical Reasoning in the Health Professions, second ed. Butterworth – Heinemann.

Gifford, L., 2000. Topical Issues in Pain 2. CNS Press Ltd, Falmouth.

Gifford, L., 2014. Graded Exposure/Case Histories. CNS Press, Falmouth.

Gleave, J.R.W., Macfarlane, R., 2002. Cauda equina syndrome: what is the relationship between timing of surgery and outcome? Br. J. Neurosurg. 16 (3), 325–328.

Greenhalgh, S., Selfe, J., 2006. Red Flags: A Guide to Identifying Serious Pathology of the Spine. Churchill Livingstone, Elsevier.

Greenhalgh, S., Selfe, J., 2010. Red Flags II: A Clinical Guide to Solving Serious Spinal Pathology. Churchill Livingstone, Elsevier.

Greenhalgh, S., Truman, C., Webster, V., Selfe, J., 2015. An Investigation into the Patient Experience of Cauda Equina Syndrome (CES). Physiother. Pract. Res. 36, 23–31.

Harding, I.J., Davies, E., Buchanan, E., Fairbank, J.T., 2005. The symptom of night pain in a back pain triage clinic. Spine 30 (17), 1985–1988.

Henschke, N., Williams, C.M., Maher, C.G., van Tulder, M.W., Koes, B.W., Macaskill, P., et al., 2010. Red flags to screen for vertebral fracture in patients presenting with low-back pain. Cochrane Database Syst. Rev. (8), Art. No.: CD008643, doi: 10.1002/14651858.CD008643.

Iles, R.A., Davidson, M., Taylor, N.F., O'Halloran, P., 2009. Systematic review of the ability of recovery expectations to predict outcomes in non-chronic non-specific low back pain. J. Occup. Rehabil. 19, 25–40.

Jones, G.T., Macfarlane, G.J., 2005. Epidemiology of low back pain in children and adolescents. Arch. Dis. Child. 90 (3), 312–316.

Kassirer, J., 2010. Teaching Clinical Reasoning: Case-Based and Coached Academic Medicine, Vol. 85, No. 7 / July 2010. Available on: <https://acmd615.pbworks.com/f/ClinicalReasoning.pdf>.

Klaber-Moffett, J., McClean, S., Roberts, L., 2006. Red Flags need more evaluation: Reply. Rheumatology 45, 921.

Krismer, M., van Tulder, M., 2007. Strategies for prevention and management of musculoskeletal conditions. Low back pain (non-specific). Best Pract. Res. Clin. Rheumatol. 21, 77–91.

Levack, P., Graham, J., Collie, D., et al., 2002. Don't wait for a sensory level-listen to the symptoms: a prospective audit of the delays in diagnosis of malignant cord compression. Clin. Oncol. 14, 472–480.

Littlewood, C., Malliaras, P., Bateman, M., Stace, R., May, S., Walters, S., 2013. The Central Nervous System – An additional consideration in 'rotator cuff tendinopathy' and a potential basis for understanding response to loaded therapeutic exercise. Man. Ther. 18 (6), 1–5.

Lyratzopoulos, G., Wardle, J., Rubin, G., 2014. Rethinking diagnostic delay in cancer: how difficult is the diagnosis? BMJ 349, g7400. doi: 10.1136/BMJ.g7400.

Mannion, A.F., Dolan, P., Adams, M.A., 1996. Psychological questionnaires: do "abnormal" scores precede or follow first-time low back pain? Spine 21, 2603–2611.

Markham, D.E., 2004. Cauda equina syndrome: diagnosis, delay and litigation risk. J. Orthop. Med. 26, 102–105.

Melzack, R., Wall, P.D., 1965. Pain mechanisms: a new theory. Science 150 (3699), 971–979. doi: 10.1126/science.150.3699.971; PMID 5320816.

Mercer, C., Jackson, A., Hettinga, D., Barlos, P., Ferguson, S., Greenhalgh, S., et al., 2006. Clinical guidelines for the Physiotherapy management of persistent low back pain, part 1: exercise. Chartered Society of Physiotherapy, London.

Metastatic breast cancer network <http://mbcn.org/education/category/incidence-and-incidence-rates> (accessed 13.07.15.).

Mitchell, E., Rubin, G., Macleod, U., 2012. Improving diagnosis of cancer: A toolkit for general practice. Royal College of General Practitioners.

NHS Choices, <http://www.nhs.uk/Conditions/Depression/Pages/Symptoms.aspx> (accessed 10.07.15.).

NHS England, (2013) The NHS belongs to the people, a call for action. <http://www.england.nhs.uk/wp-content/uploads/2013/07/nhs_belongs.pdf> (accessed 19.10.15.).

National Institute for Health and Care Excellence, (2008) Metastatic Spinal Cord Compression: Diagnosis and management of patients at risk of or with metastatic spinal cord compression. Cardiff: National Collaborating Centre for Cancer, cg75. (Online). Available: <http://publications.nice.org.uk/metastatic-spinal-cord-compression-cg75> (accessed 22.10.15.).

National Institute for Health and Care Excellence, (2015) Neuropathic pain drug treatment <http://cks.nice.org.uk/neuropathic-pain-drug-treatment> (accessed 19.10.15.).

Quinn, J., De Angelis, L., 2000. Neurological Emergencies in the Cancer Patient. Semin. Oncol. 27, 311–321.

Sackett, D.L., Rosenberg, W.C., Muir Gray, J.A., Haynes, B.R., Richardson, W.S., 1996. Evidence based medicine: what it is and what it isn't. BMJ 312, 71–72.

Southerst, D., Dufton, J., Stern, P., 2012. Multiple myeloma presenting as sacroiliac joint pain: a case report. J. Can. Chiropr. Assoc. 56 (2), 94–101.

Streiner, D., Norman, G., 2001. Health Measurement Scales a Practical Guide to Their Development and Use, second ed. Oxford University Press, Oxford.

Swain, J., 2004. Interpersonal communication. In: French, Sally, Sim, Julius (Eds.), Physiotherapy a Psychosocial Approach, third ed. Butterworth-Heinemann, Edinburgh, pp. 205–219.

The Global Burden of Disease, 2013: Generating Evidence, Guiding Policy – European Union and Free Trade Association Regional Edition. Institute for Health Metrics and Evaluation 2301 Fifth Ave., Suite 600, Seattle, WA 98121, USA.

Turnpenney, J., Greenhalgh, S., Richards, L., Crabtree, A., Selfe, J., 2013. Developing an early alert system for metastatic spinal cord compression. Prim. Health Care Res. Dev. DOI: <http://dx.doi.org/10.1017/S1463423613000376> Published online: 05 September.

Waddell, G., 2004. The Back Pain Revolution, second ed. Churchill Livingstone, Edinburgh.

World Health Organization, 2001. International Classification of Functioning, Disability and Health, World Health Organization, Geneva.

WHO. Analgesic Ladder. <http://www.who.int/cancer/palliative/painladder/en/> (accessed 14.10.15.).

Woods, E., Greenhalgh, S., Selfe, J., 2015. Cauda Equina Syndrome and the challenge of diagnosis for physiotherapists: a review. Physiother. Pract. Res. 36 (2015), 81–86.

# 4

## PSYCHOSOCIAL ASPECTS OF PRACTITIONERS
### Adapting Our Interactions With Others to Form Empowering Relationships

JENNIFER E GREEN-WILSON

## CHAPTER CONTENTS

## INTRODUCTION

Physiotherapists influence behavioural change. Individuals who work with physiotherapists need to, or may want to, change their behaviours for various reasons. For example, if competitive athletes sustain multiple injuries over time they may have to modify how they compete, how they train and perhaps even the sports in which they compete. If individuals discover that they have high blood pressure, high cholesterol and are overweight during their annual wellness check-up, they may have to modify what they eat, their level of activity and perhaps other lifestyle decisions. Yet changing behaviour and making sustainable behavioural change tends to be difficult. In order for physiotherapists to be effective in influencing behavioural change, and hopefully sustainable

behavioural change, it is important to understand what motivates human behaviour. It is also essential to acknowledge the important role physiotherapists have in influencing others and to identify how to influence others effectively.

## CHANGING BEHAVIOUR STARTS WITH THE PHYSIOTHERAPIST

Physiotherapists deal with many situations in which they would like patients/clients to change certain behaviours. These clinicians could begin to address the opportunity for change by just telling individuals what the problem is and how they might change (Quinn, 1996). If the change is small or to the other person's liking, this telling/directing approach may be effective in achieving change. However, often, this directive approach may fail to achieve the actual change because the other person may have little interest or desire in responding to the request made by the physiotherapist (Quinn, 1996). Perhaps, when physiotherapists discover that their patients/clients have not made the necessary changes or have not been compliant, for example, with the prescribed home exercise programs (HEP), then in some cases the physiotherapists may use more of a forceful or coercive style, adding some consequence if the behaviour does not change. Seldom will the physiotherapists assume that the change did not occur because they failed to influence effectively.

Generally, in trying to change others, it may be difficult for physiotherapists to see their own role as being a part of the solution or problem. The following example illustrates a possible scenario. Thelma (the physiotherapist) became discouraged because she was not able to make her patient Paul follow through on several essential behavioural changes he needed to make in order to progress with his treatment. Thelma asked her colleague for advice. During the conversation with her colleague, Thelma reflected upon what she did – how she interacted with Paul, what she said and what she did not say – to try to influence Paul in changing his behaviours. Then Thelma assessed the outcome from her interactions with Paul and discovered that she was contributing directly and indirectly to the less-than-desired results. Thelma realized that if she had changed her own style of interacting with Paul she may have been more effective at influencing him in a completely different way.

Physiotherapists need to understand the critical role they play in order to influence, engage and empower others. But before discussing how to influence the behaviours of others, it is important to clarify that physiotherapists can only truly change their own behaviour. In other words, they cannot force another person to change. Therefore physiotherapists first need to choose to change, adapt and modify their own behaviours in how they interact with different people. Then, once they adapt their approach, they will ultimately engage differently and hopefully elicit different responses or behaviours from others.

## ASSUMPTIONS ABOUT HUMAN BEHAVIOUR

Understanding assumptions about human behaviour can help physiotherapists learn how to influence others more effectively. For example, McGregor in 1960 (Heil et al., 2000) identified 'theory X' and 'theory Y', or rather, two different sets of assumptions about human behaviour after examining the behaviour of individuals at work. Theory X assumes that people dislike work; they want to avoid it and do not want to take responsibility (McGregor). Because of their dislike for work, most people must be controlled, told what to do and possibly manipulated before they will work intensely or, in the case of this discussion, actually change their own behaviour. Conversely, theory Y assumes that individuals will direct themselves if they are committed to their goals because they are self-motivated and thrive on responsibility (McGregor). These individuals understand that it takes physical and mental effort in order to achieve goals or change behaviours and lifestyle habits.

Most likely how physiotherapists interact with their patients/clients will be influenced by their beliefs and assumptions about what motivates people. Therefore using these theories – theory X and theory Y – as an example, as well as the other theories about motivation, may help physiotherapists uncover how they perceive key factors that motivate behaviour in certain ways. When physiotherapists understand that their assumptions about human behaviour and motivation influence their style of interaction with others, then they can learn how to adapt the ways in which they approach different people in order to influence behavioural change most effectively. For example, if physiotherapists believe that individuals dislike working, exercising or changing, then they may tend to use more of a directive or authoritarian style of interaction. In this case the physiotherapist would tell their patients/clients exactly what to do without a lot of discussion. Conversely, if physiotherapists assume that individuals take pride in working towards a good outcome, then they will adopt a more participative and engaging style of interacting. In this particular scenario, physiotherapists assume that because their patients/clients accept responsibility, they will be motivated to fulfill the goals they have established jointly and will not need much direction. It is worthy to note that when physiotherapists use a more participative approach to problem solving (based on theory Y assumptions) they may expect better results, greater creativity and imagination, compared with just telling others what needs to change.

Another assumption about human behaviour is that people tend to resist change – consciously or unconsciously – when they are initially asked to change. Change may create feelings of discomfort, anxiety, fear and uncertainty. Therefore understanding and acknowledging this common reaction to change may help physiotherapists be more effective in influencing behavioural change. Physiotherapists can reduce this natural resistance to change by involving the individuals who are being asked to change in the process of change. For example, physiotherapists can create opportunities to talk about what needs to change and why and allow individuals to provide input into how the change may occur. Also it is important to recognize that resistance to change can be minimized when physiotherapists have invested proactively in creating a trusting, patient-centred, supportive relationship before introducing the change. If others perceive their physiotherapists as honest and trustworthy, then they will be more likely to be open to new ways of thinking and to adopt new ways of behaving.

## MOTIVATION

Motivation is what causes or drives people to act; it describes 'why' a person does something (Cherry, 2015). Motivation, the process that starts, directs and sustains goal-oriented behaviours, involves biological, emotional, cognitive and social forces that activate behaviour (Cherry). Motives help to explain what people do (Nevid, 2013). Motives may be either the instincts, needs or wants that drive behaviour and can be referred to as the 'whys' behind observed behaviour. For example, some biological instincts, such as fear, may activate survival or flight behaviours, whereas other biological needs, such as hunger, thirst or exhaustion may activate behaviours such as eating, drinking and sleeping. Yet just having the need or desire to accomplish something may not be enough. Achieving a goal requires the ability to persist through obstacles or barriers as well as the endurance to keep going despite complications. Therefore activation, persistence and intensity are three essential components for motivation to be effective and sustainable (Nevid, 2013). Activation involves the decision to initiate a behaviour, such as starting to exercise. Persistence is the continued effort towards a goal even through obstacles and the possible requirement of a significant investment of energy, time and other resources. For example, persistence could mean doing more activities throughout the day to break up a sedentary lifestyle. Intensity can be seen in the concentration and vigor that goes into pursuing a goal. For example, one person might walk slowly and occasionally around a neighbourhood (low intensity), whereas another person might walk/jog on a daily basis or even twice a day (greater intensity).

Different types of motivation have been categorized as either extrinsic or intrinsic and both can affect behaviour. To comprehend how these approaches can be utilized best, it is important for physiotherapists to understand some of the key differences between the two types of motivation including the overall affect each can have on influencing behavioural change. Extrinsic motivation occurs when people are motivated to perform a behaviour or engage in an activity to earn a reward, gain a benefit or avoid an adverse outcome or consequence. Extrinsic motivation arises from outside of the individual and may include: rewards, trophies or medals, money, social recognition or praise. Alterna-

tively, intrinsic motivation arises from within an individual. Intrinsic motivation involves engaging in certain behaviours because it is personally rewarding; essentially, someone is intrinsically motivated to perform an activity for its own sake rather than for some external reward. The primary difference between these two types of motivation is that extrinsic motivation arises from outside of the individual, whereas intrinsic motivation arises from within and both can differ in how effective they are at driving behaviour in certain situations.

Deci and Ryan (1985) suggest that self-motivation, rather than external motivation, is at the heart of creativity, responsibility, healthy behaviour and lasting change. Furthermore, offering excessive external rewards for an already internally rewarding behaviour may lead to a reduction in intrinsic motivation. Therefore extrinsic motivators should be avoided in situations in which individuals already find certain activities intrinsically rewarding. Nevertheless, extrinsic motivation can be beneficial in some situations. External rewards can cause interest and participation in something in which the individual has no initial interest and in some situations, can be used to motivate people to acquire new skills or knowledge. However, once these new skills have been learned, people may then become more intrinsically motivated to continue to pursue this activity. External rewards can also be used as a source of feedback, allowing people to know when their performance has achieved a certain level worthy of reinforcement or praise. Interestingly, physiotherapists may be able to improve intrinsic motivation by offering positive praise and feedback when people do something better. However, intrinsic motivation may actually decrease if external rewards are given to patients/clients when they have demonstrated only a minimal amount of the required behavioural change.

Another way to view motivation is captured by Fred Lee (2004) in his book, *If Disney Ran Your Hospital: 9½ Things You Would Do Differently*. Specifically, this author identified the four levels of motivation as: compliance (level 1), willpower (level 2), imagination (level 3) and habit (level 4), and he organized these levels according to their power to affect actions or behavioural change. Upon reviewing these different levels of motivation, it becomes clear that if physiotherapists connect more with 'willpower' and 'imagination' during their initial interactions with others, then they may become more effective at igniting intrinsic motivation and ultimately, behavioural change. Although the first level of motivation or compliance is related to some expert or external authority who has the power to give or withhold rewards and consequences, it means that a person only does something because someone is making them do it. The motive for action is extrinsic. Therefore this level of motivation is weak because a person will stay in compliance only as long as the external authority, such as a physiotherapist, is present and continues to give extrinsic rewards or consequences. Alternatively the next level of motivation is 'willpower' or self-discipline. This level of motivation is intrinsic and occurs when people do things on their own because they believe they should do it; no one is making them do anything. This level of motivation builds self-esteem, confidence and a sense of competence. Likewise level 3 motivation is

'imagination'. At this level people do what they want to do because they feel like doing it! Imagination influences feelings and feelings are the source of desire. When feelings make people want to do something (as opposed to not doing something), then the motivation is powerful. Noteworthy is Lee's suggestion that empathy is generated from an ability to imagine what someone else is going through and acts of kindness, caring and compassion stem from imagination. Level 4 is 'habit' and this level occurs eventually when people are doing what comes naturally through deliberate practice or doing what they do without thinking. Level 4 provides the opportunity for ultimately achieving sustainable behavioural change.

Motivational interviewing has been identified as a strategy for physiotherapists to use in their interactions with others. This patient-centred method can enhance intrinsic motivation to change by exploring and resolving ambivalence, where ambivalence produces an inability for someone to make a choice or to take action (Miller and Rollnick, 1991). This motivational approach assumes the following: change occurs naturally; change is influenced by the interactions between people; the expression of empathy is a means of effecting change; the best predictor of change is confidence, on the part of the patient/client or the practitioner, that the patient/client will change; and more patients/clients who say they are motivated to change actually do change (Lussier and Richard, 2007). If practitioners use this approach, then they will focus more on the willingness of patients/clients to change, or on reducing their ambivalence to change rather than focusing on resistance to change. In this way physiotherapists may be able to stimulate and build upon a patient's/client's predisposition towards change.

## REFRAMING THE ROLE OF THE PHYSIOTHERAPIST AS A LEADER

Effective leaders are able to inspire others to take action. Effective leaders understand they need to connect to the 'why' behind a certain change that needs to occur in order to motivate and inspire others successfully (Sinek, 2009). These leaders ignite a sense of purpose, relatedness or connectedness within people that is not dependent on external incentives or potential benefits (Sinek, 2009). Physiotherapists need to motivate others towards action for some reason or another. Therefore an opportunity exists to broaden the mindset of practicing clinicians so that clinicians see themselves simultaneously as clinician/leaders who need to inspire others to act. Overall, leadership means social influence, in which the relationships between the leaders (ie, physiotherapists) and their followers (ie, patients/clients) are crucial. Viewing leadership as a dynamic relationship between people who work together cooperatively to achieve shared outcomes applies well to physiotherapist practice.

Trust is fundamental to building and sustaining relationships, and in the long run, effective 'followership' (Covey, 2006). Trust develops in relationships when motives are clear, honest and based on mutual benefit. A leader's credibility or authenticity is also fundamental for effective leadership and for engaging in productive, dynamic relationships. People need to believe in their leaders and must believe that their words can be trusted. When it comes to deciding whether a leader is believable, people first listen to their words, then they watch their actions. Leaders who are credible do what they say they will do (Kouzes and Posner, 2012). Additionally, credible leaders: follow through on promises, practice what they preach and ensure that their actions are consistent with their words (Kouzes and Posner, 2012). Fundamentally, credible leaders 'walk the talk'.

Highly effective leaders have a high degree of emotional intelligence (EQ) where, emotional intelligence focuses on how leaders handle themselves and their relationships (Goleman et al., 2004). EQ is the capacity to deal strategically and proficiently with all sorts of emotions, especially one's own emotions and the emotions of others. Learning to lead requires that physiotherapists focus on developing their own personal competence first, and it starts with developing self-awareness. Self-awareness requires physiotherapists to become aware of their own emotions and then paying attention to how their emotions and their emotional responses affect others. Next is the opportunity for physiotherapists to learn how to manage and modify their responses in a way so that they can become more influential while working with others. Ultimately their goal is 'resonant leadership' or when leaders become so attuned to other people's feelings that they can essentially shape and direct those feelings in particular ways to facilitate effective collaborative change (Boyatzis and McKee, 2005). By reframing the role of the physiotherapist as a leader, it becomes critical for physiotherapists to learn how to influence others – or rather, how to interact with different people more successfully – in order to achieve common goals and common interests.

## THE POWER OF INFLUENCE IN MOTIVATING OTHERS

Fundamentally physiotherapists influence others to make behavioural changes happen and can learn strategies to become more effective at influencing others. Influence is the power or fuel to change or affect someone or something. Influence triggers changes without directly forcing them to happen. Physiotherapists can choose to influence and motivate people through inspiration, as an effective 'leader', versus manipulation (Sinek, 2009). Inspiration and influence starts with clarity. Physiotherapists, working with others, need to focus on and decide what they are trying to change – what key behaviours they want to influence – before they can actually influence change. In other words, it is important to proactively and intentionally determine what others must actually do in order to improve their current situation. For example, for extrinsic motivation to work as a motivator, there must be clarity about what behaviours are expected and what outcomes will result from those behaviours.

Before people change their behaviour they have to want to do so and this means they have to think differently. People need to know 'why' they have to do what they have to do (Sinek, 2009). People will attempt to change their behaviour if they believe it will be worth it and they have the ability to do what is required. Often physiotherapists can use verbal persuasion fairly easily to influence how people view situations in different ways. Verbal persuasion can be an effective influencing strategy in many situations especially when people trust a physiotherapist's knowledge and motives. At times, however, influence requires more than just the right sequence of words. Sometimes physiotherapists need be more of a storyteller in order to tell compelling, vibrant and credible stories that relate directly to the situation requiring change (Patterson et al., 2008). In this way the stories become influential by stirring emotions, connecting with feelings and fueling imagination. If told well, these stories or simulated events can inspire others by painting a picture for future potential outcomes.

Yet when working with people who are highly resistant, verbal persuasion may not be effective. In these situations, physiotherapists will not be successful if they try to gain control over people with logic and a rational debate/argument. Instead, physiotherapists can talk with these individuals about what they want for themselves and allow time for them to discover on their own the connections between their current behaviour and what they really want. Or if possible, physiotherapists could create an opportunity for these individuals to actually experience the desired change for themselves and then help them to reflect on this experience to fuel sustainable action. Providing choice is a central feature in supporting a person's autonomy and autonomy is essential for inspiring intrinsic motivation (Deci and Ryan, 1985). Therefore, whenever possible, it is critical for physiotherapists to engage patients/clients in planning their own treatment regime or future state. When physiotherapists provide meaningful choice, it will engender willingness in others (Deci and Flaste, 1995). Noteworthy, when choice is offered, it is essential that physiotherapists provide all of the information necessary for others to make meaningful decisions.

Physiotherapists can be more influential when they empower others by giving power and control away. Creating a climate in which people are fully engaged and feel in control of their own lives is at the heart of strengthening others (Kouzes and Posner, 2012). Physiotherapists, through influence, can empower people to commit to being responsible for their own success, by listening to their ideas and acting on them (incorporating them), and by involving them in meaningful decisions (Kouzes and Posner, 2012). Physiotherapists, through influence, can build an environment that develops people's abilities or their competence to perform certain tasks as well as their self-confidence. In a climate of competence and confidence, people hold themselves personally accountable for results and they will feel ownership for their achievements. Physiotherapists through influence can strengthen others by acknowledging and giving credit/praise for their accomplishments. As people gain competence and confidence, they will become more autonomous and independent and, therefore, they will perform more effectively and display a greater sense of wellbeing. The key is empowerment and when physiotherapists give people more control and responsibility, they achieve greater results overall.

Physiotherapists can also increase their ability to influence others by developing their 'engaged listening' skills and listening to people in an engaged way is important for effecting change (Kahnweiler, 2013). Engaged listening allows physiotherapists to increase their understanding of situations, deepen their empathy, gain credibility and build engage-ment (Kahnweiler, 2013). Physiotherapists can create the right conditions for engaged listening by: slowing down the conversation, getting face to face, making sincere eye contact, focusing, being present and not multitasking. Silence is another powerful tool that physiotherapists can use for influencing others. By being present and silent, other people may talk themselves into a right decision or out of a wrong decision without the physiotherapist saying a word (Kahnweiler, 2013).

Physiotherapists need to develop their ability to influence others in order to change thought patterns as well as to inspire others to take specific action. Meaningful and important behavioural change requires energy, time and effort. Boyatzis and McKee have identified an 'intentional change model' that can be used to help people engage in personal transformation successfully (Fig. 4.1). These authors propose that sustainable change occurs when people focus on five major discoveries, including: ideal self, real self, learning agenda, experimenting with and practicing new behaviours/habits and developing and maintaining close, personal relationships. Physiotherapists, by establishing mutually beneficial and dynamic relationships with others ('discovery number five'), can help individuals cycle through these other four discoveries to achieve personal transformation or behavioural change. Through these supportive relationships, physiotherapists provide hope and compassion as the drivers and enablers for others as they experiment with and practice new behaviours. Specifically, physiotherapists could assist others in determining their 'ideal self', their unique personal vision – what behaviours they want to change and why. Then by providing

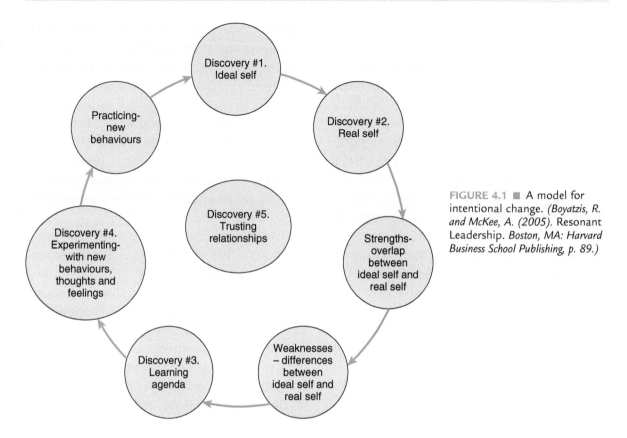

FIGURE 4.1 ■ A model for intentional change. *(Boyatzis, R. and McKee, A. (2005).* Resonant Leadership. *Boston, MA: Harvard Business School Publishing, p. 89.)*

feedback, physiotherapists could help others further by identifying their 'real self' by discussing behaviours they have actually observed. Next, when people compare their 'real self' to their 'ideal self', physiotherapists could help people isolate specific strengths and weaknesses. Learning agendas could then be created cooperatively between the physiotherapists and their patients/clients in a way that leverages strengths and moves individuals closer towards achieving their behavioural goals.

## SUMMARY

Physiotherapists influence others to make behavioural changes happen and can learn strategies to become more effective at influencing. Physiotherapists need to understand the critical role they play in order to influence, engage and empower others. In order for physiotherapists to be effective at influencing behavioural change, and hopefully sustainable behavioural change, it is important for physiotherapists to understand how their assumptions about human behaviour and motivation influence their style of interacting with others. In addition, through a process of developing greater self-awareness of their own styles, they can learn how to adapt their approach in order to influence behavioural change most effectively.

Reframing the mindset of practicing clinicians so that clinicians see themselves as 'leaders' who need to inspire others towards action applies well to physiotherapist practice. Also viewing leadership as the dynamic leader–follower relationship between physiotherapists (the 'leader') and their patients/clients (the 'follower') who work together cooperatively to achieve shared outcomes is relevant for clinical practice. Physiotherapists can be more influential when they empower their patients/clients by giving power and control away. Creating a climate in which people are fully engaged and feel in control of their own lives is at the heart of strengthening others (Kouzes and Posner, 2012). Overall, in order to facilitate actual behavioural change, physiotherapists need to help patients/clients to be ready, willing and able (feel confident) to experiment and practice new behaviours throughout all of their many interactions.

## References

Boyatzis, R., McKee, A., 2005. Resonant Leadership. Harvard Business School Publishing, Boston, MA.

Cherry, K. What is Motivation. (2015) Available at: <http://psychology.about.com/od/mindex/g/motivation-definition.htm>. (accessed 03.04.16.).

Covey, M.R., 2006. The Speed of Trust: The One Thing That Changes Everything. Free Press, New York, NY.

Deci, E.L., Flaste, R., 1995. Why We Do What We Do: Understanding Self-Motivation. Penguin Books, New York, NY.

Deci, E.L., Ryan, R.M., 1985. Intrinsic Motivation and Self-Determination in Human Behavior. Plenum, New York, NY.

Goleman, D., Boyatzis, R., McKee, A., 2004. Primal Leadership: Learning to Lead with Emotional Intelligence. Harvard Business Review Press, Boston, MA.

Heil, G., Bennis, W.G., Stephens, D.C., 2000. Douglas McGregor Revisited: Managing the Human Side of the Enterprise. John Wiley & Sons, New York, NY.

Kahnweiler, J.B., 2013. Quiet Influence: The Introvert's Guide to Making a Difference. Berrett-Koehler Publishers, Inc, San Francisco, CA.

Kouzes, J., Posner, B., 2012. The Leadership Challenge, fifth ed. Jossey-Bass, San Francisco, CA.

Lee, F., 2004. If Disney Ran Your Hospital: 9 1/2 Things You Would Do Differently. Second River Healthcare Press, Bozeman, MT.

Lussier, M.T., Richard, C., 2007. The Motivational Interview in Practice. Can. Fam. Physician 53 (12), 2117–2118.

McGregor, D., 1960. The Human Side of Enterprise. McGraw-Hill, New York, NY.

Miller, R., Rollnick, S., 1991. Motivational Interviewing: Preparing People to Change Addictive Behavior. The Guilford Press, New York, NY.

Nevid, J., 2013. Essentials of Psychology: Concepts and Applications, fourth ed. Cengage Learning, Stamford, CT.

Patterson, K., Grenny, J., Maxfield, D., McMillan, R., Switzler, A., 2008. Influencer: The Power To Change Anything. McGraw-Hill, New York, NY.

Quinn, R.E., 1996. Deep Change: Discovering the Leader Within. Jossey-Bass, San Francisco, CA.

Sinek, S., 2009. Start With Why: How Great Leaders Inspire Everyone to Take Action. Penguin Group, New York, NY.

# 5

# STRESS, PAIN AND RECOVERY
## Neuro-Immune-Endocrine Interactions and Clinical Practice

LESTER E JONES

La Trobe University, Melbourne, Physiotherapy, Allied Health Science, Higher Education MScMed(PM)

## CHAPTER CONTENTS

This chapter will explore the effects of psychological and social stressors on the warning system of the body and on the body's capacity to recover from tissue trauma or disease. The opening discussion of the body's capacity to adapt to external and internal stressors – through the integration of neural, immune and endocrine systems – will provide important background to the experimental and clinical evidence of how psychological and social factors modify neuro-immune-endocrine function to influence health.

## THE BODY'S PROTECTION SYSTEM

### Introduction and Overview

The knowledge and understanding of the body's protection system is improving all the time.

*'Only recently have we fully appreciated that the classically separated domains of neurology, endocrinology, immunology and microbiology, with their various organs – the brain, glands, gut, immune cells and microbiota, could actually be joined to each other in a multidirectional network of communication, in order to maintain homoeostasis.'*

### (El Aidy et al., 2014, p. 1)

The integration of highly evolved systems – the endocrine system, nervous system and immune system – is reflected in innumerable processes essential for the maintenance of homoeostasis (Chapman et al., 2008; El Aidy et al., 2014). The workings of the body's protection system are necessarily complex and a detailed description is beyond the scope of this chapter. However, understanding terminology, processes and responses related to this system when health is challenged is important for physiotherapists.

Integral to discussion about body protection is the stress response. Stress can be described as the condition or situation where the equilibrium of normal functioning of bodily systems or normal cellular functions is threatened (for review see Chrousos, 2009). Importantly factors that threaten normal functioning can be physical, psychological or environmental and so a biopsychosocial framework is important in understanding the effect and response. Fortunately human bodies have a great capacity for adaptation at multiple levels. Recent research into the plasticity of the nervous system – that enables adaptation to injury and modification of physical and cognitive function – suggests that a person has a great ability to adapt to adverse or challenging conditions (Gillick and Zirpel, 2012; Kleim, 2011). Such stress-related plasticity is an adaptive quality with much potential benefit for preserving homoeostasis, including when psychological and social contexts are considered (Deppermann et al., 2014). Also, therapeutic interventions are likely to be enhanced by focusing on how peripherally located interventions might diminish central processing. In particular, how neuro-immune-endocrine communication allows for detection of a threat and the promotion of safety and recovery through peripheral and central mechanisms (Gillick and Zirpel, 2012; Snodgrass et al., 2014).

Although the stress response has a positive effect on preserving homoeostasis, it has the potential to be harmful if normal regulatory processes are inhibited or not functioning (Chrousos, 2009; Liezmann et al., 2012). Dysregulation of the stress response can influence the effectiveness of homeostatic responses (Chrousos, 2009; Deppermann et al., 2014) and there is evidence that psychological and social factors are important in both the perseverance and remediation of the dysfunction (for review see Chapman et al., 2008). The magnitude and especially the chronicity of the stress may also be important with regards to the magnitude of the effect on homoeostasis and health (Kaltsas and Chrousos, 2007). Evidence suggests that early childhood stress, persistent stressful triggers and experience of a major adverse event can all result in negative health outcomes (Chrousos, 2009; Schalinski et al., 2015).

## Endocrine Control and Stress

*'The stress system integrates and responds to a great diversity of distinct circadian, neuro-sensory, blood borne and limbic signals.'*

### Kaltsas and Chrousos, 2007, p. 305

Hormones are classified into three groups: (1) steroid hormones – for example cortisol, (2) those derived from tyrosine – for example dopamine, adrenaline and noradrenaline (ie, catecholamines), and (3) peptide and protein hormones – for example oxytocin and vasopressin. They can act systemically or on specific targets and are often involved in feedback loops that inhibit (negative feedback loop) or enhance (positive feedback loop) activity in target tissues. Important endocrine structures include the hypothalamus, pituitary gland and adrenal gland, consisting of two functionally distinct parts – the adrenal cortex and the adrenal medulla. The hypothalamus and pituitary gland are commonly described with the adrenal cortex as the hypothalamic-pituitary-adrenocortical axis (HPA axis). The hypothalamus and pituitary gland are located at the base of the brain above the brainstem and the two adrenal glands are located above each kidney. The locus coeruleus, located in the brainstem (ie, pons), is an important structure for influencing endocrine function. This is because of the connections and influence it has with the so-called emotional centre of the brain, the limbic system (ie, amygdala, hippocampus, hypothalamus, anterior cingulate cortex) (Benarroch, 2009; Samuels and Szabadi, 2008). See Box 5.1 for extra notes on limbic system.

The stress system can be described as having central and peripheral components. Principally, the central components include the nuclei of the hypothalamus, producing corticotrophin-releasing hormone, and the locus coeruleus, a major source of noradrenaline. The peripheral component includes the HPA axis, the end product being cortisol, and the sympatheticoadrenomedullary system

**BOX 5.1**
**SCEPTICISM OF THE LIMBIC SYSTEM**

It is worth noting that there has recently been some scepticism about the limbic system, from a functional, structural and evolutionary perspective (LeDoux, 2012). It seems clear that the amygdala has an important role in body protection and the stress response, and is structurally complex with many nuclei. However, the assumptions, particularly from animal studies, about its role in emotional responses, may be overstated (for commentary on this see LeDoux, 2012). Convention will prevail for now and the following text will continue to refer to a limbic system that is seen to be involved in communicating emotional input.

(SAM) that produces adrenaline and noradrenaline (Nicolaides et al, 2015).

The key role of the stress system is to maintain homoeostasis and it relies on communication between brain regions such as the limbic system and locus coeruleus and the integration of nervous, immune and endocrine systems (McEwen et al., 2016). The nervous and immune system are the sentinels for the body's protection system, detecting potential threats and activating the stress system (Grace et al., 2014; Watkins et al., 2007). During a real or perceived threat, endocrine responses alter blood flow and enhance energy availability to ensure that the brain and musculoskeletal system can navigate the person to a more favourable situation (Chrousos, 2009; Nicolaides et al., 2015). This means body functions related to digestion, growth, reproduction and certain aspects of immunity are suppressed at times of stress in order to optimize the use of energy resources required to resolve the situation (for detailed reviews see Kaltsas and Chrousos, 2007 and Nicolaides et al., 2015).

There is also a hypoalgesic effect of acute stress, mediated by β-endorphin which is released by the pituitary gland (Chapman et al., 2008; Jänig et al., 2006; Melzack, 2005). Beta-endorphin is a powerful analgesic substance that binds to μ-opioid receptors and is released from the pituitary gland as a part of HPA axis activation during times of stress. Intriguingly there is some evidence that the initial effect is not analgesic (Johansen et al., 2003), although there is also some evidence that it has roles in reducing cortisol, substance p (ie, a neuromediator that sensitizes nociceptors) and promoting dopamine levels (ie, pleasure) therefore attenuating the stress response (Melzack, 2005; Sprouse-Blum et al., 2010).

*Emotion-Provoked Stress Response*

It is very difficult to identify a single starting point of the stress response because of parallel activation and complex feedback systems that trigger and attenuate the various components. Ganzel and colleagues suggest that the activation of the emotional centres is the primary controller of the stress response – and that physiological and behavioural responses are secondary (Ganzel et al., 2010). There is no doubt that the amygdala is well placed for this role with cortical and subcortical connections to stress hormone producers – the hypothalamus and locus coeruleus. Amygdala connections to the prefrontal cortex, hippocampus and anterior cingulate cortex provide potential avenues for activation in response to psychological and social threats (Muscatell et al., 2015; Öhman, 2005).

Interestingly, some novel experiments have investigated how behaviours associated with emotions might modify the stress response. A small study examining laughter found that participants who watched a humorous video had reduced serum cortisol levels compared with controls (Berk et al., 1989). Two studies examining the effects of swearing on pain found that participants who were asked to swear repeatedly during submersion of their hand in icy water had an increased heart rate and were able to keep their hand submerged for longer – suggesting the acute stress response was enhanced (Stephens et al., 2009; Stephens and Umland, 2011).

*The Sympathoadrenomedullary Pathway and Catecholamines*

A quick and early response to stress occurs via the SAM pathway. Catecholamines are important in the stress response as they act to prepare the body for physical responses through the modification of physiological process, ie, increased heart rate, blood pressure. Adrenaline, noradrenaline and dopamine are all catecholamines. The adrenal medulla is the primary source for adrenaline. Noradrenaline is primarily produced by the sympathetic nervous system and in the brain (ie, the locus coeruleus in the pons). It has multiple roles via its action as a neurotransmitter, primarily in the sympathetic nervous system, and as a hormone. Its effects include increased alertness and vigilance, increased restlessness and anxiety and enhancement of memory and memory retrieval (Berridge et al., 2012; Chrousos, 2009; Watkins and Maier, 2000; Watkins et al., 1995). Dopamine is the precursor molecule for adrenaline and noradrenaline. It has been described as a neuroimmune transmitter (Levite, 2015) because of its role in modulation of immune function via lymphocytes (Buttarelli et al., 2011; Sarkar et al., 2010; Yan et al., 2015). The actions of catecholamines also lead to a reduction in the available resources needed to repair and maintain tissues, including suppressing the release of proinflammatory cytokines (see following section on 'Cytokines' (or similar)).

### The HPA Axis and Cortisol

Corticotropin-releasing-hormone (CRH) is produced by the hypothalamus – and peripheral nerves and immune cells – and triggers the release of adrenocorticotropic hormone (ACTH) from the pituitary gland (Nicolaides et al., 2015). The hormone also acts on the adrenal cortex, modifying gene expression and promoting the synthesis and release of cortisol from the adrenal cortex. Cortisol has many effects on a broad range of tissues in the body. A key action of cortisol is to reduce the production of CRH by the hypothalamus and ACTH by the pituitary gland, therefore completing a negative feedback loop to decrease the HPA axis stress response (Kaltsas and Chrousos, 2007).

Important to this discussion is the influence of cortisol on immune and inflammatory processes (Chrousos, 2009). Cortisol has antiinflammatory and immunosuppressive effects, although some actions are further reliant on intracellular gene transcription factors (Nicolaides et al., 2015). Cortisol also has a role in consolidation of memory (Drexler et al., 2015), presumably by its action on the hippocampus (McEwen et al., 2016). Some of the molecular actions of cortisol initiated by HPA axis activation can take days to complete (see Nicolaides et al., 2015 for a comprehensive review of stress and glucocorticoids).

### Neuroplasticity as an Adaptation for Health

*'Environmental events and behavioural experience induce epigenetic changes at particular gene loci that help shape neuronal plasticity and function.'*

*Gold, 2015, p. 37*

The capacity of the nervous system to change has been underestimated for many years. In particular, brain changes – such as those observed in the rehabilitation of stroke survivors – were often attributed to a specific response to disease or tissue damage rather than as part of a normal ongoing process of adaptation (Pomeroy and Tallis, 2002). Other evidence of plasticity has been explained by sensitive phases of growth and development (Trojan and Pokorny, 1999). Arguably this is because the subtle day-to-day adaptations our systems undertake do not attract the same attention as the impressive shift in function and activity required following a neurological event or during transformative periods of growth and development.

It now seems unequivocal that the central nervous system has the capacity to change throughout one's lifespan and that these constant adaptations have a role in homoeostasis (Deppermann et al., 2014; Gillick and Zirpel, 2012). It is apparent that change in synaptic strength and the rate of transmission is responsive to patterns of activity in the elements of the nervous system (Butz et al., 2009; Garland and Howard, 2009; Pittenger and Duman, 2008; Woolf, 2011). The importance of the functional changes seen in the amygdala and hippocampus in response to stress have been written about (McEwen, 2001; 2015), but the role plasticity has in development may also influence the resilience or vulnerability of an individual in response to stressors.

## Activity-Dependent Neuroplasticity

Evidence suggests that neuroplasticity can enhance and refine advantageous and life preserving processes through several mechanisms (Butz et al., 2009; McEwen, 2012; Trojan and Pokorny, 1999). It is likely that different mechanisms predominate depending on the context. These contexts might include normal development, including physical, cognitive and emotional development (evolutionary plasticity), development of a new skill or other learning (reactive or adaptive plasticity) and recovery from injury (reparation plasticity) (Trojan and Pokorny, 1999). The general principle across these contexts is that changes to the nervous system are shaped and reinforced by the amount of activity transmitted in neurons and nerve cell bodies (Butz et al., 2009; Trojan and Pokorny, 1999).

Metabolic changes, the concentration of neurotransmitters and populations of receptors at pre- and postsynaptic membranes influence the neural changes that occur and are influenced by proinflammatory and anti-inflammatory substances and other products and mediators of the stress response (Chrousos, 2009; McEwen, 2001; Trojan and Pokorny, 1999). These changes in physiology can be attributed to changes in gene expression. In other words the psychological, environmental and physical experiences trigger nerve activity that in turn lead to changes in genetic influences on neurobiological processes (Garland and Howard, 2009; Wüst et al., 2004). It is also clear that the environmental context and concentration of stress-mediating chemicals can affect the inhibition or enhancement of neurogenesis (for comprehensive reviews see McEwen, 2007 and McEwen et al., 2016).

An important mechanism influencing early development is the systematic reduction in neuronal populations targeting redundant neurons (Casano and Peri, 2015) – that is neurons not involved in the essential activity of the nervous system. This results in the reinforcement of pathways carrying neural activity that is specific to a movement and results in increasingly refined action (Casano and Peri, 2015). Overall this adaptation contributes to the increased precision of essential tasks, such as putting food in your mouth, where neurons that are directly contributing to the desired outcome – hand to mouth – are reinforced and those that create 'noise' to the movement are subject to cell death. In line with this, early life experiences that provide stimulation and appropriate levels of challenge are likely to lead to more adaptive functioning (Boersma et al., 2014; Underwood, 2011).

As we explore this complexity it is clear that focusing on neural plasticity without attention to the adaptations taking place in other systems is inadequate and other terms may capture this better. The term bioplasticity has been used by Moseley and others (Moseley and Butler, 2015), but perhaps neuroimmune plasticity (Rosas-Ballina and Tracey, 2009) or neuroendocrine-immune plasticity (Liezmann et al., 2012) may better represent the processes of interest in this chapter.

## The Immune System and the Stress Response

*'Physical and psychological stressors activate the same bidirectional immune-brain circuits including autonomic nervous system and hypothalamo-pituitary-adrenal axis.'*

**Maier and Watkins, 1998, p. 84**

## TABLE 5.1
### Summary of Key Neuro-Immune-Endocrine Cells and Mediators

| Type | Key Cells/Mediators | Context | Action |
|------|---------------------|---------|--------|
| Glucocorticoid | Cortisol | Activated HPA axis | Prepare for fight/flight<br>Reduce inflammation<br>Immunosuppression<br>Consolidate memory |
| Catecholamine | Noradrenaline, adrenaline | Activated SAM pathway | Increase alertness, restlessness<br>Increase heart rate, blood pressure<br>Reduce inflammation<br>Suppress proinflammatory cytokines |
| Glia | Microglia | Internal danger | Detect damage in local environment<br>Prime nervous system<br>Produce cytokines<br>'Memory' for prior threat/danger |
| Proinflammatory cytokine | TNF-α<br>IL-1<br>IL-6 | Cell damage<br>Stressor (acute/chronic) | Stimulate nociceptors<br>Release neuromediators<br>Signalling and communication<br>Induce fever and sickness behaviour |

When the concept of an integrated body protection system is embraced, it makes sense that physical, psychological and social stressors will influence immune function (Ursin, 1994) and that the immune system's activity will influence the stress response (Webster Marketon and Glaser, 2008). Cytokines and glial cells make important contributions to immune function and play a key role in communication between the nervous and immune systems (see Table 5.1 for key neuro-immune-endocrine cells).

### Cytokines

Cytokines are peptides that have a primary role in cellular communication in immune-brain function. The roles and interactions of cytokines are complex and consist of anti-inflammatory and proinflammatory types. Released from macrophages and other cells in response to pathogen detection or stress, cytokines are a part of the initial peripheral immune response, activating nociceptors and triggering the release of immune-stimulatory substances, such as substance p, which reciprocally promote cytokine release (see further summary in Chapman et al., 2008 and Sprouse-Blum et al., 2010). The mechanisms of how peripheral immune activation effects brain function is likely to be multimodal. One important mechanism involves the stimulation of intermediary cells by cytokines (especially IL-1) and subsequent transmission of nerve impulses through the sensory components of the vagus nerve (for review see Wrona, 2006). The effects on brain function are wide ranging, including systemic, behavioural and emotional changes, for example, fever, anorexia, reduced social behaviour and a depressed mood, and are referred to as sickness or an acute-phase response (Kent et al., 1992; Maier and Watkins, 1998). Increased cytokine levels have been associated with changes in both serotonin and dopamine levels (Capuron and Miller, 2011), suggesting a mechanism for the influence on mood, sleep and appetite.

Proinflammatory cytokines include the interleukins IL-1 and IL-6, and tumour necrosis factor-α (TNF-α), and these have a role in activating the HPA axis (Sommer and Kress, 2004; Webster Marketon and Glaser, 2008). As a result, secretion of cytokines can enhance the inflammatory response and also increase levels of cortisol. As previously mentioned, cortisol has antiinflammatory effects. These are a result of binding with the glucocorticoid receptor which alters gene expression in, and interferes with, production of inflammatory cells and compounds (Padgett and Glaser, 2003; Webster Marketon and Glaser, 2008). The advantage the coordination of proinflammatory and antiinflammatory mechanisms has on the stressed organism may be to simultaneously promote alertness and healing, and is reflected in the brain activity of cytokines (Capuron and Miller, 2011). Catecholamines are also reported to modify immune function via β2-adrenergic receptors found on cytokine-producing macrophages (Padgett and Glaser, 2003). This self-limiting process is important to prevent a prolonged inflammatory response that would harm tissues (Austin and Moalem-Taylor, 2010; Stipursky et al, 2011).

## BOX 5.2
### TOLL-LIKE RECEPTORS

Toll-like receptors (TLRs) are a critical part of innate immune function and are involved in sensing pathogens and initiating inflammation processes. TLRs are expressed in both immune and nonimmune cell types and have multiple roles including in tissue repair and regeneration after injury (Chang, 2010; Uematsu and Akira, 2007). Higher levels of TLR4 messenger ribonucleic acid (mRNA) are associated with higher levels of inflammation and a low socioeconomic status in childhood and its presence early on appears to lead to higher levels of TLR4 mRNA in later life (Fagundes et al., 2013).

### Glia Including the Tripartite Synapse

Glial cells have the capacity to detect and remember chronic danger and are facilitated by toll-like receptors that respond when endogenous danger signalling molecules are detected (see Box 5.2) (Grace et al., 2014). Glial cells include Schwann cells in the periphery and microglia, astrocytes and oligodendrocytes in the central nervous system (Austin and Moalem-Taylor, 2010). Schwann cells produce proinflammatory cytokines and nerve growth factor and have connections with sensory nerves (see review by Thacker et al., 2007). In the central nervous system, the majority of synapses have a structurally and functionally integrated astrocyte. Such synapses are described as tripartite synapses with pre- and post-synaptic terminal, and the glial cell which secretes and regulates neurotransmitter concentrations at the synapse, in particular glutamate and brain-derived neurotropic factor (Milligan and Watkins, 2009; Stipursky et al., 2011). The role of the microglia is still being unravelled. These cells regulate astrocyte responses and probably contribute to synapse efficacy directly (Grace et al., 2014; Milligan and Watkins, 2009) with some suggesting the term tetrapartite –

involving four parts – is a more appropriate description than tripartite (Amantea, 2015). The glial cells' role in regulatory control is important in allostasis as outlined in the following section 'Allostasis and Allostatic Load'.

## Allostasis and Allostatic Load

An important concept in physiological adaptation is allostasis. It has been described as the process of '… achieving stability through change …' (McEwen and Wingfield, 2003, p. 3), which can be distinguished from homoeostasis '… the stability of the physiological processes essential to life …' (McEwen and Wingfield, 2003, p. 3). An interpretation of this is that the body can manage threats that are not symptomatic, but that an enhanced response is required – one that elicits symptoms such as pain – when the threats require a behavioural response to prevent harm and preserve the body's equilibrium. In other words, homoeostasis describes the relatively constant state of the system involving largely predictable cycles of external and internal challenges, where allostasis describes the process of supporting the state of homoeostasis through the management of responses to less predictable challenges and events (Schulz and Vögele, 2015). It is important to note that some authors prefer the term cacostasis rather than allostasis, emphasizing that this is a potentially harmful state (Chrousos, 2009).

The previous discussion on responses to stress may more appropriately be labelled as examples of allostasis. The primary mediators of allostasis include catecholamines and cytokines and the activity of these substances is altered in response to changes and challenges in the psychological, social or physical environments. When these levels are sustained and primary mediators are found to be in excess or inadequate, an individual can be said to be in an allostatic state (McEwen and Wingfield, 2003).

Ganzel and colleagues add to the nomenclature in this area by referring to allostatic accommodation (Ganzel et al., 2010). This is described as the physiological adjustments made, within normal ranges of functioning, in response to a stressor. One feature of this accommodation is the potential that the biological parameters necessary for homoeostasis can to some degree be reset to allow an enhanced response to future stressors. Ganzel and colleagues argue this is in part as a result of psycho-emotional influences such as anticipation, learning and memory (Ganzel et al., 2010). The important notion that this brings to the discussion about the stress response is that the context is always mediating the physiological response to the stressor (Ganzel et al., 2010; Zilioli et al., 2015).

In situations where the stressors are persistent or repeated, allostatic accommodation creates a cumulative effect that effects the individual. This can be described as allostatic load (McEwen and Wingfield, 2003). It can be expected that allostatic load will be increased in situations of poor health, disease, social disconnection and other sustained psychosocial stressors (Juster and McEwen, 2015; Juster et al., 2011). Allostatic overload can be seen as a state of failed adaptation to persistent or fluctuating stressors and can lead to dysregulation of the system (see Fig. 5.1; Mauss et al., 2015).

In clinical practice, allostatic load would seem important to consider, not just with presentations of chronic or persistent symptoms which invariably have complex psychosocial history, but also when considering

| Normal | Adaptation to stress | Failed adaptation | Cumulative | Dysregulation |
|---|---|---|---|---|
| Homeostasis | Allostasis | Allostatic load ◀▶ Allostatic overload | | Health outcomes |
| | *Primary mediators* (epinephrine (adrenaline), norepinephrine (noradrenaline), cortisol, DHEA-S, vagal tone, tumour-necrosis factor-α, interleukin-6) | Primary effects (anxiety, sleeping problems, mood changes, etc.) | *Secondary outcomes* (abnormal metabolism, cardiovascular risk factors, inflammation, common cold, etc.) | *Tertiary outcomes* (arterial hypertension, CVD, stroke, obesity, diabetes mellitus, depression, chronic pain/fatigue, cancer, Alzheimer's disease, gastrointestinal disorder, etc.) |
| | Note: help to maintain homeostasis, protective and damaging effects on the body possible | Note: organ-and tissue-specific cellular events that are regulated by primary mediators | Note: cumulative outcome of primary effects in response to primary mediators | Note: result of allostatic overload, prediction by extreme values of secondary outcomes and primary mediators |

FIGURE 5.1 ▪ Stress regulating process from homoeostasis to allostatic load. *CVD*, cardiovascular disease; *DHEA-S*, Dihydroepiandrosterone sulphate *((Mauss et al., 2015) Psychologically-Informed Physiotherapy.)*

acute presentations. The increased presence of stress and immune mediators may amplify sensitivity of the nervous system and promote a heightened vigilance and response to symptoms that may be out of proportion to the state of the tissues (Grace et al., 2014; Watkins and Maier, 2002). Importantly allostatic load should not be seen as a pathological state, but an increased allostatic load may prime the body's protection system for an enhanced or dysregulated stress response (Ganzel et al., 2010; Grace et al., 2014). Offidani and Ruini (2012) link relevant biomarkers to life events and chronic stressors, recognizing that identifying manifestations of this adversity is important in predicting negative health outcomes.

## Habituation

A common observation during repeated stress (ie, discrete repetitive stressful events) is a reduction in the individual's stress response. This is known as habituation and is presumably helpful in restricting the exposure of tissues to the potentially harmful stress hormones. It is evident in changes in cortisol reactivity and other measures of HPA axis activity (Wüst et al., 2005) and is also seen in gene expression for inflammatory mediators (McInnis et al., 2015). With mild or short-term stress, this change in reactivity seems to be associated with positive changes to cellular function (Johnstone et al., 2015; Poljšak and Milisav, 2012) and may be described as an acquired cellular resilience akin to acquired immunity (see commentary by Stone, 2016).

However, habituation is not universal and there are some individuals who show no change to repeated exposure. There are also examples of individuals being more sensitive to repeated stress exposure and, although genetic variation cannot be totally ruled out, the effectiveness of the individual's overall response to stress (ie, initially suppressed) is reported to play a role (Wüst et al., 2005). In such situations the characteristics of the stressor seem to be important. These include duration, intensity and frequency and the context of the stressor, including the level of social support (Kudielka and Wüst, 2010; Wüst et al., 2005).

Oxytocin is a neuropeptide that is released both centrally and peripherally and associated with a level of social support (Kudielka and Wüst, 2010). Centrally it is involved in regulating amygdala function and also influences activity in the dorsal horn of the spinal cord where it appears to augment the inhibitory effects of gamma-aminobutyric acid (GABA) (Rash et al., 2014). A recent exploratory study into early life adverse events suggested that oxytocin regulation may be an important adaption to stress with an effect on mood and physical symptoms (Crowley et al., 2015). Social support is said to 'buffer' against stress and promote wound healing and a feature of this is the release of oxytocin which

suppresses HPA axis activity (Detillion et al., 2004). In light of this, studies of repeated stress that show stress habituation should always take into account the role of the experimenter's presence and interaction. In clinical interactions, nurturing of the therapeutic alliance between a clinician and the person seeking their care also has the potential to lower stress and this is supported by the link between oxytocin and the level of trust established in such relationships (Benedetti, 2013).

## Dysregulation

It has been proposed that there are four contexts that might lead to dysregulation of the stress system: inability to initiate and sustain an adequate stress response, repeated exposure to stressful stimuli, poor adaption to repeated stressors and an inability to cease an active stress response when a threat has been dealt with (Kaltsas and Chrousos, 2007).

All of these contexts involve the HPA axis and the SAM pathway. Cortisol release can be dysregulated by prolonged HPA axis activation or constant reactivation of the HPA axis. Research into HPA axis activation and markers of inflammation has shown that adults who have had adversity, especially trauma as children, show enhanced responsiveness (Danese and McEwen, 2012; Levine et al., 2015). This is suggestive of an inability to decrease an active response. Paradoxically there can also be reduced cortisol levels when stress responses persist and there is evidence that early adverse life experiences may habituate the stress response so that it is less reactive later in the lifespan (Heim et al., 2000). This might be a reflection of poor adaptation. Although the mechanisms underpinning the variation in responses are not fully understood, the timing, duration and frequency of adverse events, the individual's resilience or vulnerability and the maturity of the body protection system at the time of the adversity all might play a role (Danese and McEwen, 2012).

Interoception, or the afferent processes that lead to awareness of bodily processes, is important in monitoring threats and is described as having three components: detection, attention and evaluation (Schulz and Vögele, 2015). Stress can lead to dysfunction of interoception, including enhanced or diminished functions (Schulz and Vögele, 2015) and when these components are not operating effectively, the body's protective response will be altered. For example, the increased sensitivity in the detection of physical threats may explain the sensitivity to physical stimuli seen in some people with persistent pain.

Finally there is evidence of dysregulation of neural functioning with chronic stress. Chronic stress is when a person has experienced continual stressful contexts or stressful events over a long period of time. Dysregulation of cognitive and emotional function is affected with altered memory functions and increased reactivity to novel stress (Deppermann et al., 2014; McEwen, 2012). Neuroplasticity may be one mechanism at play with endocrine and immune factors influencing neurogenesis and modification to synapses (Deppermann et al., 2014). Understanding the role of immune and endocrine mediators in neuroplasticity has helped identify specific molecular targets in the search for the treatment of posttraumatic stress disorder (PTSD) (Deppermann et al., 2014).

## The Effect of Stress on Pain

*'By recognizing the role of the stress system in pain processes, we discover that the scope of the puzzle of pain is vastly expanded and new pieces of the puzzle provide valuable clues in our quest to understand chronic pain.'*

### *Melzack, 2001, p. 1380*

Biomedical approaches to diagnosis essentially attribute pain to tissue pathology. Increasingly this approach is seen to be flawed as presentations of pain without tissue pathology and evidence of no pain despite tissue pathology is apparent in clinical practice and increasingly in the research literature. Consequently, reframing the meaning of pain is likely to be important. Previously the emphasis has been to interpret a person's pain report as an indicator of the presence and severity of tissue pathology. It may be more appropriate, however, to consider pain as a part of a warning system to protect us from injury or the potential for further damage (Jones, 2007; Moseley, 2007). A patient-centred approach is essential to capture the internal and external influences that might lead to a heightened vigilance for danger and also to identify factors that might make our warning system more sensitive to trigger (Moseley and Butler, 2015). In this section this reframed view of pain will be explored in the context of stress biology, drawing on the concept of allostatic load to identify how pain may be influenced by past experiences and how pain at times of stress may be enhanced and prolonged. See to Box 5.3 for extra notes on pain and inflammation.

The early work of Gifford, in particular the 'Mature Organism Model', is an important influence on these ideas (see Gifford, 1998) as are the informed reflections on persistent pain by Zusman (see Zusman, 2008; 2012; 2013).

### Current Concepts of Pain

'Central to understanding interpersonal features of pain is recognition that pain typically is experienced in complex social environments, with the person's distress manifestly obvious, often predicated upon the social setting, and reactions of others.'

*Hadjistavropoulos et al., 2011, p. 912*

It is now well established that pain is influenced and determined by multiple internal and external factors, yet there remains a focus on biomedical factors in much of current health practice (Briggs et al., 2013; Parsons et al., 2007; Zusman, 2013). Traditionally one factor, tissue damage, has been seen as the most important feature to explain a person's pain. This makes sense as it is common experience to sustain tissue damage and feel pain.

However, there are two things that need to be reflected upon. First, research over the last two decades has demonstrated there is a mismatch between evidence of pathoanatomical changes and pain (Girish et al., 2011; Ho-Joong Kim et al., 2013; Husarik et al., 2010; Jensen et al., 1994; Nakashima et al., 2015; Nardo et al., 2015; Sher et al., 1995; Stehling et al., 2010). Second, many persistent pain presentations cannot be attributed to any pathological tissue source (Zusman, 2012); see also the discussion on 'modern health worries' in Baliatsas et al. (2015). Integration of a biopsychosocial approach into clinical practice can help explain much of the evidence that conflicts with a tissue-based approach and was elegantly introduced to physiotherapy in a review article more than 20 years ago (Moffett and Richardson, 1995). What can be added to those early thoughts is the contemporary knowledge of psychoneuroimmunology.

### Pain and Neuro-Immune-Endocrine Function

Cytokines have an important role in modulating the pain experience, including linking the immune and nervous system through an interplay with glial cells (McMahon et al., 2005; Sommer and Kress, 2004; Watkins and Maier, 2005). TNF-α, a proinflammatory cytokine, has a role in triggering the release of other cytokines and has an effect on a range of tissues centrally and peripherally (for reviews see Capuron and Miller, 2011; Sommer and Kress, 2004). Peripheral effects include activating and sensitizing nociceptors – the body's neural sensors of dangerous chemical, mechanical and thermal stimuli. There is evidence that this can occur directly – that is, exposure of the free nerve ending to cytokines such as TNF-$\alpha$ – or indirectly – via other mediators or gene transcription (Capuron and Miller, 2011; Sommer and Kress, 2004). As mentioned previously, the proinflammatory cytokines also have a role in activating the HPA axis that stimulates the release of cortisol from the adrenal cortex (Capuron and Miller, 2011). This molecular link between the warning signal (ie, pain) and the stress response is understandable when considering pain as a part of the body protection response.

There are established links between dysregulation of the HPA axis – both hypercortisolism and hypocortisolism – and various pain-related conditions including fibromyalgia and rheumatoid arthritis (Chrousos, 2009). Supporting evidence includes a group of interesting studies looking at the role of exercise, $\beta$-endorphin, pain and cortisol, which have determined a mediating factor to be low mood (Chatzitheodorou et al., 2007; 2008; Harte et al., 1995; Hoeger Bement et al., 2010).

The cognitive process of rumination, or persistent negative thinking about past experience, has been linked to increased cortisol reactivity, an indication of hyperactivation of the HPA axis (Zoccola et al., 2010 and see detailed review by Zoccola and Dickerson, 2012). This makes sense, as cortisol enhances memory in terms of events, which is believed to be an evolved strategy for survival. Cortisol via hippocampal processes has also been shown to consolidate pain-related memory when the memory is reactivated – including rumination – although this may be only in the context of an anxious state (Ploghaus et al., 2001). In sum, memory of situations that are potentially dangerous will allow for early response to, or, perhaps more importantly, avoidance of, a future threat and this is especially so when the threat is recurrent.

Rumination, along with magnification and helplessness, is a feature of the psychological concept of catastrophizing. The attention-promoting effects of cortisol may promote catastrophizing (Crombez et al., 2004; Eccleston et al., 2004; Quartana et al., 2010). Catastrophizing is strongly linked to the human pain experience and shown to influence pain intensity, persistence and pain-related disability (Coronado et al., 2015; Crombez et al., 1998; Keefe et al., 2010; Khan et al., 2011; Vervoort et al., 2006). A strong social component may exist with this link, although a well-designed experimental study suggests pain-related fear might influence pain ratings more than catastrophizing (Hirsh et al., 2008). This is notable as a recent prospective study could not identify a biomarker link between dysregulated stress, childhood adverse life experiences and the development of multisite pain (Generaal et al., 2015). Pain-related fear and catastrophizing were not measured however, and the authors concluded that the link between adverse childhood experiences and multisite pain may be mediated by psychological factors (Generaal et al., 2015).

There has also been some variation in results from studies investigating immune biomarkers and pain severity. A study of immune activity during back pain confirmed there was an inflammatory process following intervertebral disc herniation but found that the levels of interleukins (IL-1$\beta$ and IL-6) did not distinguish pain >3.5 on a visual analogue scale (VAS) versus pain less than 3.5 (Andrade et al., 2013). In contrast, another study, again involving participants with disc herniation, showed that more than 3 on a VAS was associated with IL-6 and IL-8 at 12 months postsurgical repair (Pedersen et al., 2015). Of interest, recurrent herniation has been found to be associated with an increase in the cytokine TNF-α and the concentration of its receptor TNFR1 (Andrade et al., 2016). This variation fits with current concepts of pain and reflects the need for multidimensional assessment and treatment.

## The Effect of Stress on Healing

*'...psychological stress impairs normal cell-mediated immunity at the wound site, causing a significant delay in the healing process.'*

### Godbout and Glaser, 2006, p. 243

Wound healing can be affected by local and systemic factors (Khalil et al., 2015). Psychological and social circumstances may affect local factors such as the protection of the wound, promotion of optimal tissue conditions for healing and the risk of infection. For example, where someone is unable to stop work because of job security or financial concerns, they are more at risk of compromising the healing process. As well, if the mental health of a person leads them to neglect self-care, then again the ideal conditions for healing may not be preserved. The link between psychological and social factors in these examples is essentially behavioural – that is, the person's inadequate behavioural response to injury affects healing. These have been labelled as 'health-impairing behaviours' (Boyapati and Wang, 2007).

There has been substantial experimental research investigating more indirect influ-ences of psychological and social factors on healing, for example the levels of cortisol and cytokine production. These could be described collectively as systemic effects and involve the influence of characteristics such as age, gender, nutrition, chronic diseases and psychological and social stress. Research has examined the effect of exercise on healing in older men after they were given a skin lesion to the back of the nondominant hand (Emery et al., 2005), the effect of examination stress on healing of experimentally applied oral lesions (Marucha et al., 1998), the effect of hostile marital interactions (Kiecolt-Glaser et al., 2005) and the effect of anger control on the healing of experiment-induced blistering (Gouin et al., 2008).

The general outcomes from these studies have been that a broad range of stressors can raise cortisol, reduce the activity of proinflammatory cytokines and therefore delay healing (Godbout and Glaser, 2006). As well, relationships have been established between perceived stress, self-reported general health and healing rate (Ebrecht et al., 2004) and, interestingly, a positive association between healing rate and writing about distressing events, probably mediated by sleep (Koschwanez et al., 2013). The role of exercise on healing is likely to be multifactorial, including mediating psychological stress and improving perfusion of tissues (Emery et al., 2005). The outcomes from this research necessitates health professionals to acknowledge the role of psychological and social factors on tissue recovery, and therefore promotes the need to consider strategies – within their scope of practice – that optimize the healing environment.

## APPLICATION IN CLINICAL PRACTICE

### Therapeutic Alliance

'*...you can't get anywhere unless you know, and the patient knows, it is safe to proceed...*'

*Gifford, 2014*

The term 'therapeutic alliance' captures the partnership between a therapist and the client and can be described as collaborative and involving trust and empathy. It has been shown to positively influence treatment outcomes (Pinto et al., 2012) and some of the psychoneuroimmunoendocrinology issues are discussed in the following sections.

### Placebo-Like Effects in Clinical Practice

'*The mere ritual of the therapeutic act may generate therapeutic responses through the patient's expectations and beliefs (placebo responses), which sometimes may be as powerful as those generated by real medical treatments. Today, these placebo responses can be approached from a biological perspective, whereby the biochemical, anatomical, and physiological link between expectation.*'

*Benedetti, 2013, p. 1213*

The contributions to the placebo response include a supportive therapeutic relationship, contextual factors including environmental aspects associated with recovery (ie, conditioning), expectations and the psychological responsiveness of the patient and the severity of the symptoms (Benedetti, 2013; Finniss et al., 2010). It would seem appropriate to reserve the term placebo for experimental and clinical trials as it often requires an element of concealment. Ethically there is no place for deception in clinical practice. It is accepted, however, that the influences and mechanisms will be present in placebo-like effects in clinical interventions. Exploiting the knowledge of these nonspecific treatment benefits would seem appropriate and give support to the importance of a healthy therapeutic alliance and of educating the patient about the great healing powers that the body possesses.

The current knowledge of the underpinning psychoneuroimmunoendocrinology for placebo-like responses has been well described (Benedetti, 2013). This includes a detailed review of the steps involved in health professional–patient interaction. First the patient needs to feel she or he is unwell, which is triggered by cytokine activity (Watkins and Maier, 2005). Then there is a need to seek relief and this involves a positive expectation that might reduce stress when action is taken (eg, arrive at the doctor's and start to feel better). Meeting the health professional can have a profound influence over activity in the amygdala (ie, fear and emotion promoting stress), mediated by oxytocin and the level of trustworthiness the patient perceives in the health professional's appearance and manner (Benedetti, 2013). The language used and empathy of the health professional also influences the neuro-immune-endocrine mechanisms that might be triggered (Benedetti, 2013). For example, there is now impressive evidence that imaging reports can alter outcomes (Jarvik et al., 2015) and a potential mechanism for this is increased anxiety and elements of catastrophizing, resulting in HPA axis activation and catecholamine activity.

## Patient-Centred Care

Patient-centred care is a key feature of a positive therapeutic alliance (Pinto et al., 2012). Patient-centred care is respectful of a person's values and needs, and works towards goals that are reflective of the person's preferences and expectations (Hoffmann and Tooth, 2009). A key principle of patient-centred care is to make the person feel safe. This requires good interpersonal skills, well-targeted education and may involve shared-decision making (Hoffmann and Tooth, 2009). When the physiotherapist engages in this way with the person they are treating, they are creating a safe space that should reduce stress, and therefore reduce pain and enhance healing.

One small qualitative study captured the perspective of the patient involved in the clinical interaction and identified five health professional characteristics that were valued: good communication, confidence, knowledge and professionalism, ability to relate to and understand people, and transparency with information about clinical progression and outcomes (Kidd et al., 2011). This reflects the need for a respectful interaction that makes the person feel safe and builds trust and it would be expected that these elements would facilitate placebo-like responses in association with the person's treatment.

Another exploratory study identified what strategies nursing staff used to facilitate patient-centred care including promoting shared decision making, promoting meaningful, enjoyable and pleasurable living and valuing people through engagement with their life story (Edvardsson et al., 2013). A patient-centred approach demands an emphasis on the person beyond the affected body part or the presenting condition.

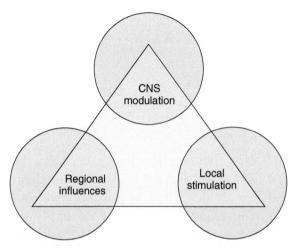

FIGURE 5.2 ▪ The pain and movement reasoning model categories – local stimulation, regional influences, central modulation (Jones and O'Shaughnessy, 2014). *('Pain and movement reasoning model' by Des O'Shaughnessy and Lester Jones is licensed under a Creative Commons Attribution-NonCommercial 3.0 Unported License.)*

## Pain and Movement Reasoning Model

*'Pain perception takes place in a context of an individual's environment, including the physical, social and emotional contexts, and then is managed in a clinical context influenced by the values and beliefs of the therapist.'*

### Jones and O'Shaughnessy, 2014, p. 270

For assessment to be patient-centred it needs to incorporate psychological, emotional and social factors and current and past history. The pain and movement reasoning model is a clinical reasoning tool that was designed to capture the complexity of pain by categorizing the range of pain mechanisms (Jones and O'Shaughnessy, 2014) (see Figure 5.2). The three categories include mechanisms that trigger or sensitize the nociceptors (ie, local stimulation), mechanisms that contribute to the pain but are remote to the location of pain (ie, regional influences) and mechanisms that alter the processing of pain in the spinal cord or brain (ie, central modulation). Although the local stimulation and regional influences categories explicitly incorporate neuro-immune interactions, the central modulation incorporates shared neuro-immune-endocrine mechanisms, influenced by psychological, emotional and social factors that are involved in both pain and stress. This includes the sensitivity to pain and stress that has been associated with early or persistent stressors across time, as well as the effect of current cognitive strategies (eg, rumination), mood (eg, anger or depression) and emotions (eg, fear or loneliness). When using the model as a clinical reasoning tool, it is expected that the clinician engage with all categories – and therefore all the potential influences of pain – and this demands an extension of assessment beyond traditional pathoanatomical approaches (Jones and O'Shaughnessy, 2014).

The 'central modulation' category of the pain and movement reasoning model allows the moderators and mediators of pain to be captured in the assessment and clinical reasoning process. Moderators can be considered to be factors that preexist yet influence subsequent signs and symptoms of an intervention or event (Turner et al., 2007). An example would be if someone has had early life traumatic experiences (moderator) then the pain of an injury may be enhanced as a result of sensitized neuro-immune processes (Fleischman et al., 2014). Or equally, if someone has persistent back pain (moderator) and gets an infection that enhances neuro-immune activity, the back pain might become worse (Grace et al., 2014). Mediators are factors that accompany or are subsequent to an event and modify the effect and outcomes of the event

(Turner et al., 2007). For example, if someone becomes concerned after reading the imaging report (mediator) of their spine, then they may magnify and ruminate on potential negative outcomes leading to heightened HPA axis activity (Gianferante et al., 2014; Jarvik et al., 2015; Webster and Cifuentes, 2010). Or if someone is unable to sleep because their pain is poorly controlled, then allostatic load might be increased and the person may become even more sensitive to movement (Juster and McEwen, 2015). Importantly, if someone had poor sleep hygiene before an injury it could be considered a moderator as a result of the bidirectional effects of sleep and pain (Straube and Heesen, 2015). Disrupted sleep contributes to allostatic load suggesting the sleep deprived person is primed for activation of the body's protection system (McEwen and Karatsoreos, 2015).

After exploring the categories of the pain and movement reasoning model the clinician is able to come up with a formulation. Formulation is a term from psychology practice which can be described as the clinician's hypotheses about the causes and influences of the person's problem, and incorporates relevant theoretical knowledge (Johnstone and Dallos, 2013). It may be useful to consider it as a step before diagnosis and planning of treatment, when the clinician uses her/his expertise to reflect on assessment findings. The model promotes a formulation process that integrates current concepts of pain and neuro-immune function within a biopsychosocial framework (Jones and O'Shaughnessy, 2014). Physiotherapists can then make decisions about treatment priorities and the need for incorporating experts from other disciplines.

Arguably this broad assessment of the person, that enables the moderators and mediators of the pain experience to be captured, promotes an enhanced interaction between the person and the health professional. Recognizing a role for neuro-immune-endocrine interactions in pain, facilitates a greater number of treatment targets including social, psychological, biomechanical and biomedical. Valuing the person's life story then allows for contextually appropriate interventions. See Box 5.4 for a brief caution when adopting this approach.

## Stress Reducing Interventions and Physiotherapy

Research has shown promising results for a range of interventions that collectively can be considered to target stress and the stress response, and which have increasing relevance for physiotherapy practice that seeks to incorporate mind-body strategies. The research supporting mindfulness and yoga will be looked at in some detail but research also supports other interventions including Feldenkrais (Hillier and Worley, 2015), Tai Chi (Robert-McComb et al., 2015) and hypnosis (Jensen et al., 2015). Shared components of these contemplative techniques can

include cultivating body awareness (interoception), controlled and mindful movement, present awareness through the focus on breathing, learning to take effective action (empowerment) and social safety.

As confidence grows in the importance of the integration of neuro-immune and endocrine systems on health, mind-body interventions such as these that regulate the stress response may increasingly be recommended as preventative strategies.

Other areas that have potential to modify psychoneuroimmunoendocrinological factors include musical activities, with some evidence supporting benefits of group drumming, group singing, passive listening to relaxing music (Chanda and Levitin, 2013) and intensive experiences in natural settings like the concept of 'forest bathing' (Mao, Cao et al., 2012). It would be reasonable to think that these relatively economical, accessible and available experiences could be a feature of future psychologically informed health care.

### Mindfulness

Mindfulness probably has the broadest acceptance of these interventions and has been defined as:

> '...the awareness that emerges through paying attention on purpose, in the present moment, and nonjudgementally to the unfolding of experience moment by moment.'

> *Kabat-Zinn, 2003, p. 145*

Research has demonstrated that mindfulness training can reduce levels of inflammatory biomarkers (eg, IL-6, c-reactive protein) across populations as diverse as lonely older adults, unemployed job seekers, people with

---

**BOX 5.4**

**RISK OF IATROGENIC OUTCOMES WHEN EXTENDING SCOPE**

It is important to recognize that extending assessment or treatment into the realm of mind-body integration has risks. An untrained clinician can do great harm to someone who is vulnerable as a result of prior trauma. Care must be taken to ensure that health professionals are clear on their scope of practice and are aware of the consequences of confronting clients – intentionally or unintentionally – with past traumatic experiences.

advanced cancer and their caregivers and women who have experienced interpersonal trauma (Creswell et al., 2012; 2016; Gallegos et al., 2015; Lengacher et al., 2012). A reduction in cortisol, associated with a reduction in stress measures, has also been documented (Lengacher et al., 2012), but not consistently (Cash et al., 2015). Although mindfulness and immunity studies have been criticized methodologically, including that the measurement of inflammatory biomarkers is generally incorporated as a secondary and not primary outcome (Black and Slavich, 2016), mindfulness also seems to be associated with improvements in relevant psychological measures of anxiety, depression, loneliness, stress and emotional-regulation (Cash et al., 2015; Creswell et al., 2012; Gallegos et al., 2015).

Mindfulness has also been incorporated into management for people with pain conditions. A study investigated the effect of mindfulness training in women with fibromyalgia and, although it did not report improvements in pain or physical function, fatigue and sleep were both improved (Cash et al., 2015). Other research has found a reduction in pain outcomes including pain intensity (Brotto et al., 2015; Reiner et al., 2013). The effects of mindfulness on cognitive variables like anxiety, attention and catastrophizing may provide some explanation for the changes in pain perception.

A repeated commentary in the mindfulness literature suggests that the quality and quantity of training affects the level of mindfulness that is achieved, the change that occurs in other variables (eg, psychological measures and inflammatory biomarkers) and the sustainability of effect.

## Yoga

Interventions incorporating yoga have increasing research support for the treatment of pain (Tekur et al., 2012; Ward et al., 2013) and reduction of stress and anxiety (Kiecolt-Glaser et al., 2010; Sharma and Knowlden, 2012). Mechanisms of how yoga interventions improve pain and stress outcomes are not entirely understood, but key aspects may be an enhanced positive affect, and the cultivation of self-compassion and mindfulness (see the following reviews by Riley and Park, 2015 and Ward et al., 2013). Increasingly studies are measuring changes in stress hormones and other markers to identify the mechanisms and effects. For example, in a study that included novices and experts in the practice of yoga, the experts had significantly lower biological markers for inflammation (ie, IL-6) (Kiecolt-Glaser et al., 2010).

There are more clinical based studies too. Depressive illnesses have been associated with a dysregulated stress response (for a comprehensive review see Gold, 2015) and an intensive yoga intervention for people with depression was found to improve depression, state and trait anxiety scores (Tekur et al., 2012). The study location was a city in India where yoga practice is arguably more common and acceptable, and so these findings may not be generalizable to other cultural contexts. However, a reduction in depression was also achieved in a randomized control trial of a yoga intervention in American women with PTSD, and sustained in those women who continued their yoga practice at 18 months' follow-up (Rhodes et al., 2016). PTSD symptoms were also reduced. An 8-week yoga intervention improved cortisol levels in women with fibromyalgia, a condition that has been associated with hypocortisolism (Curtis et al., 2011). Studies that have investigated yoga interventions for preventing and controlling type 2 diabetes – a condition associated with hypercortisolism – have also shown promising outcomes (Sharma and Knowlden, 2012). Promising results have also been reported for using yoga and aerobic exercise to reduce stress in people with schizophrenia, although the lack of physiological measures for stress and a large dropout rate reduce confidence in these results (Vancampfort et al., 2011).

As with mindfulness, the research would suggest that those who persist with a regular yoga practice are the most likely to show health and wellbeing benefits (Rhodes et al., 2016).

## FUTURE DIRECTIONS AND CONCLUSIONS

### Future Directions

#### Epigenetics

'...development never ends and adolescents, young adults, mature and aging individuals continue to show the results of experiences, including opportunities for redirection of unhealthy tendencies through a variety of interventions.'

*McEwen et al, 2015, p. 7*

Epigenetics is a growing area of research, investigating factors that alter gene transcription and expression without changing the gene sequence (Feil and Fraga, 2012). It seems apparent that environmental influences have an effect on gene expression during gestation and throughout the lifespan (Feil, 2006; Feil and Fraga, 2012; Radley et al., 2011). Some

change can be short term, whereas other modifications can be long lasting with potential effects on susceptibility or resilience to disease (Klengel and Binder, 2015; Zannas and West, 2014).

There are a number of reviews that have looked at the role of epigenetics on the body's protection responses such as stress (Radley et al., 2011) and pain (Stone and Szyf, 2013) and some of the mechanisms have been described earlier in this chapter. The importance of the interaction of neuro-immune-endocrine activity, environmental and psychological factors , and gene expression is still being unravelled. As the mechanisms become clearer, however, there is potential to better explain health outcomes including susceptibility and resilience to chronic conditions (Klengel and Binder, 2015; Lirk et al., 2015; Zannas and West, 2014).

#### The Microbiome

. '...organisms within the gut play a role in early programming and later responsivity of the stress system'.

*Moloney et al., 2014, p. 49*

The interaction between the nervous system and our microbial population is an exciting and potentially revolutionary area of research. It is becoming apparent that homoeostasis relies on appropriate communication between the central nervous system and the gut microbiota and disease risk is heightened when there is dysregulation of these processes (El Aidy et al., 2014; Moloney et al., 2014; Sun and Chang, 2014). The links between the central nervous system, the autonomic nervous system and the enteric nervous system, underpin neural communication, with the vagus nerve providing the pathway for bidirectional communication between the gut and brain (Moloney et al., 2014). The comparisons with the immune system's role in stress, and indeed pain, are apparent and there is growing evidence of brain-gut immune disruption and autonomic dysregulation in irritable bowel syndrome (Elsenbruch, 2011; Phillips et al., 2014), and associations with other inflammatory and pain conditions (Woolf, 2011). Links between gut dysfunction and mood and behaviour change reinforce that this will be an important area to monitor in the future (El Aidy et al., 2014; Kaplan et al, 2015; Logan, 2015; Sun and Chang, 2014).

### Surgical Prehabilitation

Another area that is likely to develop in the future is an enhanced surgical prehabilitation that recognizes the role of neuro-immune-endocrine factors on healing and pain. Authors in this field have flagged the need for building 'physiological reserve', including attention to nutrition and psychological factors (Carli and Scheede-Bergdahl, 2015). Katz and colleagues have developed a sophisticated approach to the management of pain associated with surgery (Katz et al., 2015). By considering the risks at various stages – preoperative, intraoperative and postoperative – they created optimal and timely interventions to improve pain outcomes. This included assessing for mood and catastrophizing early, monitoring of adverse surgical outcomes like nerve damage or inflammation and reviewing for characteristics of PTSD in the longer term (Katz et al., 2015). This sophisticated approach to pain assessment and treatment could be seen as an application of psychoneuro-immunoendocrinology and would seem to be an important example for future practice.

### Conclusions

It is clear that it is no longer appropriate to employ unsophisticated single system approaches to clinical practice. A persistence with purely pathoanatomical models of physiotherapy will be detrimental not only to patients, but also to the profession's future growth. This chapter has attempted to provide an overview of stress biology using an integrated systems approach. By considering the body's protection system as the integration of neural, immune and endocrine systems, the complexity of many clinical presentations can be better understood. This includes the role of personal and environmental factors and the effects of prior adverse life events on pain and healing. It also emphasizes the benefits of patient-centred care, not only to capture the person's story and potential influence on health, but also to create a safe therapeutic interaction that facilitates health-promoting neuro-immune-endocrine responses. Taking a psychologically informed, or even a psychoneuroimmunoendocrinologically informed, approach to physiotherapy recognizes the power of the clinical interaction to influence health on multiple levels.

### References

Amantea, D., 2015. Editorial overview: Neuroscience: Brain and immunity: new targets for neuroprotection. Current Opinion in Pharmacology 26, v–viii.

Andrade, P., Hoogland, G., Garcia, M.A., Steinbusch, H.W., Daemen, M.A., Visser-Vandewalle, V., 2013. Elevated IL-1β and IL-6 levels in lumbar herniated discs in patients with sciatic pain. Eur. Spine J. 22, 714–720.

Andrade, P., Hoogland, G., Teernstra, O.P., Van Aalst, J., Van Maren, E., Daemen, M.A., et al., 2016. Elevated levels of tumor necrosis factor-α and TNFR1 in recurrent herni-ated lumbar discs correlate with chronicity of post-operative sciatic pain. Spine J. 16, 243–251.

Austin, P.J., Moalem-Taylor, G., 2010. The neuro-immune balance in neuropathic pain: Involvement of inflamma-tory immune cells, immune-like glial cells and cytokines. J. Neuroimmunol. 229, 26–50.

Baliatsas, C., Van Kamp, I., Hooiveld, M., Lebret, E., Yzer-mans, J., 2015. The relationship of modern health worries to non-specific physical symptoms and per-ceived environmental sensitivity: A study combining self-reported and general practice data. J. Psychosom. Res. 79, 355–361.

Benarroch, E.E., 2009. The locus coeruleus norepinephrine system Functional organization and potential clinical significance. Neurology 73, 1699–1704.

Benedetti, F., 2013. Placebo and the new physiology of the doctor-patient relationship. Physiol. Rev. 93, 1207–1246.

Berk, L.S., Tan, S.A., Fry, W.F., Napier, B.J., Lee, J.W., Hubbard, R.W., et al., 1989. Neuroendocrine and stress hormone changes during mirthful laughter. Am. J. Med. Sci. 298, 390–396.

Berridge, C.W., Schmeichel, B.E., España, R.A., 2012. Noradrenergic modulation of wakefulness/arousal. Sleep Med. Rev. 16, 187–197.

Black, D.S., Slavich, G.M., 2016. Mindfulness meditation and the immune system: a systematic review of rand-omized controlled trials. Ann. N. Y. Acad. Sci. 1373, 13–24.

Boersma, G., Bale, T., Casanello, P., Lara, H., Lucion, A., Suchecki, D., et al., 2014. Long-Term Impact of Early Life Events on Physiology and Behaviour. J. Neuroendo-crinol. 26, 587–602.

Boyapati, L., Wang, H.L., 2007. The role of stress in periodon-tal disease and wound healing. Periodontol. 2000 44, 195–210.

Briggs, A.M., Slater, H., Smith, A.J., Parkin-Smith, G.F., Watkins, K., Chua, J., 2013. Low back pain-related beliefs and likely practice behaviours among final-year cross-discipline health students. Eur. J. Pain 17, 766–775.

Brotto, L.A., Basson, R., Smith, K.B., Driscoll, M., Sadownik, L., 2015. Mindfulness-based group therapy for women with provoked vestibulodynia. Mindfulness 6, 417–432.

Buttarelli, F.R., Fanciulli, A., Pellicano, C., Pontieri, F.E., 2011. The dopaminergic system in peripheral blood lymphocytes: from physiology to pharmacology and potential applications to neuropsychiatric disorders. Curr. Neuropharmacol. 9, 278.

Butz, M., Wörgötter, F., Van Ooyen, A., 2009. Activity-dependent structural plasticity. Brain Res. Rev. 60, 287.

Capuron, L., Miller, A.H., 2011. Immune system to brain signaling: neuropsychopharmacological implications. Pharmacol. Ther. 130, 226–238.

Carli, F., Scheede-Bergdahl, C., 2015. Prehabilitation to enhance perioperative care. Anesthesiol. Clin. 33, 17–33.

Casano, A.M., Peri, F., 2015. Microglia: Multitasking Special-ists of the Brain. Dev. Cell 32, 469–477.

Cash, E., Salmon, P., Weissbecker, I., Rebholz, W.N., Bayley-Veloso, R., Zimmaro, L.A., et al., 2015. Mindfulness meditation alleviates fibromyalgia symptoms in women: Results of a randomized clinical trial. Anns Behav. Med. 49, 319–330.

Chanda, M.L., Levitin, D.J., 2013. The neurochemistry of music. Trends Cogn. Sci. 17, 179–193.

Chang, Z., 2010. Important aspects of Toll-like receptors, ligands and their signaling pathways. Inflamm. Res. 59, 791–808.

Chapman, C.R., Tuckett, R.P., Song, C.W., 2008. Pain and stress in a systems perspective: reciprocal neural, endo-crine, and immune interactions. J. Pain 9, 122–145.

Chatzitheodorou, D., Kabitsis, C., Malliou, P., Mougios, V., 2007. A pilot study of the effects of high-intensity aerobic exercise versus passive interventions on pain, disability, psychological strain, and serum cortisol con-centrations in people with chronic low back pain. Phys. Ther. 87, 304–312.

Chatzitheodorou, D., Mavromoustakos, S., Milioti, S., 2008. The effect of exercise on adrenocortical responsiveness of patients with chronic low back pain, controlled for psychological strain. Clin. Rehabil. 22, 319–328.

Chrousos, G.P., 2009. Stress and disorders of the stress system. Nat. Rev. Endocrinol. 5, 374–381.

Coronado, R.A., George, S.Z., Devin, C.J., Wegener, S.T., Archer, K.R., 2015. Pain sensitivity and pain catastro-phizing are associated with persistent pain and disability after lumbar spine surgery. Arch. Phys. Med. Rehabil. 96, 1763–1770.

Creswell, J.D., Irwin, M.R., Burklund, L.J., Lieberman, M.D., Arevalo, J.M., Ma, J., et al., 2012. Mindfulness-based stress reduction training reduces loneliness and pro-inflammatory gene expression in older adults: a small randomized controlled trial. Brain Behav. Immun. 26, 1095–1101.

Creswell, J.D., Taren, A.A., Lindsay, E.K., Greco, C.M., Gianaros, P.J., Fairgrieve, A., et al. In Press. Alterations in resting state functional connectivity link mindfulness meditation with reduced interleukin-6: a randomized controlled trial. Biol. Psychiatry 80, 53–61.

Crombez, G., Eccleston, C., Baeyens, F., Eelen, P., 1998. When somatic information threatens, catastrophic thinking enhances attentional interference. Pain 75, 187–198.

Crombez, G., Eccleston, C., Van Den Broeck, A., Goubert, L., Van Houdenhove, B., 2004. Hypervigilance to pain in fibromyalgia: the mediating role of pain intensity and catastrophic thinking about pain. Clin. J. Pain 20, 98–102.

Crowley, S.K., Pedersen, C.A., Leserman, J., Girdler, S.S., 2015. The influence of early life sexual abuse on oxytocin concentrations and premenstrual symptomatology in women with a menstrually related mood disorder. Biol. Psychol. 109, 1–9.

Curtis, K., Osadchuk, A., Katz, J., 2011. An eight-week yoga intervention is associated with improvements in pain, psychological functioning and mindfulness, and changes in cortisol levels in women with fibromyalgia. J. Pain Res. 4, 189–201.

Danese, A., McEwen, B.S., 2012. Adverse childhood experiences, allostasis, allostatic load, and age-related disease. Physiol. Behav. 106, 29–39.

Deppermann, S., Storchak, H., Fallgatter, A.J., Ehlis, A.-C., 2014. Stress-induced neuroplasticity: (Mal)adaptation to adverse life events in patients with PTSD–A critical overview. Neuroscience 283, 166–177.

Detillion, C.E., Craft, T.K., Glasper, E.R., Prendergast, B.J., Devries, A.C., 2004. Social facilitation of wound healing. Psychoneuroendocrinology 29, 1004–1011.

Diegelmann, R.F., Evans, M.C., 2004. Wound healing: an overview of acute, fibrotic and delayed healing. Front. Biosci. 9, 283–289.

Drexler, S.M., Merz, C.J., Hamacher-Dang, T.C., Tegenthoff, M., Wolf, O.T., 2015. Effects of cortisol on reconsolidation of reactivated fear memories. Neuropsychopharmacology 40, 3036–3043.

Ebrecht, M., Hextall, J., Kirtley, L.-G., Taylor, A., Dyson, M., Weinman, J., 2004. Perceived stress and cortisol levels predict speed of wound healing in healthy male adults. Psychoneuroendocrinology 29, 798–809.

Eccleston, C., Crombez, G., Scotford, A., Clinch, J., Connell, H., 2004. Adolescent chronic pain: patterns and predictors of emotional distress in adolescents with chronic pain and their parents. Pain 108, 221–229.

Edvardsson, D., Varrailhon, P., Edvardsson, K., 2013. Promoting person-centeredness in long-term care: An exploratory study. J. Gerontol. Nurs. 40, 46–53.

El Aidy, S., Dinan, T.G., Cryan, J.F., 2014. Immune modulation of the brain-gut-microbe axis. Front. Microbiol. 5, 146. doi:10.3389/fmicb.2014.00146.

Elsenbruch, S., 2011. Abdominal pain in irritable bowel syndrome: a review of putative psychological, neural and neuro-immune mechanisms. Brain Behav. Immun. 25, 386–394.

Emery, C.F., Kiecolt-Glaser, J.K., Glaser, R., Malarkey, W.B., Frid, D.J., 2005. Exercise accelerates wound healing among healthy older adults: a preliminary investigation. J. Gerontol. A. Biol Sci. Med. Sci. 60, 1432–1436.

Fagundes, C.P., Glaser, R., Kiecolt-Glaser, J.K., 2013. Stressful early life experiences and immune dysregulation across the lifespan. Brain Behav. Immun. 27, 8–12.

Feil, R., 2006. Environmental and nutritional effects on the epigenetic regulation of genes. Mutat. Res. 600, 46–57.

Feil, R., Fraga, M.F., 2012. Epigenetics and the environment: emerging patterns and implications. Nat. Rev. Genet. 13, 97–109.

Finniss, D.G., Kaptchuk, T.J., Miller, F., Benedetti, F., 2010. Biological, clinical, and ethical advances of placebo effects. Lancet 375, 686–695.

Fleischman, D.S., Bunevicius, A., Leserman, J., Girdler, S.S., 2014. Menstrually related mood disorders and a history of abuse: moderators of pain sensitivity. Health Psychol. 33, 147.

Gallegos, A.M., Lytle, M.C., Moynihan, J.A., Talbot, N.L., 2015. Mindfulness-based stress reduction to enhance psychological functioning and improve inflammatory biomarkers in trauma-exposed women: A pilot study. Psychol. Trauma 7, 525.

Ganzel, B.L., Morris, P.A., Wethington, E., 2010. Allostasis and the human brain: Integrating models of stress from the social and life sciences. Psychol. Rev. 117, 134.

Garland, E.L., Howard, M.O., 2009. Neuroplasticity, psychosocial genomics, and the biopsychosocial paradigm in the 21st century. Health Soc. Work 34, 191–199.

Generaal, E., Vogelzangs, N., Macfarlane, G.J., Geenen, R., Smit, J.H., De Geus, E.J., et al., 2015. Biological stress systems, adverse life events and the onset of chronic multisite musculoskeletal pain: a 6-year cohort study. Ann. Rheum. Dis. 75, 847–854.

Gianferante, D., Thoma, M.V., Hanlin, L., Chen, X., Breines, J.G., Zoccola, P.M., et al., 2014. Post-stress rumination predicts HPA axis responses to repeated acute stress. Psychoneuroendocrinology 49, 244–252.

Gifford, L., 1998. Pain, the tissues and the nervous system: A conceptual model. Physiotherapy 84, 27–36.

Gifford, L., 2014. Aches and Pains. Aches and Pains Ltd, Falmouth.

Gillick, B.T., Zirpel, L., 2012. Neuroplasticity: an appreciation from synapse to system. Arch. Phys. Med. Rehabil. 93, 1846–1855.

Girish, G., Lobo, L.G., Jacobson, J.A., Morag, Y., Miller, B., Jamadar, D.A., 2011. Ultrasound of the shoulder: asymptomatic findings in men. AJR Am J. Roentgenol. 197, W713–W719.

Godbout, J.P., Glaser, R., 2006. Stress-induced immune dysregulation: implications for wound healing, infectious disease and cancer. J. Neuroimmune Pharmacol. 1, 421–427.

Gold, P., 2015. The organization of the stress system and its dysregulation in depressive illness. Mol. Psychiatry 20, 32–47.

Gouin, J.-P., Kiecolt-Glaser, J.K., Malarkey, W.B., Glaser, R., 2008. The influence of anger expression on wound healing. Brain Behav. Immun. 22, 699–708.

Grace, P.M., Hutchinson, M.R., Maier, S.F., Watkins, L.R., 2014. Pathological pain and the neuroimmune interface. Nat. Rev. Immunol. 14, 217–231.

Hadjistavropoulos, T., Craig, K.D., Duck, S., Cano, A., Goubert, L., Jackson, P.L., et al., 2011. A biopsychosocial formulation of pain communication. Psychol. Bull. 137, 910.

Harte, J.L., Eifert, G.H., Smith, R., 1995. The effects of running and meditation on beta-endorphin, corticotropin-releasing hormone and cortisol in plasma, and on mood. Biol. Psychol. 40, 251–265.

Heim, C., Ehlert, U., Hellhammer, D.H., 2000. The potential role of hypocortisolism in the pathophysiology of stress-related bodily disorders. Psychoneuroendocrinology 25, 1–35.

Hillier, S., Worley, A., 2015. The effectiveness of the feldenkrais method: a systematic review of the evidence. Evid. Based Complement. Alternat. Med. doi:10.1155/2015/752160.

Hirsh, A.T., George, S.Z., Bialosky, J.E., Robinson, M.E., 2008. Fear of pain, pain catastrophizing, and acute pain perception: relative prediction and timing of assessment. J. Pain 9, 806–812.

Ho-Joong Kim, M., Bo-Gun Suh, M., Dong-Bong Lee, M., Gun-Woo Lee, M., Dong-Whan Kim, M., Kyoung-Tak Kang, M., et al., 2013. The influence of pain sensitivity on the symptom severity in patients with lumbar spinal stenosis. Pain Physician 16, 135–144.

Hoeger Bement, M., Weyer, A., Keller, M., Harkins, A.L., Hunter, S.K., 2010. Anxiety and stress can predict pain perception following a cognitive stress. Physiol. Behav. 101, 87–92.

Hoffmann, T., Tooth, L., 2009. Talking with clients about evidence. In: Hoffmann, T., Bennett, S., Del Mar, C. (Eds.), Evidence-based Practice Across the Health Professions. Elsevier Australia, Sydney.

Husarik, D.B., Saupe, N., Pfirrmann, C.W., Jost, B., Hodler, J., Zanetti, M., 2010. Ligaments and plicae of the elbow: normal MR imaging variability in 60 asymptomatic subjects 1. Radiology 257, 185–194.

Jänig, W., Chapman, C., Green, P., 2006. Pain and body protection: sensory, autonomic, neuroendocrine, and behavioral mechanisms in the control of inflammation and hyperalgesia. In: Proceedings of the 11th World Congress on Pain. IASP Press, Seattle, pp. 331–347.

Jarvik, J.G., Gold, L.S., Comstock, B.A., Heagerty, P.J., Rundell, S.D., Turner, J.A., et al., 2015. Association of early imaging for back pain with clinical outcomes in older adults. JAMA 313, 1143–1153.

Jensen, M.C., Brant-Zawadzki, M.N., Obuchowski, N., Modic, M.T., Malkasian, D., Ross, J.S., 1994. Magnetic resonance imaging of the lumbar spine in people without back pain. NEJM 331, 69–73.

Jensen, M.P., Adachi, T., Tomes-Peres, C., Lee, J., et al., 2015. Mechanisms of hypnosis: toward the development of a biopsychosocial model. Int. J. Clin. Exp. Hypn. 63, 34–75.

Johansen, O., Brox, J., Flaten, M.A., 2003. Placebo and nocebo responses, cortisol, and circulating beta-endorphin. Psychosom. Med. 65, 786–790.

Johnstone, D.M., Mitrofanis, J., Stone, J., 2015. Targeting the body to protect the brain: inducing neuroprotection with remotely-applied near infrared light. Neural Regen. Res. 10, 349.

Johnstone, L., Dallos, R. (Eds.), 2013. Formulation in Psychology and Psychotherapy: Making Sense of People's Problems. Routledge, London.

Jones, L., 2007. Introduction to current concepts of pain. In: Partridge, C. (Ed.), Recent Advances of Physiotherapy. Wiley, London.

Jones, L.E., O'Shaughnessy, D.F., 2014. The pain and movement reasoning model: introduction to a simple tool for integrated pain assessment. Man. Ther. 19, 270–276.

Juster, R.-P., McEwen, B.S., 2015. Sleep and chronic stress: new directions for allostatic load research. Sleep Med. 16, 7–8.

Juster, R.-P., Sindi, S., Marin, M.-F., Perna, A., Hashemi, A., Pruessner, J.C., et al., 2011. A clinical allostatic load index is associated with burnout symptoms and hypocortisolemic profiles in healthy workers. Psychoneuroendocrinology 36, 797–805.

Kabat-Zinn, J., 2003. Mindfulness-based interventions in context: past, present, and future. Clin. Psychol. Sci. Pract. 10, 144–156.

Kaltsas, G.A., Chrousos, G.P., 2007. The neuroendocrinology of stress. In: Cacioppo, J., Tassinary, L., Bernston, G. (Eds.), Handbook of Psychophysiology. Cambridge University Press.

Kaplan, B.J., Rucklidge, J.J., Romijn, A., Mcleod, K., 2015. The emerging field of nutritional mental health inflammation, the microbiome, oxidative stress, and mitochondrial function. Clin. Psychol. Sci. 3, 964–980.

Katz, J., Weinrib, A., Fashler, S.R., Katznelzon, R., Shah, B.R., Ladak, S.S., et al., 2015. The Toronto General Hospital transitional pain service: development and implementation of a multidisciplinary program to prevent chronic postsurgical pain. J. Pain Res. 8, 695–702.

Keefe, F.J., Shelby, R.A., Somers, T.J., 2010. Catastrophizing and pain coping: moving forward. Pain 149, 165–166.

Kent, S., Bluthé, R.-M., Kelley, K.W., Dantzer, R., 1992. Sickness behavior as a new target for drug development. Trends Pharmacol. Sci. 13, 24–28.

Khalil, H., Cullen, M., Chambers, H., Carroll, M., Walker, J., 2015. Elements affecting wound healing time: an evidence based analysis. Wound Repair Regen. 23, 550–556.

Khan, R.S., Ahmed, K., Blakeway, E., Skapinakis, P., Nihoyannopoulos, L., Macleod, K., et al., 2011. Catastrophizing:

a predictive factor for postoperative pain. Am. J. Surg. 201, 122–131.

Kidd, M.O., Bond, C.H., Bell, M.L., 2011. Patients' perspectives of patient-centredness as important in musculoskeletal physiotherapy interactions: a qualitative study. Physiotherapy 97, 154–162.

Kiecolt-Glaser, J.K., Christian, L., Preston, H., Houts, C.R., Malarkey, W.B., Emery, C.F., et al., 2010. Stress, inflammation, and yoga practice. Psychosom. Med. 72, 113.

Kiecolt-Glaser, J.K., Loving, T.J., Stowell, J.R., Malarkey, W.B., Lemeshow, S., Dickinson, S.L., et al., 2005. Hostile marital interactions, proinflammatory cytokine production, and wound healing. Arch. Gen. Psychiatry 62, 1377–1384.

Kleim, J.A., 2011. Neural plasticity and neurorehabilitation: teaching the new brain old tricks. J. Commun. Disord. 44, 521–528.

Klengel, T., Binder, E.B., 2015. Epigenetics of stress-related psychiatric disorders and gene× environment interactions. Neuron 86, 1343–1357.

Koschwanez, H.E., Kerse, N., Darragh, M., Jarrett, P., Booth, R.J., Broadbent, E., 2013. Expressive writing and wound healing in older adults: a randomized controlled trial. Psychosom. Med. 75, 581–590.

Kudielka, B.M., Wüst, S., 2010. Human models in acute and chronic stress: assessing determinants of individual hypothalamus–pituitary–adrenal axis activity and reactivity. Stress 13, 1–14.

LeDoux, J.E., 2012. Evolution of human emotion: a view through fear. Prog. Brain Res. 195, 431.

Lengacher, C.A., Kip, K.E., Barta, M., Post-White, J., Jacobsen, P.B., Groer, M., et al., 2012. A pilot study evaluating the effect of mindfulness-based stress reduction on psychological status, physical status, salivary cortisol, and interleukin-6 among advanced-stage cancer patients and their caregivers. J. Holist. Nurs. 30, 170–185.

Levine, M., Cole, S., Weir, D., Crimmins, E., 2015. Childhood and later life stressors and increased inflammatory gene expression at older ages. Soc. Sci. Med. 130, 16–22.

Levite, M., 2015. Dopamine and T Cells: Receptors, direct and potent effects, endogenous production and abnormalities in autoimmune, neurological and psychiatric diseases. Acta Physiol. 216, 42–89.

Liezmann, C., Stock, D., Peters, E.M., 2012. Stress induced neuroendocrine-immune plasticity: A role for the spleen in peripheral inflammatory disease and inflammaging? Dermatoendocrinol. 4, 271–279.

Lirk, P., Fiegl, H., Weber, N., Hollmann, M., 2015. Epigenetics in the perioperative period. Br. J. Pharmacol. 172, 2748–2755.

Logan, A.C., 2015. Dysbiotic drift: mental health, environmental grey space, and microbiota. Dementia 8, 9.

Maier, S.F., Watkins, L.R., 1998. Cytokines for psychologists: implications of bidirectional immune-to-brain communication for understanding behavior, mood, and cognition. Psychol. Rev. 105, 83.

Mao, G.-X., Lang, X.G., Cao, Y.B., He, Z.H., Lu, Y.D., et al., 2012. Therapeutic effect of forest bathing on human hypertension in the elderly. J. Cardiol. 60, 495–502.

Marucha, P.T., Kiecolt-Glaser, J.K., Favagehi, M., 1998. Mucosal wound healing is impaired by examination stress. Psychosom. Med. 60, 362–365.

Mauss, D., Jian, L., Schmidt, B., Angerer, P., Jarczok, M.N., 2015. Measuring allostatic load in the workforce: a systematic review. Ind. Health 53, 5.

McEwen, B.S., 2001. Plasticity of the hippocampus: adaptation to chronic stress and allostatic load. Ann. N. Y. Acad. Sci. 933, 265–277.

McEwen, B.S., 2007. Physiology and neurobiology of stress and adaptation: central role of the brain. Physiol. Rev. 87, 873–904.

McEwen, B.S., 2012. Brain on stress: how the social environment gets under the skin. Proc. Natl. Acad. Sci. U. S. A. 109, 17180–17185.

McEwen, B.S., 2015. Preserving neuroplasticity: role of glucocorticoids and neurotrophins via phosphorylation. Proc. Natl. Acad. Sci. U. S. A. 112, 15544–15545.

McEwen, B.S., Gray, J.D., Nasca, C., 2015. Recognizing resilience: learning from the effects of stress on the brain. Neurobiol. Stress 1, 1–11.

McEwen, B.S., Karatsoreos, I.N., 2015. Sleep deprivation and circadian disruption: stress, allostasis, and allostatic load. Sleep Med. Clin. 10, 1–10.

McEwen, B.S., Nasca, C., Gray, J.D., 2016. Stress effects on neuronal structure: hippocampus, amygdala, and prefrontal cortex. Neuropsychopharmacology 41, 3–23.

McEwen, B.S., Wingfield, J.C., 2003. The concept of allostasis in biology and biomedicine. Horm. Behav. 43, 2–15.

Mcinnis, C.M., Wang, D., Gianferante, D., Hanlin, L., Chen, X., Thoma, M.V., et al., 2015. Response and habituation of pro-and anti-inflammatory gene expression to repeated acute stress. Brain Behav. Immun. 46, 237–248.

McMahon, S.B., Cafferty, W.B., Marchand, F., 2005. Immune and glial cell factors as pain mediators and modulators. Exp. Neurol. 192, 444–462.

Melzack, R., 2001. Pain and the neuromatrix in the brain. J. Dent. Educ. 65, 1378–1382.

Melzack, R., 2005. Evolution of the Neuromatrix Theory of Pain. The Prithvi Raj Lecture: Presented at the Third World Congress of World Institute of Pain, Barcelona 2004. Pain Pract. 5, 85–94.

Milligan, E.D., Watkins, L.R., 2009. Pathological and protective roles of glia in chronic pain. Nat. Rev. Neurosci. 10, 23–36.

Moffett, J.A.K., Richardson, P.H., 1995. The influence of psychological variables on the development and perception of musculoskeletal pain. Physiother. Theory Pract. 11, 3–11.

Moloney, R.D., Desbonnet, L., Clarke, G., Dinan, T.G., Cryan, J.F., 2014. The microbiome: stress, health and disease. Mamm. Genome 25, 49–74.

Moseley, G., Butler, D., 2015. The Explain Pain Handbook: Protectometer. Noigroup Publications, Adelaide.

Moseley, G.L., 2007. Reconceptualising pain according to its underlying biology. Phys. Ther. Rev. 12, 169–178.

Muscatell, K.A., et al., 2015. Greater amygdala activity and dorsomedial prefrontal–amygdala coupling are associated with enhanced inflammatory responses to stress. Brain Behav. Immun. 43, 46–53.

Nakashima, H., Yukawa, Y., Suda, K., Yamagata, M., Ueta, T., Kato, F., 2015. Abnormal findings on magnetic resonance images of the cervical spines in 1211 asymptomatic subjects. Spine 40, 392–398.

Nardo, L., Parimi, N., Liu, F., Lee, S., Jungmann, P.M., Nevitt, M.C., et al., 2015. Femoroacetabular impingement: prevalent and often asymptomatic in older men: the osteoporotic fractures in men study. Clin. Orthop. Relat. Res. 1–9.

Nicolaides, N.C., Kyratzi, E., Lamprokostopoulou, A., Chrousos, G.P., Charmandari, E., 2015. Stress, the stress system and the role of glucocorticoids. Neuroimmunomodulation 22, 6–19.

Offidani, E., Ruini, C., 2012. Psychobiological correlates of allostatic overload in a healthy population. Brain Behav. Immun. 26, 284–291.

Öhman, A., 2005. The role of the amygdala in human fear: automatic detection of threat. Psychoneuroendocrinology 30, 953–958.

Padgett, D.A., Glaser, R., 2003. How stress influences the immune response. Trends Immunol. 24, 444–448.

Parsons, S., Harding, G., Breen, A., Foster, N., Pincus, T., Vogel, S., et al., 2007. The influence of patients' and primary care practitioners' beliefs and expectations about chronic musculoskeletal pain on the process of care: a systematic review of qualitative studies. Clin. J. Pain 23, 91–98.

Pedersen, L.M., Schistad, E., Jacobsen, L.M., Røe, C., Gjerstad, J., 2015. Serum levels of the pro-inflammatory interleukins 6 (IL-6) and-8 (IL-8) in patients with lumbar radicular pain due to disc herniation: a 12-month prospective study. Brain Behav. Immun. 46, 132–136.

Phillips, K., Wright, B.J., Kent, S., 2014. Irritable bowel syndrome and symptom severity: Evidence of negative attention bias, diminished vigour, and autonomic dysregulation. J. Psychosom. Res. 77, 13–19.

Pinto, R.Z., Ferreira, M.L., Oliveira, V.C., Franco, M.R., Adams, R., Maher, C.G., et al., 2012. Patient-centred communication is associated with positive therapeutic alliance: a systematic review. J. Physiother. 58, 77–87.

Pittenger, C., Duman, R.S., 2008. Stress, depression, and neuroplasticity: a convergence of mechanisms. Neuropsychopharmacology 33, 88–109.

Ploghaus, A., Narain, C., Beckmann, C.F., Clare, S., Bantick, S., Wise, R., et al., 2001. Exacerbation of pain by anxiety is associated with activity in a hippocampal network. J. Neurosci. 21, 9896–9903.

Poljšak, B., Milisav, I., 2012. Clinical implications of cellular stress responses. Bosn. J. Basic Med. Sci. 12, 122–126.

Pomeroy, V., Tallis, R., 2002. Restoring movement and functional ability after stroke: now and the future. Physiotherapy 88, 3–17.

Quartana, P.J., Buenaver, L.F., Edwards, R.R., Klick, B., Haythornthwaite, J.A., Smith, M.T., 2010. Pain catastrophizing and salivary cortisol responses to laboratory pain testing in temporomandibular disorder and healthy participants. J. Pain 11, 186–194.

Radley, J.J., Kabbaj, M., Jacobson, L., Heydendael, W., Yehuda, R., Herman, J.P., 2011. Stress risk factors and stress-related pathology: neuroplasticity, epigenetics and endophenotypes. Stress 14, 481–497.

Rash, J.A., Aguirre-Camacho, A., Campbell, T.S., 2014. Oxytocin and pain: a systematic review and synthesis of findings. Clin. J. Pain 30, 453–462.

Reiner, K., Tibi, L., Lipsitz, J.D., 2013. Do Mindfulness-Based Interventions Reduce Pain Intensity? A Critical Review of the Literature. Pain Med. 14, 230–242.

Rhodes, A., Spinazzola, J., Van Der Kolk, B., 2016. Yoga for adult women with chronic PTSD: A long-term follow-up study. J. Altern. Complement. Med. 22, 189–196.

Riley, K.E., Park, C.L., 2015. How does yoga reduce stress? A systematic review of mechanisms of change and guide to future inquiry. Health Psychol. Rev. 9, 379–396.

Robert-McComb, J.J., Chyu, M.-C., Tacon, A., Norman, R., 2015. The effects of tai chi on measures of stress and coping style. Focus Altern. Complement. Ther. 20, 89–96.

Rosas-Ballina, M., Tracey, K.J., 2009. The neurology of the immune system: neural reflexes regulate immunity. Neuron 64, 28–32.

Samuels, E., Szabadi, E., 2008. Functional neuroanatomy of the noradrenergic locus coeruleus: its roles in the regulation of arousal and autonomic function part I: principles of functional organisation. Curr. Neuropharmacol. 6, 235.

Sarkar, C., Basu, B., Chakroborty, D., Dasgupta, P.S., Basu, S., 2010. The immunoregulatory role of dopamine: an update. Brain Behav. Immun. 24, 525–528.

Schaible, H.-G., Ebersberger, A., Natura, G., 2011. Update on peripheral mechanisms of pain: beyond prostaglandins and cytokines. Arthritis Res. Ther. 13, 210.

Schalinski, I., Elbert, T., Steudte-Schmiedgen, S., Kirschbaum, C., 2015. The cortisol paradox of trauma-related disorders: lower phasic responses but higher tonic levels of cortisol are associated with sexual abuse in childhood. PLoS ONE 10, e0136921 doi:10.1371/journal.pone .0136921.

Schulz, A., Vögele, C., 2015. Interoception and stress. Front. Psychol. 6, 993.

Sharma, M., Knowlden, A.P., 2012. Role of yoga in preventing and controlling type 2 diabetes mellitus. J. Evid. Based Complement. Altern. Med. 17, 88–95.

Sher, J.S., Uribe, J.W., Posada, A., Murphy, B.J., Zlatkin, M.B., 1995. Abnormal findings on magnetic resonance images of asymptomatic shoulders. J. Bone Joint Surg. Am. 77, 10–15.

Snodgrass, S.J., Heneghan, N.R., Tsao, H., Stanwell, P.T., Rivett, D.A., Van Vliet, P.M., 2014. Recognising neuroplasticity in musculoskeletal rehabilitation: a basis for greater collaboration between musculoskeletal and neurological physiotherapists. Man. Ther. 19, 614–617.

Sommer, C., Kress, M., 2004. Recent findings on how proinflammatory cytokines cause pain: peripheral mechanisms in inflammatory and neuropathic hyperalgesia. Neurosci. Lett. 361, 184–187.

Sprouse-Blum, A.S., Smith, G., Sugai, D., Parsa, F.D., 2010. Understanding endorphins and their importance in pain management. Hawaii Med. J. 69, 70.

Stehling, C., Lane, N., Nevitt, M., Lynch, J., Mcculloch, C., Link, T., 2010. Subjects with higher physical activity levels have more severe focal knee lesions diagnosed with 3T MRI: analysis of a non-symptomatic cohort of the osteoarthritis initiative. Osteoarthritis Cartilage 18, 776–786.

Stephens, R., Atkins, J., Kingston, A., 2009. Swearing as a response to pain. Neuroreport 20, 1056–1060.

Stephens, R., Umland, C., 2011. Swearing as a response to pain—effect of daily swearing frequency. J. Pain 12, 1274–1281.

Stipursky, J., Romão, L., Tortelli, V., Neto, V.M., Gomes, F.C.A., 2011. Neuron–glia signaling: Implications for astrocyte differentiation and synapse formation. Life Sci. 89, 524–531.

Stone, J., 2016. The heart, dementia and why stress can be good for you. In: Ockham's Razor. 2016: Australian Broadcasting Commission.

Stone, L.S., Szyf, M., 2013. The emerging field of pain epigenetics. Pain 154, 1–2.

Straube, S., Heesen, M., 2015. Pain and sleep. Pain 156, 1371–1372.

Sun, J., Chang, E.B., 2014. Exploring gut microbes in human health and disease: pushing the envelope. Genes Dis. 1, 132–139.

Tekur, P., Nagarathna, R., Chametcha, S., Hankey, A., Nagendra, H., 2012. A comprehensive yoga programs improves pain, anxiety and depression in chronic low back pain patients more than exercise: an RCT. Complement. Ther. Med. 20, 107–118.

Thacker, M.A., Clark, A.K., Marchand, F., McMahon, S.B., 2007. Pathophysiology of peripheral neuropathic pain: immune cells and molecules. Anesth. Analg. 105, 838–847.

Trojan, S., Pokorny, J., 1999. Theoretical aspects of neuroplasticity. Physiol. Res. 48, 87–98.

Turner, J.A., Holtzman, S., Mancl, L., 2007. Mediators, moderators, and predictors of therapeutic change in cognitive–behavioral therapy for chronic pain. Pain 127, 276–286.

Uematsu, S., Akira, S., 2007. Toll-like receptors and Type I interferons. J. Biol. Chem. 282, 15319–15323.

Underwood, C., 2011. Getting students moving. Res. Dev. 24, 3.

Ursin, H., 1994. Stress, distress, and immunity. Ann. N. Y. Acad. Sci. 741, 204–211.

Vancampfort, D., De Hert, M., Knapen, J., Wampers, M., Demunter, H., Deckx, S., et al., 2011. State anxiety, psychological stress and positive well-being responses to yoga and aerobic exercise in people with schizophrenia: a pilot study. Disabil. Rehabil. 33, 684–689.

Vervoort, T., Goubert, L., Eccleston, C., Bijttebier, P., Crombez, G., 2006. Catastrophic thinking about pain is independently associated with pain severity, disability, and somatic complaints in school children and children with chronic pain. J. Pediatr. Psychol. 31, 674–683.

Ward, L., Stebbings, S., Cherkin, D., Baxter, G.D., 2013. Yoga for functional ability, pain and psychosocial outcomes in musculoskeletal conditions: a systematic review and meta-analysis. Musculoskeletal Care 11, 203–217.

Watkins, L., Maier, S., 2000. The pain of being sick: implications of immune-to-brain communication for understanding pain. Annu. Rev. Psychol. 51, 29–57.

Watkins, L., Maier, S., 2005. Immune regulation of central nervous system functions: from sickness responses to pathological pain. J. Intern. Med. 257, 139–155.

Watkins, L.R., Hutchinson, M.R., Milligan, E.D., Maier, S.F., 2007. "Listening" and "talking" to neurons: Implications of immune activation for pain control and increasing the efficacy of opioids. Brain Res. Rev. 56, 148–169.

Watkins, L.R., Maier, S.F., 2002. Beyond neurons: evidence that immune and glial cells contribute to pathological pain states. Physiol. Rev. 82, 981–1011.

Watkins, L.R., Maier, S.F., Goehler, L.E., 1995. Immune activation: the role of pro-inflammatory cytokines in inflammation, illness responses and pathological pain states. Pain 63, 289–302.

Webster, B.S., Cifuentes, M., 2010. Relationship of early magnetic resonance imaging for work-related acute low back pain with disability and medical utilization outcomes. J. Occup. Environ. Med. 52, 900–907.

Webster Marketon, J.I., Glaser, R., 2008. Stress hormones and immune function. Cell. Immunol. 252, 16–26.

Woolf, C.J., 2011. Central sensitization: Implications for the diagnosis and treatment of pain. Pain 152, S2–S15.

Wrona, D., 2006. Neural–immune interactions: an integrative view of the bidirectional relationship between the brain and immune systems. J. Neuroimmunol. 172, 38–58.

Wüst, S., Federenko, I.S., Rossum, E.F., Koper, J.W., Kumsta, R., Entringer, S., et al., 2004. A psychobiological perspective on genetic determinants of hypothalamus-pituitary-adrenal axis activity. Ann. N. Y. Acad. Sci. 1032, 52–62.

Wüst, S., Federenko, I.S., Van Rossum, E.F., Koper, J.W., Hellhammer, D.H., 2005. Habituation of cortisol responses to repeated psychosocial stress—further characterization and impact of genetic factors. Psychoneuroendocrinology 30, 199–211.

Yan, Y., Jiang, W., Liu, L., Wang, X., Ding, C., Tian, Z., et al., 2015. Dopamine controls systemic inflammation through inhibition of NLRP3 inflammasome. Cell 160, 62–73.

Zannas, A.S., West, A.E., 2014. Epigenetics and the regulation of stress vulnerability and resilience. Neuroscience 264, 157–170.

Zilioli, S., Slatcher, R.B., Ong, A.D., Gruenewald, T.L., 2015. Purpose in life predicts allostatic load ten years later. J. Psychosom. Res. 79, 451–457.

Zoccola, P.M., Dickerson, S.S., 2012. Assessing the relationship between rumination and cortisol: A review. J. Psychosom. Res. 73, 1–9.

Zoccola, P.M., Quas, J.A., Yim, I.S., 2010. Salivary cortisol responses to a psychosocial laboratory stressor and later verbal recall of the stressor: The role of trait and state rumination. Stress 13, 435–443.

Zusman, M., 2008. Associative memory for movement-evoked chronic back pain and its extinction with musculoskeletal physiotherapy. Phys. Ther. Rev. 13, 57–68.

Zusman, M., 2012. A review of the proposal that innocuous proprioceptive input may maintain movement-evoked joint pain. Phys. Ther. Rev. 17, 346–349.

Zusman, M., 2013. Belief reinforcement: one reason why costs for low back pain have not decreased. J. Multidiscip. Healthc. 6, 197.

# 6

# CARE OF THE ANXIOUS PATIENT
## Understanding and Managing Anxiety Through Cognitive and Patient-Centred Strategies

ANDREW L EVANS ■ ANTHONY J HICKEY

## CHAPTER CONTENTS

## INTRODUCTION

In 2010 alone there were approximately 8.2 million cases of anxiety reported in the United Kingdom (UK; Fineberg et al., 2013). Research also suggests that anxiety is prevalent following injury and during physiotherapy sessions. For example, Wiseman et al. (2015) found that 54% of traumatically injured patients reported above normal anxiety scores on at least one of the three occasions they were interviewed (ie, during hospital admission, 3 months post injury, and 6 months post injury). Anxiety experienced following injury and during physical rehabilitation can be attributed to a number of factors. During the early stages of rehabilitation, Johnston and Carroll (1998) found that negative emotion (eg, anxiety) reported by athletes suffering serious injury (eg, a fractured scaphoid) resulted from the disruption the injury caused to their normal physical functioning. During the middle stages of rehabilitation, negative emotion was provoked by negative cognitive appraisal (and reappraisal) of the physical rehabilitation progress. At the end of rehabilitation, negative emotion primarily stemmed from impatience towards returning to sport.

Dealing with anxious patients would therefore appear to be commonplace when working as a physiotherapist. The aims of the current chapter are four-fold. First, this chapter aims to explain the role of cognition in the generation of emotion and behaviour. Second, this chapter aims to explore irrational and rational beliefs by focusing on the nature, origins and effects of irrational and rational beliefs in a rehabilitation context. Third, this chapter aims to explain the role of two key psychological strategies (ie, self-talk and imagery) in injury and rehabilitation. Finally, this chapter aims to explore a patient-centred approach to managing anxiety within patients by focusing on core conditions (eg, psychological contact) and key skills (eg, positive asset searching). After reading this chapter, we hope that physiotherapists will be able to recognize the components of the ABC framework underpinning cognitive behaviour therapy (CBT) when working with patients experiencing anxiety. We also hope that physiotherapists will be able to: (a) identify irrational and rational beliefs when working with patients, (b) understand the importance of referral and the ABCDE framework of rational emotive behaviour therapy (REBT), (c) use simple techniques to ascertain the irrationality and rationality of patients and (d) promote rationality towards injury and rehabilitation through oral communication. To understand what happens during referral, we explain the psychologist's role in disputing irrational beliefs. After reading this chapter, we hope that physiotherapists will be able to encourage and integrate the use of self-talk and imagery into rehabilitation programmes. Finally, we hope that physiotherapists will be able to develop a patient-centred approach to

consulting through increased awareness and use of core counselling conditions and skills in applied practice.

## COGNITIVE BEHAVIOURAL THERAPY

Typically, individuals will describe that an emotion and/or behaviour is being caused by a specific event or situation (see Fig. 6.1; pathway A). For example, in sport, a football athlete may describe feeling anxious (emotion) and avoid touching the football during a football match (behaviour) because they are being evaluated by a coach (situation). Yet if an event automatically stimulated an emotion and behaviour in such a direct manner then the same event will produce the same emotional and behavioural response for any individual encountering that event (Westbrook et al., 2011). According to the cognitive appraisal paradigm (see Lazarus, 1991), emotional and behavioural responses are influenced by primary and secondary forms of cognitive appraisal. During primary appraisal, individuals appraise an event in terms of the relevance of that event to their goals. For example, if an athlete where to experience injury (event) and that injury has relevance to their goals (eg, participating in sporting competition), then primary appraisal would lead to the experience of more negative forms of emotion (eg, anxiety). Conversely, if an athlete were to experience injury (same event) and that injury has limited relevance to their goals, then primary appraisal would lead to the experience of more positive forms of emotion. During secondary appraisal, individuals will appraise an event in terms of their potential to cope with the demands associated with an

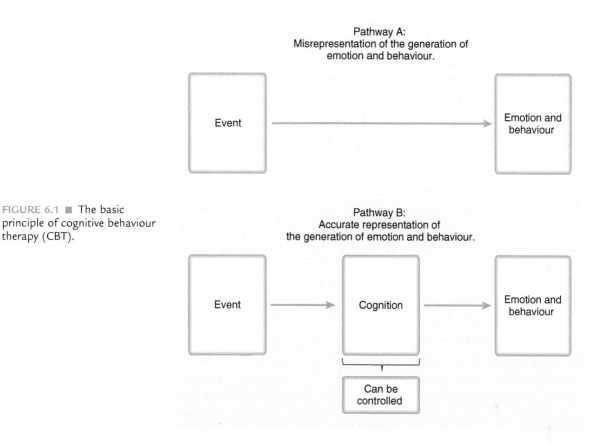

Pathway A:
Misrepresentation of the generation of
emotion and behaviour.

Event

Emotion and
behaviour

FIGURE 6.1 ■ The basic principle of cognitive behaviour therapy (CBT).

Pathway B:
Accurate representation of
the generation of emotion and behaviour.

Event

Cognition

Emotion and
behaviour

Can be
controlled

event. So, an individual with limited coping potential will experience more negative forms of emotion, whereas an individual with high coping potential will experience more positive forms of emotion. In psychological literature, research on emotion supports the notion that individuals can (and will) react differently to the same event. For example, Jones et al. (1994) found that the intensity of cognitive and somatic anxiety experienced by nonelite swimming athletes differed depending on whether nonelite swimming athletes perceived anxiety to be helpful or unhelpful for swimming performance. Similarly, Moore et al. (2012) found that participants who exhibited a threat response (where demand appraisal exceeds resource appraisal) towards a golf putting task reported more unfavourable emotions (eg, cognitive anxiety) than participants who exhibited a challenge response (where resource appraisal meets or exceeds demand appraisal). Such research suggests that individuals do not respond in a unified manner when encountering an event and highlights the role of cognition in the generation of emotion and behaviour. Thus the main premise behind CBT is that an individual's perception of the world is subjective and cognitively mediated (Hemmings and Holder, 2009). Put simply, what individuals think (cognition) about an event or in a situation will influence what they feel (emotion) and how they behave (behaviour: see Fig. 6.1; pathway B). To illustrate the principle of CBT consider the following example of two athletes faced with the same event. Athlete A describes experiencing high levels of anxiety and frustration (emotion) towards their anterior cruciate ligament (ACL) injury (event) because they think they will not be able to cope with being injured and missing out on an important upcoming cup competition (cognitive appraisal). Alternatively, athlete B describes experiencing low levels of anxiety and frustration (emotion) towards their ACL injury (same event) because they will be able to cope with being injured and missing out on an important upcoming cup competition (cognitive appraisal). Therefore the difference in the emotional experience of athlete A and B can be explained by the discrepancy in the cognitive appraisal of their injury.

## IRRATIONAL AND RATIONAL BELIEFS

REBT (see Ellis, 1957) is an approach to CBT that suggests psychological disturbances (eg, anxiety) are caused by a patient's judgement of an event (eg, injury) rather than the event itself (Aurelius et al., 1945). In other words, REBT emphasizes that the effect of an event (A) on emotion and behaviour (C) will be mediated by a patient's beliefs regarding factors such as pain, failure, rejection and poor treatment (B; Ellis and Dryden, 1997). Research supports the ABC framework of REBT by demonstrating that the patient's beliefs about events such as pain, injury, rehabilitation and treatment procedures predict subsequent emotion and patient functioning (eg, Jensen et al., 1999; Turner

et al., 2002). According to REBT, patients can hold irrational or rational beliefs about an event. Dryden (2009) proposed that irrational and rational beliefs comprise one primary belief and three secondary beliefs about an event that are derived from the primary belief in question. A primary irrational belief is rigid, extreme, and illogical whereby an assertion of a preference is transmitted into a demand (eg, 'I want to succeed and therefore I must'; Turner et al., 2014). Secondary irrational beliefs are characterized by awfulizing (or catastrophizing; eg, nothing good can come from a bad event), low frustration tolerance (eg, adversity cannot be tolerated), and depreciation (eg, self and/or others are rated unfavourably on an outcome or behaviour). For example, in response to injury, a patient could believe that 'it is awful to be injured' (awfulizing), 'I cannot stand being injured' (low frustration tolerance), and 'I am useless now that I am injured' (depreciation). Alternatively, a primary rational belief is flexible, nonextreme and logical whereby a preference is asserted and a demand is negated (eg, 'I want to succeed but that does not mean I must'; Turner et al., 2014). Secondary rational beliefs are characterized by anti-awfulizing (eg, something good can come from a bad event), high frustration tolerance (eg, adversity can be tolerated), and acceptance (eg, unconditionally accepting that self and others are fallible, unique, and unrateable). For instance, in response to injury, a patient could believe that 'although it is bad to be injured it is not awful' (antiawfulizing), 'although it will be tough, I can stand being injured' (high frustration tolerance), and 'injury does not mean I am useless; anyone can experience injury' (acceptance). Research generally supports the view that irrational beliefs lead to dysfunctional emotions and maladaptive behaviour that can hinder well-being and long-term goal attainment (Dryden, 2009). For example, Anderson and Emery (2014) found that adherence to cardiac rehabilitation in 61 patients was significantly and negatively predicted by irrational beliefs towards health. Specifically, endorsing beliefs about health that were not grounded in medical evidence (eg, illogical) were associated with poorer adherence to cardiac rehabilitation. Furthermore, Buer and Linton (2002) found a dose-response pattern in relation to catastrophizing about pain and pain intensity. In particular, Buer and Linton (2002) found that greater levels of catastrophizing led to greater pain intensity around nonchronic spinal pain. Research also supports the proposition that rational beliefs lead to functional emotions and adaptive behaviour that can aid wellbeing and long-term goal attainment (Dryden, 2009). For example, Cramer and Buckland (1995) found that participants who read rational statements about a person completing a performance task experienced significantly less anxiety during a problem solving task compared with participants who read irrational statements. Overall, it would seem that harbouring rational beliefs is a healthy way of thinking, whereas holding irrational beliefs is an unhealthy way of thinking in terms of emotional and behavioural responding.

## Origins of Irrational and Rational Beliefs

The precise origins of rational and irrational beliefs are not clearly defined within REBT research. In sport, Turner and Barker (2013)

suggested that a shift from rational to irrational thinking often stems from the pressure of competing, an obsession with results and the view that success and self-worth are positively related (eg, 'winning makes me a better person'). Many athletes also have high-quality support and training facilities available, which may generate the belief that the world absolutely must be fair to them as their developmental experiences have depicted (Turner and Barker, 2013). In patient samples, irrational beliefs (in particular catastrophizing) usually originate from factors including the perception of being vulnerable, being subject to danger and having insufficient control over an event (Turner and Aaron, 2001). For example, a patient may catastrophize about chronic back pain because the pain will be intolerable and terrible: 'I will lose my job and not be able to support my family (which is awful)'. Further, the irrational belief 'life must always be fair' may lead to anger through a patient's inability to tolerate the frustration and pain associated with their injury. According to Ellis (1976) there are hundreds of irrationalities that exist within societies (eg, politics, economy, health) and in virtually all humans within those societies. Ellis (1976) therefore suggests that everyone is irrational some of the time which points to a biological and genetic basis for irrationality. Research has also shown how irrational and rational thinking can be influenced by sport psychologists through education and counselling approaches. For example, Turner et al. (2014) delivered a workshop about the ABC framework of REBT which involved educating 15 male elite academy football athletes. Practitioners also worked with athletes to recognize and dispute demands and awfulizing around being dese-lected from their academy, making a mistake leading to a goal being conceded and approaching the biggest match of their season. Turner et al. showed that educating athletes about REBT principles significantly reduced total irrational beliefs in the short term. Emerging research has also docu-mented the influence of promoting irrational and rational beliefs communicated through language on subsequent event appraisal and behavioural responding. Evans et al. (under review) employed two confederates to deliver a rational or irrational team-talk to two equally matched football teams during the half-time interval of a competitive football match. The irrational team-talk contained statements such as 'failure to win the second-half would be completely intolerable' (ie, low frustration tolerance). The rational team-talk included statements such as 'losing the second-half would be tough to handle, but it is bearable and would be tolerable' (ie, high frustration tolerance). Athletes who received the irrational team-talk reported significantly higher threat appraisal (ie, a negative response to an event; see Jones et al., 2009, for a review) in relation to their second-half football per-formance than athletes who received the rational team-talk. Athletes in the irrational team-talk group also reported higher avoid-ance goal orientation (ie, seeking to avoid a negative outcome to an event; see Morris and Kavussanu, 2008) for their second-half football performance than athletes within the rational team-talk group. Such data cor-roborate past research documenting that demandingness is positively associated with avoidance (Watson et al., 1998) and awfuliz-ing is positively correlated with submis-siveness (Goldberg, 1990). What is more, avoidance tendencies are positively related to anxiety (see Stenling et al., 2014). Interest-ingly, athletes in each condition were equally (and highly) motivated to perform during their upcoming second-half performance after receiving their respective team-talk. This finding suggests that promoting rational beliefs will not demotivate engagement in activities given that communicating rational beliefs encourages individuals to adopt strong preferences about an event, not to devalue the importance of performance (Turner and Barker, 2013).

## The Psychologist's Role: Referral and Disputation

Primarily, the use of REBT principles requires adequate training and experience (Dryden and Branch, 2008; Turner and Barker, 2014), meaning psychologists are well-placed to explore rational and irrational thinking with a patient in more detail. Therefore physio-therapists should aim to refer patients har-bouring irrational beliefs to psychologists. The ultimate goal of REBT is to identify and replace irrational beliefs with rational beliefs with the aim of reducing dysfunctional emo-tions including anxiety, unhealthy anger and depression (Turner et al., 2014). In the initial stages of REBT, a psychologist will encourage a patient or group to appreciate that it is their irrational beliefs (B), and no the event (A) itself, that are causing maladaptive emotional and behavioural responses (C) (Turner et al., 2014). A practitioner would subsequently work with a patient or group to dispute (D) their irrational beliefs and replace them with rational alternatives (E). The overall purpose of the disputation phase is to enable a patient or group to understand that their irrational beliefs are false, illogical and unhelpful, whereas rational alternatives are true, logical and helpful (Dryden, 2009). According to MacLaren et al. (2016), there are five primary disputation techniques included in REBT including being pragmatic (eg, 'how is B helping you?'), thinking empirically (eg, 'where is the evidence that B is true?'), being logical (eg, 'does B make sense?'), being philosophical (eg, 'can you live a satisfying life if B persists?'), and referring to a friend (eg, 'what would you tell a friend in your situation?'). Following successful disputation of irrational beliefs, rational alternatives are exposed to the same disputation process but are emphasized as being true, logical and helpful. The ABCDE framework of REBT is summarized in Figure 6.2. The aforementioned, research by Turner et al. found a temporary significant reduction in total irrational beliefs following one REBT workshop involving disputing (and replacing) irrational beliefs in a sample of football athletes. Nevertheless, no significant difference in total irrationality was found between preworkshop and follow-up phases (6 weeks after the workshop), indicating that the effects of one REBT workshop on total irrational beliefs were not maintained. In a

follow-up study, Turner et al. (2015) conducted multiple REBT education workshops as part of an REBT programme with elite football academy athletes. Turner et al. (2015) found that all elements of irrational beliefs measured by the shortened general attitudes beliefs scale (SGABS; Lindner et al., 1999) reduced at the intervention onset. Furthermore, elements of irrational beliefs including need for achievement and demand for fairness remained reduced in the long term. Thus the process of reducing irrational thinking would appear to require a prolonged period of education and disputation.

During disputation, a psychologist can emphasize that, although a situation (eg, injury) can be extremely bad, it is highly unlikely that a situation can be awful (Turner et al., 2014). According to Aurelius et al. (1945), it is the feeling of awfulness that causes the dysfunctional emotion and/or maladaptive behaviour presented by a patient. Additionally, when patients believe that a situation (eg, pain) is unbearable a psychologist can highlight that until the point of nonexistence or some other form of escape a patient can stand anything (Herse, 2005). Finally, when a patient expresses a demand about an event a psychologist can use empirical lines of questioning to challenge patients to present

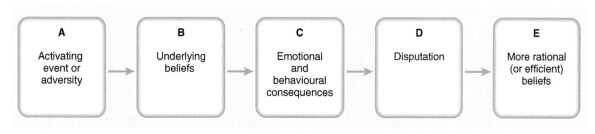

FIGURE 6.2 ■ The ABCDE framework of rational emotive behaviour therapy (REBT).

evidence to support their demand. In particular, a psychologist can highlight that the word 'must' is a rigid demand that implies necessity, requirement, certainty, inevitably, or something that is absolutely required or indispensable. However, the things absolutely required to exist as a patient (and human being) are factors including food, water, oxygen and prescribed medication. Therefore a key strategy used during reflection involves educating patients on the classic ABC process underpinning CBT. A psychologist can suggest to a patient that if they can think differently (B) about an event (A) then they can feel differently (C) about that event. During reflection, a psychologist should also highlight the role of words and language in the development of irrational and rational thinking. General semantics theory (Korzybski, 1933) suggests that language can guide cognition, emotion and behaviour. For example, imprecise language (eg, 'I cannot stand pain') can augment imprecise thinking (Dryden, 2014), whereas negative language (eg, 'being in pain is rubbish') can trigger the release of cortisol which the body interprets as anxiety (Kross et al., 2014). Conversely, precise language (eg, 'I can stand pain') can augment precise thinking (Dryden, 2014), whereas positive language (eg, 'I am in control of pain experienced') can provide the body with instruction and encourage adaptive responding (eg, challenge appraisal: a positive approach to an event; Kross et al., 2014).

## Communicating Rationality and Gaging Perspective

For physiotherapists, it would therefore appear important to communicate rational perspectives following injury and during rehabilitation to encourage patients to positively appraise injury to experience positive emotion and adopt adaptive behaviour (eg, an approach focus for rehabilitation). Based on Turner et al. (2015), communicating rational beliefs as a physiotherapist may also increase the likelihood of reducing irrational thinking by patients during the rehabilitation process. For example, to promote antiawfulizing, a physiotherapist could emphasize to a patient that: 'we (patient and practitioner) cannot say with confidence that no good can come from being injured'. Here, a physiotherapist could make reference to previous and similar cases of an injury whereby patients have recovered fully to render potential awfulizing as illogical. Similarly, to promote high frustration tolerance, a physiotherapist could explain to a patient that: 'although you (the patient) may experience pain during rehabilitation, there is no evidence to suggest that you cannot tolerate pain'. Indeed, a patient is likely to be tolerating pain given they are injured which again can be used as a means of encouraging high frustration tolerance. Ultimately it would be beneficial for physiotherapists to use language during consultations aligned to the primary and secondary beliefs characteristic of rational beliefs to promote patients to adopt rational perspectives towards injury and rehabilitation.

Physiotherapists could also use a simple technique to gage patient perspective on events encountered within a rehabilitation context. For example, practitioners could ask patients to rate their initial pain on a Badness Scale (Turner and Barker, 2014) ranging from 0% bad to 101% bad (representing awful) to highlight levels of catastrophizing towards current pain. Practitioners could then ask patients to rate other types of pain (eg, chronic, acute) or scenarios (eg, experiencing continued pain for 6 weeks) using the same Badness Scale to allow patients to compare their assessment of pain. The Badness Scale could also be used to highlight levels of frustration tolerance. For example, practitioners could ask patients to rate the extent to which they can tolerate their current pain. Practitioners could then ask patients to rate the extent to which they tolerate other types of pain. Statements such as: 'I cannot stand being in pain' would provide evidence of low frustration tolerance towards pain. By using the Badness Scale, a practitioner would be able to ask patients whether it is true, helpful and logical to describe events in their current way of thinking to encourage patients to gain rational perspective about injury-related events and rehabilitation. An illustration of the Badness Scale can be found in Figure 6.3. Figure 6.3 also depicts the use of the Badness Scale in applied practice.

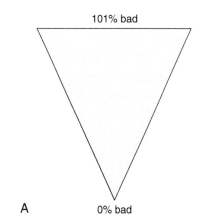

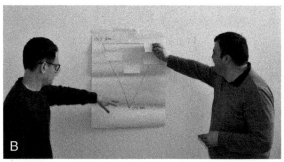

FIGURE 6.3 ■ (A) An illustration of the Badness Scale used to identify secondary irrational (eg, awfulizing) and rational beliefs (eg, antiawfulizing) harboured by patients. (B) Using the Badness Scale in applied practice.

## SELF-TALK

Self-talk represents 'the dialogue in which an individual interprets feelings and perceptions, regulates changes, evaluations, and convictions, and gives themselves instructions and reinforcement' (Hackfort and Schwenkmezger, 1993, p. 355). Crucially, self-talk is much more than simply having a conversation with oneself – self-talk has a distinct purpose and is intentional. According to Hardy (2006), the structure of self-talk can range from single cue words (eg, 'control'), to specific phrases (eg, 'be prepared'), and full intact sentences (eg, 'I am feeling calm and relaxed today'). On the one hand, individuals may practice self-talk in an overt manner (ie, verbalizing self-talk through speech). On the other hand, individuals may practice self-talk in a covert fashion (ie, self-talk through inner speech) using the voice within the mind. Early research studies suggested that the content of self-talk can either be positive or negative. For example, self-talk used as a form of praise or means of maintaining an athlete's attention to the present (rather than on the future or past mistakes) has been commonly conceptualized as positive self-talk (Hardy, 2006). Alternatively, self-talk used as a form of criticism or that is inappropriate, irrational, counterproductive or anxiety-provoking has been termed negative self-talk (Hardy, 2006). However, self-talk contains an interpretative element meaning that the effectiveness of self-talk statements can differ from person to person (Tod et al., 2011). Thus it seems more accurate to conceptualize self-talk as facilitative or debilitative (rather than positive and negative). To highlight the conceptualization of self-talk as facilitative or debilitative, consider the following scenario of two injured athletes reinforcing the same self-talk statement: 'this is tough!' during a rehabilitation programme. Typically, athlete A is not resilient and does not respond well to adversity. For athlete A, a self-talk statement indicating they are experiencing adversity predetermines a maladaptive approach to rehabilitation (eg, withdrawal of effort). Therefore athlete A would negatively interpret the self-talk statement: 'this is tough!' because the statement suggests they are experiencing adversity (which is unhelpful). In contrast, athlete B is resilient and typically responds well to adversity. For athlete B, a self-talk statement indicating they are experiencing adversity predetermines an adaptive approach to rehabilitation (eg, persistence of effort). Therefore athlete B would positively interpret the self-talk statement: 'this is tough!' because the statement indicates they are experiencing adversity (which is helpful). For a physiotherapist, the key to understanding which forms of self-talk would be effective for patients lies in the ability to appreciate how individuals interpret self-talk.

## Functions of Self-Talk

Individuals report using self-talk for motivational and instructional purposes. Motiva-tional self-talk can be split into three specific motivational functions – arousal, mastery and drive (Hardy, 2006). The motivational arousal function relates the use of self-talk to assist individuals in manipulating arousal levels (eg, psyching up or relaxing). To illustrate, Hatzigeorgiadis et al. (2009) found that cognitive anxiety experienced by 72 tennis athletes during a forehand drive test decreased from baseline to postintervention following the use of motivational arousal self-talk (eg, 'strong'). Examples of motivational arousal self-talk that could be used by a patient to lower arousal during rehabilitation include: 'I am in control' and 'relax'. The motivational mastery function refers to the use of self-talk to master challenging situations and is associated with psychological factors including mental toughness, concentration and self-confidence. For instance, Hatzigeorgiadis et al. (2009) found that self-confidence experienced during a forehand drive test by tennis athletes significantly increased from baseline to postintervention following the use of motivational mastery self-talk (ie, 'I can'). Examples of motivational mastery self-talk that could be used by a patient during rehabilitation include: 'I can cope' or 'I have been here before and succeeded'. Finally, the motivational drive function relates to the use of self-talk for goal achievement and is associated with manipulating effort and persistence. As an example, Blanchfield et al. (2014) found that ratings of perceived exertion during a cycling time to exhaustion task were significantly lower for participants who used motivational drive self-talk (eg, early-mid stage: 'feeling good') throughout the task compared with participants within a control condition. Examples of motivational drive self-talk that could be used by a patient during rehabilitation include: 'push through' or 'dig in and keep going'. Instructional self-talk can be divided into two functions – specific and general. Instructional specific self-talk represents the use of self-talk to focus attention on technical aspects of skilled performance (eg, golf-putt). Instructional general self-talk relates to the use of self-talk to focus attention towards a general performance strategy (eg, approaching a competitive match). Research studies have supported the notion that instructional self-talk should be useful for activities that require precision. For example, Hatzigeorgiadis et al. (2004) found that the performance of fine motor tasks requiring skill, timing and accuracy where enhanced to a greater extent by instructional, compared with motivational, self-talk. Examples of instructional self-talk that could be used by a patient (specifically or generally) during rehabilitation include: 'wrist firm' or 'straight and slow'. Based on the functions of self-talk, a matching hypothesis has been proposed which suggests that the use of self-talk should be matched to individual needs and task requirements (see Theodorakis et al., 2000). Reflecting on empirical evidence, it would appear most beneficial to encourage patients to use motivational forms of self-talk when experiencing a psychological (eg, debilitating anxiety) or behavioural issue (eg, low exertion of effort) following injury and during rehabilitation. Alternatively, it would seem most beneficial to encourage patients to use instructional forms of self-talk when learning the key points associated with practicing a skill or strategy during rehabilitation.

## Case Example and Ascertaining Current Self-Talk

During a recent applied experience, an elite female ice skater developed a series of motivational self-talk statements aimed at controlling anxiety and elevating self-confidence in preparation for competitive ice skating. However, after 6 weeks of practicing self-talk, the athlete explained that it had been ineffective in helping her to control anxiety and build self-confidence in readiness for competition. The athlete further explained that she had been struggling to believe what she had been saying to herself, despite understanding what she should be saying to herself precompetition. Therefore the use of self-talk would appear to be ineffective when it contradicts the underlying beliefs harboured by individuals. To increase the effectiveness of motivational self-talk, it would appear beneficial to confirm or develop a rational perspective on an activating event through REBT before developing self-talk to reinforce rational beliefs within individuals. Indeed, Turner and Barker (2014) suggested that some athletes incorporate rational beliefs within their self-talk to promote rationality upon approaching an impending event. To ascertain current self-talk practice, a practitioner could (for example) present a patient with a diary during the early stages of rehabilitation. The diary could be completed by the patient over the course of a week of typical rehabilitation. The patient should be encouraged to write down words, phrases or statements within their diary that they reinforce (either overtly or covertly) before, during or after completing rehabilitation activities. The patient should also be encouraged to write down their cognitive appraisal of injury throughout the week. A follow-up discussion between practitioner and patient could take place to explore the content and provide an interpretation of the self-talk. Accordingly a practitioner could work with a patient to develop functional self-talk statements based on the individual needs or task requirements encountered during a rehabilitation programme.

## IMAGERY

Imagery is the process of creating or recreating an experience in the mind using multiple senses (sight, sound, touch, smell, taste). Imagery is also performed under volitional control and can occur in the absence of the real stimulus normally associated with an actual experience (see Morris et al., 2005). Research evidence suggests that the use of imagery during rehabilitation is underutilized compared with imagery used in training and competition. For example, Sordoni et al. (2000) found that athletes use imagery less frequently when injured compared with training and competition which implies that athletes struggle to transfer their imagery use in training and competition to injury and rehabilitation. One explanation for the difficulties athletes experience in applying imagery to injury could be that they do not view rehabilitation exercises (eg, active plantar flexion of the ankle) as skills in the same way they view sporting activities (eg, taking a free kick in football). Additionally, the poor adherence rates to rehabilitation programmes documented in extant literature (see, Brewer, 1998) implies that patients do not frequently use imagery because they are not physically practicing rehabilitation activities. The role

of a physiotherapist should therefore involve encouraging athletes to transfer principles of imagery used during training and competition to injury and rehabilitation (Sordoni et al., 2000).

### Perspective and Ability

Two types of imagery perspectives exist. Internal imagery (or first person perspective; 1PP) refers to imaginal experiences conducted through the mind's eye. External imagery (or third person perspective; 3PP) refers to imaginal experiences performed as if watching oneself through the eyes of others. Morris and Spittle (2012) documented that individuals typically default to 1PP because 3PP depends on experience or the presentation of external sensory cues or experiences. However, using a combination of 1PP and 3PP can be advantageous when engaging in imagery. For example, 1PP can provide individuals with important kinaesthetic information, whereas 3PP can provide individuals with important information regarding the form of bodily movement. Thus being able to use a combination of imagery perspectives would increase the content of imagery, meaning imagery becomes a more vivid experience. For example, when learning a rehabilitation exercise, 1PP would provide a patient with information as to how the exercise should feel, whereas 3PP would provide a patient with information as to how the exercise should be performed. To assess an individual's ability to switch perspectives, an imagery ability questionnaire can be completed. Imagery ability also measures the vividness and controllability of images when using 1PP, 3PP and kinaesthetic imagery. An example of an imagery ability questionnaire is the vividness of movement imagery questionnaire-2 (VMIQ-2; Roberts et al., 2008) which requires individuals to rate the clarity and vividness of 12 different movements (eg, running, walking) when using 1PP, 3PP and kinaesthetic imagery. Each movement is rated from one (perfectly clear and vivid) to five (no image at all) before all 12 items are added together to provide an overall score for each form of imagery. Scores above 36 mean that individuals are not proficient in using 1PP, 3PP or kinaesthetic imagery. Individuals can be provided with imagery ability training when a score of 36 or greater is presented to improve imagery ability. Encouraging individuals to consult video resources has been suggested to develop 3PP imagery ability (Morris and Spittle, 2012). The use of written imagery scripts have also been found to train 1PP imagery ability (Spittle and Morris, 2011). An example activity to develop imagery control involves asking individuals to picture an image of a person in their mind (see Bump, 1989). The individual imagines sprinkling a potion over the head of their imagined person which allows the size of the imagined person to be manipulated. The individual is then asked to gradually shrink the size of their imagined person to the size of a can of drink (coke) whilst being prompted to focus on gradual changes (eg, features). Once the imagined person has been shrunk, the individual should gradually return the imagined person back to their normal size. Accordingly the individual is asked to gradually increase the size of their imagined person to the size of a giant. Once the imagined person has been returned to their normal size, the practitioner and individual can reflect on the individual's ability to control images within their mind.

## Functions of Imagery

Empirical evidence highlights that athletes use three types of imagery during injury and rehabilitation: cognitive imagery, motivational imagery and healing imagery (Sordoni et al., 2002). Cognitive imagery involves imagining general strategies (cognitive general imagery) or specific skills (cognitive specific imagery). Motivational imagery involves imagining goal-oriented behaviour (motivational specific imagery), effective coping and mastery of challenging situations (motivational general-mastery imagery), or changes in emotion (motivational general-arousal imagery). Finally healing imagery involves imagining physiological processes (eg, imagining tissue mending itself). For a physiotherapist it would appear to be beneficial to understand the functions of imagery so that the correct type can be recommended to patients based on the physical or psychological issue presented. For example, if a patient is experiencing anxiety around returning to training following injury then motivational general-arousal imagery could be advised to encourage the patient to imagine remaining calm and controlling their anxiety. Using a qualitative methodology; Driediger et al. (2006) sought to explore the functions of each type of imagery used by 10 injured athletes receiving physiotherapy treatment. Driediger et al. (2006) found that cognitive imagery was used to learn and properly perform rehabilitation exercises during rehabilitation. Motivational imagery was used during rehabilitation for a variety of purposes, including enhancing mental toughness, maintaining concentration and fostering a positive attitude towards rehabilitation. Healing imagery was also used for a number of reasons such as managing pain (eg, imagining the pain in an ankle joint dispersing), blocking pain and dealing with expected pain in the future. More recently, Wesch et al. (2016) explored the effects of an imagery intervention incorporating cognitive, motivational and healing forms of imagery on task efficacy and coping efficacy before physiotherapy treatment of five athletes with a type B malleolar fracture. An example of the cognitive imagery used by athletes involved imagining drawing out the letter A with their repaired ankle. An example of the motivational imagery used by athletes involved imagining feeling energized whilst performing. An example of healing imagery used by athletes involved imagining pain seeping away similarly to water seeping away out of a small hole in a container. Interview data revealed that all participants perceived the imagery intervention to be effective beyond the general information provided by a practitioner. Observable and statistically significant increases in task efficacy and coping efficacy were noted in two and three of the participants respectively. Overall imagery appears to be an effective psychological skill for athletes seeking to improve skill learning, manipulate emotional states (eg, anxiety) and/or cope with pain during rehabilitation.

## Fundamental Theories of Imagery

According to psychoneuromuscular theory (see Hale, 1982), imagery activates the same neuromuscular pathways used during physical movement and provides feedback from Golgi tendons to the brain. Bakker et al. (1996) provided support for the psychoneuromuscular theory by comparing electromyographical (EMG) activity of both biceps brachii muscles in the active and passive arm

of 39 participants during imagined lifting of a 4.5 kg and 9 kg dumbbell weight. Participants were presented with instructions to guide imagined dumbbell lifts that either contained stimulus propositions or response propositions. Stimulus propositions describe the specific content of a scenario to be imagined (eg, an object's movement). Alternatively response propositions contain assertions about behaviour including verbal responses (eg, being congratulated), somatomotor events (eg, muscle tension) and visceral events (eg, heart rate). Bakker et al. (1996) found that imagery emphasizing response propositions produced significantly greater EMG activity in the active arm than imagery emphasizing stimulus propositions. EMG activity in the active arm was also significantly greater than EMG activity in the passive arm. Finally EMG activity in the active arm was significantly greater during the imagined 9 kg dumbbell lift compared with the imagined 4.5 kg dumbbell lift. Findings confirm that imagery activates the same neuromuscular pathways used during physical movement. Findings also suggest that neuromuscular pathways will be activated to a greater magnitude when the imaginal experiences of athletes include response propositions compared with stimulus propositions. The importance of response propositions is also highlighted in Lang's (1985) bioinformational theory. Initial research by Lang et al. (1980) demonstrated that images of emotional scenes and images of emotionally neutral action scenes containing response propositions resulted in greater muscle tension and heart rate in participants compared with images containing predominantly stimulus propositions. Based on bioinformational theory, it would appear that imagery can alter responses (eg, anxiety) to environmental stimuli by changing the meaning associated with images coded in the brain.

## Guidelines for Imagery Use

For imagery to be effective then, patients should seek to incorporate response propositions within their imaginal experiences. To support imagery use, patients can generate imagery resources (eg, written scripts, videos). Wilson et al. (2010) explored whether imagery resulted in greater imagery ability and EMG activity when an imagery script was generated by a participant compared with an experimenter. During condition one, 19 participants performed 16 dumbbell curls with their right arm. Accordingly participants received response training which involved participants focusing on their actual physiological and psychological responses during the performance of a dumbbell curl. Responses were recorded and used to construct personalized imagery scripts. During condition two, participants were instructed to mentally recreate the responses during response training. During condition three, participants were instructed to read an experimenter-generated imagery script. Imagery ability and EMG activity in the biceps and triceps muscles within the left (passive) and right (active) arm were measured during a relaxed baseline, a physical trial, a participant-generated imagery condition and an experimenter-generated imagery condition. Wilson et al. (2010) found that self-reported imagery ability and EMG activity in the biceps muscle of the right arm was greatest when participants generated their own imagery scripts compared with imagery scripts developed by an experimenter. Therefore practitioners should encourage patients to develop their

### BOX 6.1

An example extract from a motivational imagery script used by a football athlete to control anxiety upon return to competition following injury:

'As the start of the match approaches take a moment to focus on your surroundings (10 seconds). See the sports kit you are wearing (5 seconds). Hear the clatter of football boots within the changing room (5 seconds). Hear your teammates talk about tactics for the upcoming match (5 seconds). As you focus on your surroundings you feel prepared and calm. Your rehabilitation and training has gone well. You are physically strong and ready to perform. Say to yourself: "I feel calm and in control" (5 seconds). Take a few moments to focus on the sense of control you have (10 seconds).'

own imagery scripts to support their imagery use during rehabilitation. An example extract from a motivational imagery script used to control anxiety is displayed in Box 6.1. Wesch et al. (2016) also provide further examples of cognitive, motivational and healing imagery scripts for injury and rehabilitation.

Findings from neuroscience research document that physical movement, observation and imagery share the same neuron system – a phenomenon called functional equivalence. Therefore Holmes and Collins (2001) developed the PETTLEP model (physical, environmental, task, timing, learning, emotional, and perspective) to ensure that imagery is a close representation of physical practice (making imagery functionally equivalent). Elements of the PETTLEP (Physical, Environment, Task, Timing, Learning, Emotion, and Perspective) model are based upon the psychoneuromuscular and bioinformational theories of imagery. Table 6.1 provides an example of applying the PETTLEP model to a patient using motivational general arousal imagery to control anxiety about returning from injury to training and competition. Research by Smith et al. (2008) demonstrated that

| TABLE 6.1 |
| --- |
| **Applying the PETTLEP Model in an Athlete Using Motivational General Arousal Imagery to Manage Anxiety About Returning From Injury to Training and Competition** |

| Element | Brief Description With Examples |
| --- | --- |
| **P**hysical | Adopt physical components of a skill or event (eg, wearing appropriate sports kit, adopting correct posture) |
| **E**nvironment | The imagined environment should be as similar as possible to the actual performing environment (eg, crowd noise) |
| **T**ask | Match the task content of imagery to the athlete (eg, the preferred thoughts, feelings, and actions as during actual performance) |
| **T**iming | Imagine skills or events at the same pace as actual performance (eg, including response propositions for each stimulus) |
| **L**earning | Tailor imagery content to the stage of learning (eg, focusing on the feel of movement during the autonomous stage of learning) |
| **E**motion | Incorporate emotional responses into the imaginal experience (eg, feeling calm, feeling in control) |
| **P**erspective | Use a combination of 1PP and 3PP. |

that golf-putting performance improved to the greatest extent in participants who completed PETTLEP imagery and physical practice, compared with participants who completed either PETTLEP imagery, physical practice or nothing (a control group). Interestingly participants who merely completed PETTLEP imagery exhibited a significant improvement in golf-putting performance which further highlights that imagery is a useful psychological strategy to engage in during injury when physical practice cannot be completed.

Overall, the following framework provides practitioners with a method of integrating imagery into injury and rehabilitation. First, based on Richardson and Latuda (1995) and Arvinen-Barrow et al. (2013), practitioners should introduce imagery to patients by providing education about the potential benefits of imagery use within injury and rehabilitation. Second, a patient's imagery ability should be assessed formally through an imagery ability questionnaire and informally through questioning (eg, 'how frequently have you used imagery?' and 'how effective has your previous use of imagery been?'). Third, patients should be supported with developing basic imagery skills (eg, being able to create vivid, controllable images) depending on their imagery ability. Richardson and Latuda (1995) advocated that 15-minute training sessions should be practiced twice daily to develop imagery skills. Fourth, in addition to the current guidelines proposed, practitioners should recognize the types of imagery applicable to a patient's needs and work with a patient to apply the types of imagery to a variety of settings within injury and rehabilitation (eg, before rehabilitation exercises). Finally imagery can be incorporated into the rehabilitation programme of a patient providing the skill has been practiced sufficiently during personal time.

## PATIENT-CENTRED THERAPY

Patient-centred therapy (PCT) first emerged in the 1950s based on the theorizing of Carl Rogers (1951). PCT is an approach to supporting people psychologically and holds an assumptive position that people have the potential to self-direct (Rogers, 1986). Recently in the UK, there has been strong emphasis placed on the value of providing patient-centred care within a variety of disciplines associated with caring professions. For example, approaches to medical education have evolved from being predominantly didactic and delivered by doctors to approaches that have the patient at the centre of their learning (Bleakley and Bligh, 2008). Empirically, research suggests that patients cite authoritarian approaches to physiotherapy as harmful to adherence (Redmond and Parrish, 2008). Instead, patients prefer physiotherapy programmes where participation is optional and where they are involved in target-setting and formulating rehabilitation activities (Redmond and Parrish, 2008). Patient-centred approaches focus on understanding each patient as an individual whilst designing and delivering bespoke care adapted to a patient's unique needs (The Health Foundation, 2014). Indeed, current guidelines suggest that patient care must be sensitive to each patient's particular requirements, preferences (in terms of their care and treatment) and resources (National Institute for Clinical Excellence, 2011). Although such guidelines were primarily targeted at mental health care professionals, the philosophy and conditions underpinning patient-centred care (eg, cultivating trust, demonstrating unconditional positive regard; see Rogers, 1980) are transferable and applicable to other fields, such as psychotherapy. It is noteworthy, even within the guidelines provided by National Institute for Clinical Excellence (2011), that the practitioner–patient relationship should be focused on working with a patient and incorporating a more holistic approach that considers the patient as a human being. Indeed, Section 4 of the Chartered Society of Physiotherapists' (2012) Quality Assurance Standards informs members of the importance of viewing relationships with patients as partnerships. Section 4 also notifies members that individuals using a service (ie, physiotherapy) should be respected at all times and fully involved in their own care. Research has indicated that adopting a patient-centred conceptual framework to professional practice enables people to exercise autonomy (McCormack and McCance, 2006) which, according to self-determination theory (see Ryan and Deci, 2000), is a basic psychological need that underpins intrinsic motivation and goal-striving. Furthermore, the self-concordance model (see Sheldon and Elliot, 1999) suggests that changes in psychological wellbeing occur when activities satisfy basic psychological needs. Therefore adopting a patient-centred approach affords practitioners the opportunity to consider themes, such as the patient's self-concept, which could inhibit change (Coghlan, 1993) and their self-actualizing tendency, which Rogers (1961) described as the propensity within human-beings for realizing their potential.

Patients presenting for physiotherapy will be in a state of dissonance with their physiological condition and in need of professional support. When anxiety occurs, a patient's state of dissonance will be altered further, which causes disruptions in experience, awareness and perceptions of internal, physiological and external worlds (Hunt et al, 2006; Lueck, 2007; Tod, 2014). The intensity of cognition, emotion and physiological responses that can occur and destabilize a patient's sense of reality and the world around them can subsequently affect the connection between a physiotherapist and patient. For example, a patient whose attention is consumed by thoughts about feeling unsafe to stand or the pain that standing might cause them could begin to become less aware of their environment and practitioner. A wide array of factors can influence the development of anxiety experienced by a patient. For example, patients may have encountered previous episodes of physiotherapy that involved intense pain therefore creating a negative association between physiotherapy and pain within their mind (Gaskin et al., 2012). Patients may also experience white coat syndrome which results in hypertension just from the presence of medical practitioners or those treating patients wearing white coats (Laundray and Lip, 1999). According to the cognitive appraisal paradigm (see Lazarus, 1991), anxiety can also arise in patients as a result of poor coping potential, the relevance of physical rehabilitation to goals and the effect that physiotherapy will have on future expectations (eg, changes in identity). During physiotherapy, patients will present emotional reactions to stimuli providing the patient and practitioner with opportunities to learn about a patient's emotional responses. For example, a patient may exhibit symptoms of anxiety when being greeted by a physiotherapist during an initial consultation through rapid speech and breathing. Being able to identify emotional responses of patients would appear important so that emotions can be validated and redirected to support physiological change that can enhance the likelihood of achieving the goals of physiotherapy. Empiri-

cally, Danielsson et al. (2013) found that steadily developing awareness about somatic sensations in physiotherapy created opportunities for patients to learn about, reappraise and manage the energy they were experiencing as anxiety. Thus goal-awareness can have a significant effect on supporting patients with their anxiety as a physiotherapist's ability to empathize with the desired outcome can help support the patient in gaining a sense of control. Indeed, stress appraisal theories (eg, the Theory of Challenge and Threat States in Athletes; Jones et al., 2009) suggest that increased perception of control is a key resource appraisal that can enable athletes to meet or exceed the demands of an event. Goal-awareness can also help patients redirect energy that is creating anxiety towards taking appropriate steps to reach their goal. For example, Gaskin et al. (2012) explained how a patient found the enthusiasm to conform to their physiotherapy regime so they could walk at their graduation event.

## Core Conditions

To progress towards the goals of physiotherapy, a physiotherapist should seek to obtain psychological contact with a patient so that a therapeutic alliance can be created. Psychological contact refers to an acknowledged relationship between patient and practitioner which Rogers (1957) argued needs to exist for therapeutic change to occur. For psychological contact to happen, a client will be in a state of incongruence (eg, vulnerable or anxious) whilst a practitioner will be in a state of congruence and integrated into the relationship. Incongruence is caused by a discrepancy between a patient's self-concept and reality. To highlight the notion of incongruence, consider the case of Carl – a 36-year-old male experiencing back pain. Carl believes he is resilient and able to cope with any situation (self-concept). However, Carl's physiotherapist (Jo) noticed that Carl did not make eye contact and talked quickly during the initial stages of their first consultation (reality). In other words, Carl's self-concept (ie, being resilient) is not consistent with reality (ie, being anxious and avoidant). Therefore the role of a physiotherapist involves assisting patients in making a therapeutic change by discovering congruence between their self-concept and reality. To facilitate therapeutic change, Rogers (1957) identified other core conditions that a practitioner must demonstrate in their relationship with their patient. First, a practitioner should experience unconditional positive regard for their patient at all times. Unconditional positive regard is achieved when a practitioner maintains a positive attitude towards a patient even when a practitioner does not necessarily approve of a patient's thoughts or actions (nonjudgemental warmth). Second, a practitioner should demonstrate empathetic understanding. Empathy relates to the ability of a practitioner to understand what a patient is feeling with regards to a situation or event (Rogers, 1961). In certain scenarios, empathetic understanding might be difficult to demonstrate to a patient. For instance, a practitioner may have never experienced a situation that a patient finds themselves encountering. However, a practitioner is likely to have experienced the emotional and behavioural responses that a patient is experiencing in an alternative scenario which means that a practitioner can show empathy by understanding how the patient is feeling and behaving. Ultimately Rogers (1957) suggests that unconditional positive regard, empathy and congruence are essential for facilitating change in a patient.

## Other Key Conditions and Skills

During a consultation it can be advantageous for a physiotherapist to reflect upon a patient's emotional experience through attending to nonverbal (eg, folded arms) and verbal communication (eg, 'I am worried and confused'). Reflecting a patient's emotion can enable more information to be gathered about an emotional experience (eg, antecedents, consequences) which helps bring an emotion into sharper focus. Reflecting a patient's emotion can also facilitate a development in psychological contact so that a patient feels sufficiently supported and can begin to explore their emotional experience more intimately. A patient may join in the reflective process either audibly or through internal dialogue as a result of the growth in trust established by the physiotherapist's apparent genuineness and dependability. Accordingly opportunities are created for the physiotherapist and patient to benefit from learning at a deeper level about the patient's emotional experience (Henriksen and Ringsted, 2011). To exemplify the importance of emotional listening and reflection, consider the following dialogue between a physiotherapist and patient during the initial stages of a consultation:

**Patient:** 'I just feel really anxious at the moment about my return from injury to competition'.

**Physiotherapist:** 'Anxious?'

**Patient:** 'Yes. Anxious. I find myself worrying that I will not be the same performer when I return to competition'.

Here the physiotherapist has reflected an emotion back to the patient which allowed the patient to elaborate upon their emotional experience. Consequently the physiotherapist was able to gather more information about the patient's emotional experience. Additionally a physiotherapist could use lines of questioning to clarify the intensity of an emotional experience. For example, upon learning that a patient is experiencing anxiety, a practitioner could ask: 'would you say that you feel extremely anxious then?' Using scaling questions (eg, a little, very much, not at all) to establish incremental change can also assist a practitioner when assessing the intensity of emotions and validating the effectiveness of subsequent intervention procedures (Sharf, 2015).

During a consultation, other engagement techniques can be used to gather information and help a patient achieve congruence. First, it can be useful to appear welcoming and help a patient settle during the initial stages of a consultation. Examples of welcoming a patient include providing an introduction to yourself and your service. Addressing patients by their preferred name and introducing yourself by your first name can also help a patient feel accepted whilst breaking down potential barriers of inequality (Sutton and Stewart, 2002). Examples of settling include having an initial conversation about something other than the patient's issue (eg, the weather). Ultimately welcoming and settling are important to enable a patient to feel comfortable with potentially unfamiliar surroundings and services. Being comfortable with a practitioner and their surroundings allows patients to talk freely which can result in a number of patient outcomes including

satisfaction and trust (Hayes, 2007). Sutton and Stewart (2002) explained that practitioners should not restrict the patient by placing emphasis on difficulties, problems and issues. In sport psychology literature, practitioners also work to maximize strengths to develop human potential (eg, Gordon and Gucciardi, 2011). Counselling and psychotherapy literature have also documented that focusing on strengths through problem-free talk can be invigorating for patients (Hanton, 2011). Therefore practitioners should incorporate positive asset searching into consultations. For example, a practitioner could ask a patient: 'what do you excel at when you experience adversity such as being injured?' Consequently, a practitioner can evidence resources that a patient has already used during previous events that can be applied to their current situation. Drawing on the cognitive appraisal paradigm (see Lazarus, 1991), evidencing resources would increase coping potential which would increase the likelihood of patients' experiencing more positive forms of emotion. Challenging and confronting patients about their current thinking can be useful for unearthing resources that exist within a patient's coping repertoire. For example, a patient may explain during a consultation that they are feeling anxious about being injured. A practitioner could challenge a patient's emotional response to injury by asking: 'do you think it is helpful to feel anxious?' Alternatively a patient may explain that they feel anxious but smile as though they are feeling content. A practitioner could confront this distortion of feeling by asking: 'you say you feel anxious, yet you are smiling as you speak as though you feel content'. Such examples of challenging and confronting during consultations are similar to disputation techniques used within REBT (see Dryden, 2009). However, practitioners should remain cautious when using challenging and confronting techniques as a statement iterated by a practitioner may not be what a client wants to hear (Sutton and Stewart, 2002). Thus it would be best to use challenging and confronting with great sensitivity and care following the successful creation of trustworthiness between practitioner and patient. In addition to showing interest in issues pertaining to physical rehabilitation, it can also be useful to show interest in a patient's broader identity. For instance, asking a patient about their broader identity (eg, family life) shows genuineness and can help a practitioner build rapport by learning more about a patient. Knowing more about a patient's broader identity can also assist in the planning and integration of rehabilitation activities outside of consultations. Being able to integrate rehabilitation activities into a weekly schedule has been found to be an important factor in explaining adherence to physical rehabilitation (Medina-Mirapeix et al., 2009). Finally, asking patients about their preferred future through the use of miracle questioning can be useful to provide a focus and an end-point for physiotherapy (Sharf, 2015). Example miracle questions include: 'where would you like to be in 5 months' time?' and 'how will you notice when the problem has gone?'

## CONCLUDING REMARKS

This chapter has highlighted that events do not predetermine the way patients feel and behave. Rather, CBT suggests that patients' cognitions mediate the influence of an event upon emotion and behaviour. In particular, irrational and rational beliefs harboured by patients about events will influence subsequent emotional and behavioural responding. Irrational beliefs are characterized by demandingness, awfulizing (or catastrophizing), low frustration tolerance and depreciation. Rational beliefs are characterized by strong preference, antiawfulizing, high frustration tolerance and appreciation. It is important for physiotherapists to recognize irrational and rational beliefs harboured by patients given the association between core beliefs and subsequent wellbeing, goal attainment, emotion and behaviour. Although physiotherapists should be aware of referral, physiotherapists should seek to communicate rational beliefs during consultations to encourage patients to formulate rational perspectives towards injury and rehabilitation. To gage patient perspective, physiotherapists can also use a Badness Scale to explore primary and secondary irrational and rational beliefs. Overall it is strongly recommended that physiotherapists work with psychologists when attempting to alleviate irrational thinking in patients. This chapter has also highlighted that rational beliefs can be reinforced through self-talk. Specifically self-talk has motivational and cognitive functions which can be integrated into rehabilitation programmes to manipulate a host of psychological (eg, anxiety) and physical performance factors. Perhaps the most important point to consider when developing self-talk for injury and rehabilitation is to understand a patient's interpretation of self-talk to ensure its use is effective during rehabilitation. Additionally this chapter has provided a framework and guidelines for incorporating imagery into injury and rehabilitation. In short, practitioners should introduce patients to imagery (through education), check imagery ability and develop basic imagery skills. Practitioners can then suggest the most appropriate motivational or cognitive form of imagery and assist a patient in incorporating imagery into rehabilitation (eg, using PETTLEP, including response propositions in imagery resources). Finally, this chapter has explained the role and importance of PCT within rehabilitation contexts. To successfully help patients manage anxiety, an array of conditions (eg, psychological contact) and skills (eg, challenging current thinking) should be evidenced by a practitioner during consultations. To this end we hope this chapter has provided physiotherapists with an understanding of the emergence of anxiety from the perspective of CBT and REBT. We hope physiotherapists are now in a position to communicate rational perspectives, apply principles of self-talk and imagery use, and adopt a patient-centred approach to help patients manage anxiety in response to injury and rehabilitation.

## References

Anderson, D.R., Emery, C.F., 2014. Irrational health beliefs predict adherence to cardiac rehabilitation: A pilot study. Health Psychol. 33 (12), 1614–1617. doi:10.1037/hea0000017.

Arvinen-Barrow, M., Clement, D., Hemmings, B., 2013. Imagery in sport injury rehabilitation. In: Arvinen-Barrow, M., Walker, N. (Eds.), The Psychology of Sport Injury and Rehabilitation. Routledge, New York, pp. 71–85.

Aurelius, M., Lucian, J., Martyr, J., Pater, W., Edman, I., 1945. Marcus Aurelius and His Times. Pub for The Classics Club, New York.

Bakker, F.C., Boschker, M.S.J., Chung, T., 1996. Changes in muscular activity while imagining weight lifting using stimulus or response propositions. J. Sport Exerc. Psychol. 18 (3), 313–324.

Blanchfield, A.W., Hardy, J., De Morree, H.M., Staniano, W., Marcora, S.M., 2014. Talking yourself out of exhaustion: The effects of self-talk on endurance performance. Med. Sci. Sports Exerc. 46 (5), 998–1007. doi:10.1249/MSS.0000000000000184.

Bleakley, A., Bligh, J., 2008. Students learning from patients: Let's get real in medical education. Adv. Health Sci. Educ. Theory Pract. 13 (1), 89–107.

Brewer, B.W., 1998. Adherence to sport injury rehabilitation programs. J. Appl. Sport Psychol. 10 (1), 70–82. doi:10.1080/10413209808406378.

Buer, N., Linton, S.J., 2002. Fear-avoidance beliefs and catastrophizing: Occurrence and risk factor in back pain and ADL in the general population. Pain 99 (3), 485–491. doi:10.1016/S0304-3959(02)00265-8.

Bump, L.A., 1989. Sport Psychology Study Guide (and Workbook). Human Kinetics, Champaign, IL.

Chartered Society of Physiotherapists, 2012. Quality Assurance Standards for Physiotherapy Service Delivery. Chartered Society of Physiotherapists, London.

Coghlan, D., 1993. A person-centred approach to dealing with resistance to change. Leadership Org. Dev. J. 14 (4), 10–14. doi:10.1108/01437739310039433.

Cramer, D., Buckland, N., 1995. Effect of rational and irrational statements and demand characteristics on task anxiety. J. Psychol. 129 (3), 269–275. doi:10.1080/00223980.1995.9914964.

Danielsson, L., Scherman, M.H., Rosberg, S., 2013. To sense and make sense of anxiety: Physiotherapists' perceptions of their treatment for patients with generalized anxiety. Physiother. Theory Pract. 29 (8), 604–615. doi:10.3109/09593985.2013.778382.

Driediger, M., Hall, C., Callow, N., 2006. Imagery use by injured athletes: A qualitative analysis. J. Sports Sci. 24 (3), 261–271.

Dryden, W., 2009. How to Think and Intervene Like an REBT Therapist. Routledge, London.

Dryden, W., 2014. Rational Emotive Behaviour Theory: Distinctive Features, second ed. Routledge, East Sussex.

Dryden, W., Branch, R., 2008. The Fundamentals of Rational Emotive Behaviour Therapy: A Training Handbook, second ed. John Wiley & Sons, West Sussex.

Ellis, A., 1957. Rational psychotherapy and individual psychology. J. Individ. Psychol. 13, 38–44.

Ellis, A., 1976. The biological basis of human irrationality. J. Individ. Psychol. 32, 145–168.

Ellis, A., Dryden, W., 1997. The Practice of Rational-Emotive Behavior Therapy. Springer, New York.

Evans, A.L., Pickering, R., Turner, M.J., Powditch, R., (under review). The effects of rational and irrational team talks on cognitive appraisal and achievement goal orientation of varsity soccer athletes. Int. J. Sport Psychol.

Fineberg, N.A., Haddad, P.M., Carpenter, L., Gannon, B., Sharpe, R., Young, A.H., et al., 2013. The size, burden and cost of the disorders of the brain in the UK. J. Psychopharmacol. 27 (9), 761–770. doi:10.1177/0269881113495118.

Gaskin, C.J., Anderson, M.B., Morris, T., 2012. Physical activity in the life of a woman with cerebral palsy: Physiotherapy, social exclusion, competence, and intimacy. Disability & Society 27 (2), 205–218. doi:10.1080/09687599.2011.644931.

Goldberg, G.M., 1990. Irrational beliefs and three interpersonal styles. Psychol. Rep. 66 (3), 963–969. doi:10.2466/pr0.1990.66.3.963.

Gordon, S., Gucciardi, D.F., 2011. A strengths-based approach to coaching mental toughness. J. Sport Psychol. Action 2 (3), 143–155. doi:10.1080/21520704.2011.598222.

Hackfort, D., Schwenkmezger, P., 1993. Anxiety. In: Singer, R.N., Murphey, M., Tennant, L.K. (Eds.), Handbook of Research on Sport Psychology. Macmillan, New York, pp. 328–364.

Hale, B.D., 1982. The effects of internal and external imagery on muscular and ocular concomitants. J. Sport Psychol. 4, 379–387.

Hanton, P., 2011. Skills in Solution Focused Brief Counselling & Psychotherapy. Sage, London.

Hardy, J., 2006. Speaking clearly: A critical review of the self-talk literature. Psychol. Sport Exerc. 7 (1), 81–97. doi:10.1016/j.psychsport.2005.04.002.

Hatzigeorgiadis, A., Theodorakis, Y., Zourbanos, N., 2004. Self-talk in the swimming pool: The effects of self-talk on thought content and performance on water polo tasks. J. Appl. Sport Psychol. 16 (2), 138–150. doi:10.1080/10413200490437886.

Hatzigeorgiadis, A., Zourbanos, N., Mpoumpaki, S., Theodorakis, Y., 2009. Mechanisms underlying the self-talk-performance relationship: The effects of motivational self-talk on self-confidence and anxiety. Psychol. Sport Exerc. 10 (1), 186–192. doi:10.1016/j.psychsport.2008.07.009.

Hayes, E., 2007. Nurse practitioners and managed care: Patient satisfaction and intention to adhere to nurse practitioner plan of care. J. Am. Acad. Nurse Pract. 19 (8), 418–426. doi:10.1111/j.1745-7599.2007.00245.x.

Hemmings, B., Holder, T., 2009. Applied Sport Psychology: A Case-Based Approach. John Wiley, Oxford.

Henriksen, A.-H., Ringsted, C., 2011. Learning from patients: Students' perceptions of patient-instructors. Med. Educ. 45 (9), 913–919. doi:10.1111/j.1365-2923.2011.04041.x.

Herse, M., 2005. Encyclopedia of Behavior Modification and Cognitive Behavior Therapy: Adult Clinical Populations, vol. 1. Sage Publications, London.

Holmes, P.S., Collins, D.J., 2001. The PETTLEP approach to motor imagery: A functional equivalence model for sport psychologists. J. Appl. Sport Psychol. 13 (1), 60–83. doi:10.1080/10413200109339004.

Hunt, C., Keogh, E., French, C.C., 2006. Anxiety sensitivity: The role of conscious awareness and selective attentional bias to physical threat. Emotion 6 (3), 418–428. doi:10.1037/1528-3542.6.3.418.

Jensen, M.P., Romano, J.M., Turner, J.A., Good, A.B., Wald, L.H., 1999. Patient beliefs predict patient functioning: Further support for a cognitive-behavioural model of chronic pain. Pain 81 (1–2), 95–104. doi:10.1016/S0304-3959(99)00005-6.

Johnston, L.H., Carroll, D., 1998. The context of emotional responses to athletic injury: A qualitative analysis. J. Sport Rehabil. 7 (3), 206–220.

Jones, G., Hanton, S., Swain, A., 1994. Intensity and interpretation of anxiety symptoms in elite and non-elite sports performers. Pers. Individ. Dif. 17 (5), 657–663.

Jones, M., Meijen, C., McCarthy, P.J., Sheffield, D., 2009. A theory of challenge and threat states in athletes. Int. Rev. Sport Exerc. Psychol. 2 (2), 161–180. doi:10.1080/17509840902829331.

Korzybski, A., 1933. Science and Sanity. International Society of General Semantics, San Francisco.

Kross, E., Bruehlman-Senecal, E., Park, J., Burson, A., Dougherty, A., Shablack, H., et al., 2014. Self-talk as a regulatory mechanism: How you do it matters. J. Pers. Soc. Psychol. 106 (2), 304–324. doi:10.1037/a0035173.

Lang, P.J., 1985. The cognitive psychophysiology of emotion: Fear and anxiety. In: Tuma, A.H., Maser, J.D. (Eds.), Anxiety and the Anxiety Disorders. Erlbaum, Hillsdale, NJ, pp. 131–170.

Lang, P.J., Kozak, M.J., Miller, G.A., Levin, D.N., McLean, A., 1980. Emotional imagery: Conceptual structure and pattern of somato-visceral response. Psychophysiology 17 (2), 179–192. doi:10.1111/j.1469-8986.1980.tb00133.x.

Laundray, M.J., Lip, G.Y., 1999. White coat hypertension: A recognised syndrome with uncertain implications. J. Hum. Hypertens. 13 (1), 5–8.

Lazarus, R.S., 1991. Progress on a cognitive-motivational-relational theory of emotion. Am. Psychol. 46 (8), 819–834. doi:10.1037//0003-066X.46.8.819.

Lindner, H., Kirkby, R., Wertheim, E.H., Birch, P., 1999. A brief assessment of irrational thinking: The shortened General Attitude and Belief Scale. Cognit. Ther. Res. 23 (6), 651–663. doi:10.1023/A:1018741009293.

Lueck, M.D., 2007. Anxiety levels: Do they influence the perception of time? UWL Journal of Undergraduate Research 10, 1–5.

MacLaren, C., Doyle, K.A., DiGiuseppe, R., 2015. Rational emotive behavior therapy (REBT) theory and practice.

In: Tinsley, H.E.A., Lease, S.H., Giffin Wiersma, N.S. (Eds.), Contemporary Theory and Practice in Counseling and Psychotherapy. Sage, USA.

McCormack, B., McCance, T.V., 2006. Development of a framework for person-centred nursing. J. Adv. Nurs. 56 (5), 472–479. doi:10.1111/j.1365-2648.2006.04042.x.

Medina-Mirapeix, F., Escolar-Reina, P., Gascón-Cánovas, J.J., Montilla-Herrador, J., Collins, S.M., 2009. Personal characteristics influencing patients' adherence to home exercise during chronic pain: A qualitative study. J. Rehabil. Med. 41 (5), 347–352. doi:10.2340/16501977-0338.

Moore, L.J., Vine, S.J., Wilson, M.R., Freeman, P., 2012. The effect of challenge and threat states on performance: An examination of potential mechanisms. Psychophysiology 49 (10), 1417–1425.

Morris, T., Spittle, M., 2012. A default hypothesis of the development of internal and external imagery perspectives. Journal of Mental Imagery 36 (1&2), 1–30.

Morris, T., Spittle, M., Watt, A.P., 2005. Imagery in Sport. Human Kinetics, Champaign, IL.

Morris, R.L., Kavussanu, M., 2008. Antecedents of approach-avoidance goals in sport. J. Sports Sci. 26 (5), 465–476. doi:10.1080/02640410701579388.

National Institute for Clinical Excellence, 2011. Service user experience in adult mental health: Improving the experience of care for people using adult NHS mental health services. NICE Guidelines [CG136].

Redmond, R., Parrish, M., 2008. Variables influencing physiotherapy adherence among young adults with cerebral palsy. Qual. Health Res. 18 (11), 1501–1510. doi:10.1177/1049732308325538.

Richardson, P.A., Latuda, L.M., 1995. Therapeutic imagery and athletic injuries. J. Athl. Train. 30 (1), 10–12.

Roberts, R., Callow, N., Hardy, L., Markland, D., Bringer, J., 2008. Movement imagery ability: Development and assessment of a revised version of the vividness of movement imagery questionnaire. J. Sport Exerc. Psychol. 30 (2), 200–221.

Rogers, C.R., 1951. Client-Centered Therapy: Its Current Practice, Implications and Theory. Constable, London.

Rogers, C.R., 1957. The necessary and sufficient conditions of therapeutic personality change. J. Consult. Psychol. 21 (2), 95–103.

Rogers, C.R., 1961. On Becoming a Person. Constable, London.

Rogers, C.R., 1980. A way of Being. Houghton Mifflin, Boston, MA.

Rogers, C.R., 1986. Carl Rogers on the development of the person-centered approach. Person-Centred Review 1 (3), 257–259.

Ryan, R.M., Deci, E.L., 2000. Self-determination theory and the facilitation of intrinsic motivation, social development, and well-being. Am. Psychol. 55 (1), 68–78. doi:10.1037/0003-066X.55.1.68.

Sharf, R.S., 2015. Theories of Psychotherapy and Counselling: Concepts and Cases, sixth ed. Cengage Learning, Boston, MA.

Sheldon, K.M., Elliot, A.J., 1999. Goal striving, need satisfaction, and longitudinal well-being: The self-concordance model. J. Pers. Soc. Psychol. 76 (3), 482–497. doi:10.1037/0222-3514.76.3.482.

Smith, D., Wright, C.J., Cantwell, C., 2008. Beating the bunker: The effect of PETTLEP imagery on golf bunker shot performance. Res. Q. Exerc. Sport 79 (3), 385–391.

Sordoni, C., Hall, C., Forwell, L., 2000. The use of imagery by athletes during injury rehabilitation. J. Sport Rehabil. 9 (4), 329–338.

Sordoni, C., Hall, C., Forwell, L., 2002. The use of imagery in athletic injury rehabilitation and its relationship to self-efficacy. Physiotherapy Canada 54 (3), 177–185.

Spittle, M., Morris, T., 2011. Can internal and external imagery perspectives be trained? Journal of Mental Imagery 35 (3&4), 81–104.

Stenling, A., Hassmén, P., Holmström, S., 2014. Implicit beliefs of ability, approach-avoidance goals and cognitive anxiety among team sport athletes. Eur. J. Sport Sci. 14 (7), 720–729. doi:10.1080/17461391.2014.901419.

Sutton, J., Stewart, W., 2002. Learning to Counsel, second ed. How to Books, Oxford.

The Health Foundation, 2014. Person-Centred Care Made Simple: What Everyone Should Know About Person-Centred Care. The Health Foundation, London.

Theodorakis, Y., Weinberg, R., Natsis, P., Douma, I., Kazakas, P., 2000. The effects of motivational versus instructional self-talk on improving motor performance. Sport Psychol. 14 (3), 253–271.

Tod, D., 2014. Sport Psychology: The Basics. Routledge, London.

Tod, D., Hardy, J., Oliver, E., 2011. Effects of self-talk: A systematic review. J. Sport Exerc. Psychol. 33 (5), 666–687.

Turner, J.A., Aaron, L.A., 2001. Pain-related catastrophizing: What is it? Clin. J. Pain 17 (1), 65–71.

Turner, M.J., Barker, J.B., 2013. Examining the efficacy of rational-emotive behavior therapy (REBT) on irrational beliefs and anxiety in elite youth cricketers. J. Appl. Sport Psychol. 25 (1), 131–147. doi:10.1080/10413200.2011.574311.

Turner, M.J., Barker, J.B., 2014. Using rational emotive behavior therapy with athletes. Sport Psychol. 28 (1), 75–90.

Turner, J.A., Jensen, M.P., Warms, C.A., Cardenas, D.D., 2002. Catastrophizing is associated with pain intensity, psychological distress, and pain-related disability among individuals with chronic pain after spinal cord injury. Pain 98 (1–2), 127–134. doi:10.1016/S0304-3959(02)00045-3.

Turner, M.J., Slater, M.J., Barker, J.B., 2015. The season-long effects of rational emotive behavior therapy on the irrational beliefs of professional academy soccer athletes. Int. J. Sport Psychol. 45 (5), 429–451.

Turner, M.J., Slater, M.J., Barker, J.B., 2014. Not the end of the world: The effects of Rational Emotive Behavior Therapy on the irrational beliefs of elite academy athletes. J. Appl. Sport Psychol. 26 (2), 144–156. doi:10.1080/10413200.2013.812159.

Watson, P.J., Sherback, J., Morris, R.J., 1998. Irrational beliefs, individualism-collectivism, and adjustment. Pers. Individ. Dif. 24 (2), 173–179. doi:10.1016/S0191-8869(97)00168-2.

Wesch, N., Callow, N., Hall, C., Pope, J.P., 2016. Imagery and self-efficacy in the injury context. Psychol. Sport Exerc. 24, 72–81. doi:10.1016/j.psychsport.2015.12.007.

Westbrook, D., Kennerley, H., Kirk, J., 2011. An Introduction to Cognitive Behaviour Therapy: Skills and Applications, second ed. Sage, London.

Wiseman, T.A., Curtis, K., Lam, M., Foster, K., 2015. Incidence of depression, anxiety and stress following traumatic injury: A longitudinal study. Scand. J. Trauma Resusc. Emerg. Med. 23, 29. doi:10.1186/s13049-015-0109-z.

Wilson, C., Smith, D., Burden, A., Holmes, P., 2010. Participant-generated imagery scripts produce greater EMG activity and imagery ability. Eur. J. Sport Sci. 10 (6), 417–425. doi:10.1080/17461391003770491.

# SUPPORTING, COMPLEMENTARY, ALTERNATIVE AND EVOLVING MODELS OF PRACTICE
## Towards the Development of Your Biopsychosocial Practice

ALAN CHAMBERLAIN

## INTRODUCTION

This chapter is intended to raise further awareness and facilitate the reader's biopsychosocial practice development. Supporting, contemporary, alternative and evolving models of practice will be considered from the clinical, teaching and learning fields of knowledge with examples being used to contextualize and relate these in professional practice development.

In some contexts and clinical service provisions, patients may be referred to as clients, but they will be referred to as patients rather than clients throughout this chapter, as clients can equally be referred to and be customers and both clients and customers may also be organizations procuring a clinical service from a provider. Hence the distinction being made from the outset, in the changing face of current public and private sector service provision.

Theoretical models, paradigms and frameworks are all constructs that are designed to help structure and understand knowledge, and guide its subsequent application and thus underpin the skills in practice. Before discussing the various models of practice, it is important to understand and define what is meant by a model of practice and consider the above interchangeable terms.

## THE DEFINITION, PURPOSE AND FUNCTION OF THEORETICAL MODELS AND THEIR PSEUDONYMS

If theoretical model is concerned with the theory of a subject or field of knowledge and study rather than its practical application

(Oxford Dictionaries, 2016), then a model of theory would simply be a model that is based on a theory rather than practice or fact (McKeown and Summers, 2008, p. 280) and it can be argued that it is the application of theory in practice that establishes whether facts exist. This is explicit if theory is considered to be a set of explanatory ideas; abstract knowledge or reasoning; an idea or opinion and a model defined as a miniature representation; a pattern; or an item worthy of imitation (McKeown and Summers, 2008, p. 280). A theoretical model could therefore be considered to be a miniature representation of theory and worthy of imitation in practice to establish facts by its application and where the theoretical model may be presented in either an abstract pattern format, such as a diagram or figure, or succinctly presented in table format. In short, a theoretical model is a description or representation utilized to understand the way in which a system or process works (Oxford Dictionaries, 2016). Similarly a model of health or a model of care, for example, may be a miniature presentation of a theoretical model for application or imitation that helps us understand the way such a theory can be applied in clinical practice.

Pseudonyms for the term 'model' include paradigm, which is defined as an example or model (McKeown and Summers, 2008, p. 196). The two terms may therefore be used interchangeably and it is useful to know when the reader is searching and interrogating the literature for theoretical models in practice. Some texts may refer to a framework, which is defined as a supporting structure (McKeown and Summers, 2008, p. 111). If a theoretical model is considered to be a miniature representation of theory that helps to give support in practice, it is understandable how some texts may equally refer to a theoretical framework, which may also be interchangeably used.

The undergraduate and postgraduate practitioner will need to remain abreast of current and future theoretical models, paradigms and frameworks that drive, structure and underpin practice. In addition, knowledge, understanding and skills in practice are so co-dependent and inter-related, examples of models will be drawn from the fields of education and health, in order to demonstrate this.

Undergraduate and graduate therapists alike will already know of examples of underpinning theoretical models and some are presented in Table 7.1, together with common formal and informal acronyms that practitioners have adopted as either guidance or as an aide memoir in practice.

Table 7.1 lists several examples of models in educational and clinical practice, which is nonexhaustive. There will be many more in other subspecialties of clinical and educational practice, but for the purpose of demonstration, musculoskeletal practice examples have been listed.

## Examples of Models in Practice: Their Adoption and Adaption

As indicated earlier, models can be presented in various formats, and very often many can be adapted for application across similar or related fields of knowledge and practice.

Some examples, adapted and developed from theoretical models in practice, are discussed next and may be equally useful to the undergraduate and postgraduate reader as a practitioner and life-long learner making the

| TABLE 7.1 | |
| --- | --- |
| **A Nonexhaustive Table of Common Theoretical Models and Acronyms in Practice** | |
| **Field of Knowledge/Area of Practice** | **Model or Acronym** |
| Education, teaching, learning, reflection and professional development | Kolb's learning cycle (Bassot, 2013; Kolb, 1984; 2015)/Gibbs' reflection cycle (Bassot, 2013; Gibbs, 1998) |
| | Donald Schön's reflection model (Bassot, 2013 citing Shön, 1983) |
| | Peter Jarvis' reflection model (Bassot, 2013 citing Jarvis; Jarvis, 1987; 2006; 2010) |
| | Dreyfus model – *Novice to Expert* |
| | SWOT analysis – strengths, weaknesses, opportunities, threats (Bassot, 2013; CSP, 2001) adapted from SWOT to SNOT analysis, where N represents needs |
| | SMART goals – specific, measurable, achievable, realistic, time-scaled; adapted to SMART(ER) to include E and R for evaluation and reevaluation respectively |
| Musculoskeletal clinical practice: Examination, diagnosis and assessment | Biopsychosocial model (World Health Organization, 2013) |
| | SOAP process – subjective examination, objective examination, analysis or assessment, plan (Baxter, 2003); adapted to SOAPE to include the letter E for evaluation purposes |
| | Maitland arthrogenic approach (Hengeveld and Banks, 2005; Maitland et al., 2005) |
| | McKenzie mechanical diagnosis and therapy (McKenzie and May, 2003) |
| | Cyriax's system of orthopaedic medicine (various publications) |
| | Panjabi stabilizing system model (1992) |
| | SAID principle (Selye, 1951) |
| | ICF – International Classification Framework (World Health Organization, 2013) |
| | Problem-framing |
| | SMART goals – specific, measurable, achievable, realistic, time-scaled; as many educators have expressed, many prefer to adapt SMART to SMART(ER) to include E and R for evaluation and reevaluation respectively |
| Musculoskeletal clinical practice: Treatment, management and intervention | Biopsychosocial model (World Health Organization, 2013) |
| | SOAP process – subjective examination, objective examination, analysis or assessment, plan (Baxter, 2003); adapted to SOAPE to include the letter E for evaluation purposes |
| | Problem-framing |
| | SMART goals – specific, measurable, achievable, realistic, time-scaled; as many educators have expressed, many prefer to adapt SMART to SMART(ER) to include E and R for evaluation and reevaluation respectively |
| | PRICE – protect, rest, ice, compression, elevation (Bleakley, 2010) |
| | POLICE – protect, optimal loading, ice, compression, elevation (Bleakley, 2012) |
| | DRIFTS – duration, repetition, intensity, frequency, technique, time and sets; a further adaptation of DRIFT (Chamberlain et al., 2013) |
| | FITT – frequency, intensity, technique, time (Sanghvi, 2013) |
| | MEAT – movement, exercise, analgesics and treatment/therapy |
| | RAMP – restore, adapt, maintain, prevent |

transition to, from and between andragogy and pedagogy. The classic distinction between andragogy and pedagogy is where the learner may learn through student-centred methods or teacher-centred methods, as opposed to the original criticized distinction of the art and science of learning methods for adults and children respectively (Jarvis et al., 2003 citing Knowles, 1980). Jarvis (1985) compares the assumptions of Knowles' andragogy and pedagogy, which may be useful for the reader to consider, as they progress through their professional programmes and continue to develop. The reader should be able to identify where the most suitable method of learning is located to best meet their learning needs on the continuum from pedagogy to andragogy or whether a mix of the two methods presented in Table 7.2 is required. In other words, whether a more dependent or independent and autonomous method of learning is required at various points or stages of your career, is dependent on one's learning needs as a lifelong learner and the clinical practitioner.

The examples will contextualize and visually demonstrate the function of models across learning and clinical practice, before finally considering the evolvement, development and application of the clinical flag system and the closely related biopsychosocial model in clinical practice. Practice, whether it is learning or clinical in nature, does not exist in a politico-economical and psychosocial vacuum. It is important to understand the influences on your practice and how you the practitioner may be enabled to recognize and address your learning needs for a safe practice in what can be a complex environment.

From Table 7.1, the practitioner will recognize the commonly used SOAP (Subjective, Objective, Analysis or Assessment and Plan) model utilized in patient examination and assessment. However, during the first decade of the twenty first century, this structured documentation model that assisted

---

| | **Pedagogy** | **Andragogy** |
|---|---|---|
| **The Learner** | – Dependent<br>Teacher directs what, when and how a subject is learned and tests that it has been learned | – Moves towards independence<br>– Self-directing<br>Teacher encourages and nurtures this movement |
| **The Learner's Experience** | Of little worth<br>Hence teaching methods are didactic | A resource for learning; hence teaching methods include discussion, problem-solving, etc. |
| **Readiness to Learn** | People learn what society expects them to, so that the curriculum is standardized | People learn what they need to know, so that learning programmes are organized around life application |
| **Orientation to Learning** | Acquisition of subject matter<br>Curriculum organized by subjects | Learning experience should be based around problems, because people are performance-centred in their learning |

**TABLE 7.2 A Comparison of Knowles' Assumptions of Pedagogy and Andragogy**

(Jarvis, 1985)

the practitioner to collect data for analysis, enabling clinical-reasoned assessment and goal-setting, underwent changes where practitioners were encouraged not only to continue to conduct a subjective examination and an objective examination with a review and examination of body systems and specific tissues using tests and measures, but to also evaluate making clinical judgements based on this for the formulation of diagnosis and prognosis and the selection of an intervention (Baxter, 2003). This therefore led to the adaptation of the original SOAP model to the SOAPE (Subjective, Objective, Analysis or Assessment, Plan and Evaluation) model for examination, assessment and intervention documentation, together with a continuum of evaluation throughout the process based on data gathered from examination and re-examination. This serves to demonstrate the evolution of models, how they may be initially imitated and adopted into practice and later adapted or improved, to reflect changes or better understanding in practice.

Practitioners, as lifelong learners, will be familiar with models and tools in learning practice and a few have been included in Table 7.1. Bassot explains the use of the Johari Window developed by Joseph Luft and Harry Ingham (Bassot, 2013 citing Luft, 1984), so named by combining the first names of the authors. The Johari Window (see Fig. 7.1A) is a model that illustrates how practitioners can gain useful insight and self-awareness

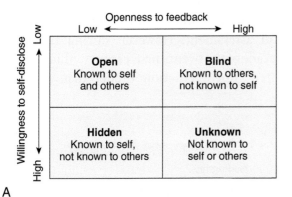

A

FIGURE 7.1 ■ **(A)** The Johari Window (Bassot, 2013 citing Luft, 1984) to gain useful insight and self-awareness for being open to and receiving feedback. **(B)** The adapted Johari Window for more independent identification and analysis of learning using the SWOT or SNOT analysis. *(Adapted from a previously published CSP Proforma (CSP, 2001).)*

| Strengths<br>What can I do well/have I done well? | Weaknesses or needs<br>What am I less good at or do I need to improve on? Where are the gaps in my knowledge, understanding and skills? |
|---|---|
| Opportunities<br>What opportunities exist or might become available to help me achieve my goals? What resources are available to me, in order to help me achieve my goals? | Threats<br>What may act to inhibit my progress or act as a barrier to my learning? Who may form a barrier and why? |

B

by being open to and receiving feedback (Bassot, 2013 citing Luft, 1984) from significant others.

Across the health and other professions, their representative professional bodies and higher education institutions, the Johari Window was adopted and adapted further for independent learner use. The Window (see Fig. 7.1B) still looks like a traditional window frame subdivided into four quarters. The window subdivision headings were adapted in a CSP (Chartered Society of Physiotherapy) publication (CSP, 2001) with each window quarter being headed 'strengths', 'weaknesses', 'opportunities' and 'threats' for the independent learner to identify and analyse their learning (SWOT analysis). The acronym of SWOT may be apt in the context of a learning environment, but because of the negative connotation of the term 'weaknesses', some clinical educators anecdotally adapted their SWOT (Strengths, Weaknesses, Opportunities and Threats) analysis further, to adopt the more positive term of 'needs'. Thus producing a further adaptation of the Johari Window and a move from SWOT to a SNOT (Strengths, Needs, Opportunities and Threats) analysis, albeit that the latter acronym could be considered a rather unpleasant term in itself, but it does allow for an element of fun in learning!

Earlier the SOAP model was adapted to include evaluation and, as a further example in clinical and learning practice, many will already be aware of another model listed in Table 7.1 known as the SMART goals model, where identified learning or clinical goals are encouraged to be specific, measureable, achievable and time-scaled. However, in the spirit of including a continuum of evaluation,

many educators advocate an adaption of the original model to reflect this using the acronym SMARTER goals, where the letter 'E' represents an evaluation of the goals identified and the letter 'R' represents reevaluation, where the same goals and outcomes will be evaluated. Further goals may be identified as earlier goals are either achieved or modified. This serves as another example of how models can evolve as they are applied in practice and knowledge and understanding is developed within a field, or theories are modified. An example visual representation of the model for application in clinical practice is provided in Figure 7.2, where SMARTER goals were discussed in an undergraduate health practitioner seminar in the promotion of athlete habilitation and rehabilitation programme adherence and compliance.

The SMARTER goals model has been adopted within teaching and learning and subsequently adopted and adapted for use in clinical practice. This serves to demonstrate how a model can be adopted across fields of knowledge and practice and not only adapted to suit the context of practice, but further developed and evolved to emphasize the crucial stage of practice evaluation and reevaluation.

An acronym formed from the initial letter(s) of other words, an abbreviation, mnemonics or phrases and rhymes, designed to give structure or aid memory and recall, are useful in practice and several acronyms are offered in Table 7.1. It is beyond the scope of this chapter to discuss each of the acronyms and models listed. However, examples of some are being offered not only to demonstrate the adoption, development, evolvement and adaption of models, but also to

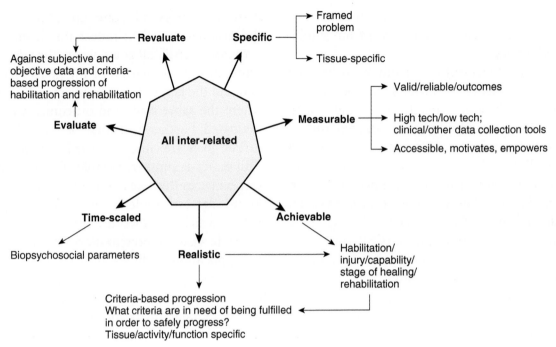

FIGURE 7.2 ■ The SMARTER Goals model applied within a seminar, in the promotion of athlete habilitation & rehabilitation programme adherence and compliance.

encourage you to consider models that may support and structure your own practice development and support and compliment other models in practice.

It has briefly been demonstrated how some models may be utilized across fields of knowledge and practice, such as the SMART goals model in education and how it has been adapted since being adopted by the field of clinical practice to form the SMARTER goals model to include evaluation and reevaluation. Some models may have more purposeful and pertinent acronyms derived to support practice such as the aptly named FITT principle formulated for exercise prescription, where the word FITT is formed from the initial letters of frequency, intensity, time and type of exercise (Sanghvi, 2013), whereas others may be less so and yet designed to

equally support the practice of more specific exercise prescription. Author frustration from some years ago still exists today, where physiotherapy practices commonly failed to adopt the science from other fields of knowledge such and as sport and exercise in their habilitation and rehabilitation technique prescription, beyond that of early intervention such as 10 repetitions of 10 second holds to be conducted 10 times per day! This frustration prompted the use of the word 'drift' where it was considered practitioners seemed to collectively 'drift' along without question, using the same low level prescription for each level of habilitation and rehabilitation technique and irrespective of the target tissues and tissue characteristics. From this frustration, the acronym DRIFT was derived where the letters were the initial letters of duration, repetition, intensity, frequency and technique (Chamberlain et al., 2013), which was designed to structure, refine and specify therapeutic technique prescription further. The letter S has since been added to DRIFT to form DRIFTS, in order to add the word 'sets' for therapeutic technique prescription. Not all letters of the acronym may be required in the prescription of a therapeutic technique, but the acronym serves to highlight consideration of all the component parts that may be required in a habilitation or rehabilitation programme.

In the fields of education and training where continuing professional development (CPD) encompasses both formal and informal learning, education and training models have been introduced, adopted, developed, evolved and adapted as the subject and context has become better understood. For example, early models espoused by the professional body the Chartered Society of Physiotherapy (CSP) have continued to be developed and revised. Figure 7.3 shows an early CPD model, which was further developed as an academic exercise (see Fig. 7.4) by the adoption and adaptation of the

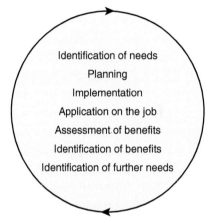

FIGURE 7.3 ■ The modified continuing professional development (CPD) process of 1996. *(O'Sullivan, 1996)*

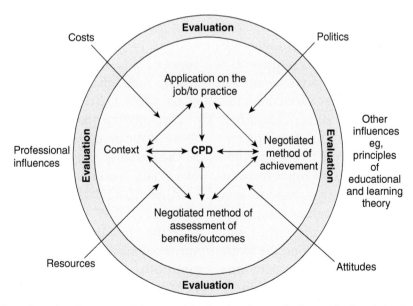

FIGURE 7.4 ■ The reformulated centre-periphery model reflecting the continuing professional development (CPD) process. *(Chamberlain, Unpublished, adapted from Griffin, 1995, p. 5.8; CSP, 1994, p. 4; and O'Sullivan, 1996, pp. 14-15.)*

centre-periphery model developed by Griffin (1995) to demonstrate the complexity, influences and the larger context of the CPD process beyond that demonstrated by the earlier models published by the CSP (see Figure 7.5) (CSP, 1994; O'Sullivan, 1996). The more recently developed CPD model published by the CSP remains devoid of the complexity and influences of the larger context in practice, resulting in scope for further development to reflect those demonstrated in Figure 7.4. The practitioner needs to remain critical in their reading and understanding and to consider where there is scope for adoption, development, evolvement and adaption of models that may be better suited to contemporary practice, as it too develops and evolves. The adoption and adaption of Griffin's (1995) centre-periphery model in Figure 7.4 facilitates the practitioner to consider the threats or barriers, motivators and opportunities that can be listed within the SNOT analysis in Figure 7.1B when planning continuing professional development. For example, resources such as time and finance for a formal CPD course may represent a threat or barrier to access, but taking annual leave and self-funding may overcome the barrier and help in the meeting of identified and necessary or desired and development learning needs. The attitudes of significant other stakeholders such as an employer, or a lack of resource support may present as a motivator and an opportunity for an employee to consider in their future career path and employment decisions. It is beyond the scope of this chapter to fully discuss the operationalization of the adapted centre-periphery model, but, along with the remainder of the previously mentioned models, it serves to demonstrate how models can be subject to constructive and balanced critique with reference to the research, literature and practice. From this process, a more comprehensive model can emerge or, conversely, a more succinct and simplified model.

## Learning and Theoretical Reflective Models of Practice

For several years, health professionals have been encouraged to be reflective in practice. In other words, analyse and evaluate. It is beyond the scope of this chapter to fully discuss the various reflective models of practice that have evolved across the professions, but as practitioners develop, they may find that some models are better suited than others at various times throughout their careers. Reflective practice is not new and is largely based on Donald Schön's '…seminal work *The Reflective Practitioner (1983)*…' where in the health professions, '…practice is messy…' 'often confusing…where there will not always be a logical solution,' and '…when working with people will not always be predictable…' (Bassot, 2013 citing Schön, 1983); however, coping with this is central to being a professional (Bassot, 2013).

Dealing with the feelings of patients and those of the practitioner can be complex and so the reader is referred to the original work of Donald Schön and other authors considered in Barbara Bassot's (2013) discussions on various models of reflective practice for reflective practice development, where a variety of models are succinctly explained and contrasted. As the practitioner needs to develop to manage the more complex needs of some patients, more tools to support the practitioner's development will be needed.

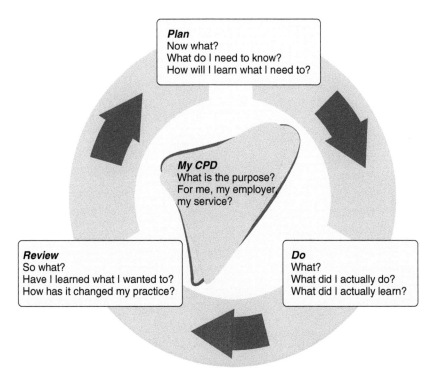

**Plan**
Now what?
What do I need to know?
How will I learn what I need to?

**My CPD**
What is the purpose?
For me, my employer,
my service?

**Review**
So what?
Have I learned what I wanted to?
How has it changed my practice?

**Do**
What?
What did I actually do?
What did I actually learn?

FIGURE 7.5 The Chartered Society of Physiotherapy continuing professional development (CSP CPD) process model. *(CSP, 2015)*

Bassot recognises how Gibbs' Reflective Cycle (Gibbs, 1988; Bassot, 2013 citing Gibbs 1988) is very useful (see Fig. 7.6) and helps the practitioner to consider and process feelings in practice. The similarity of Gibbs' Reflective Cycle to Kolb's Experiential Learning Cycle (Bassot, 2013 citing Kolb 1984) (see Fig. 7.7) is made explicit with the main difference being that of greater detail in the former than the latter, which facilitates a deeper level of critically reflective practice (Bassot, 2013). Neophyte practitioners may initially gain more from the use of Kolb's learning cycle and may progress to use Gibbs' reflective cycle as they progress through their programme and gain some experience. Eventually, as experience is gained and practitioners become more expert or advanced in their field of practice,

there may be a need for an even more detailed and sophisticated reflection model.

Originally developed and published by Jarvis (1987), after recognizing that many well-known models of learning were flawed (including Kolb's Learning Cycle) on account of the fact that they failed to consider the social context and interaction (Jarvis, 2006; 2010). Jarvis' model (see Fig. 7.8) is significantly an evolution of Kolb's Cycle more complex than others and it highlights a range of differing ways a learner can respond to an experience, including not necessarily learning from every situation (Bassot, 2013).

Both Jarvis (2006) and Bassot (2013) explain the main reasons for nonlearning and the reader is referred to these texts for more detail on the reasons offered for nonlearning.

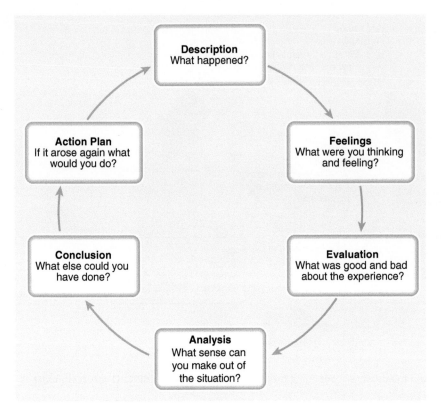

FIGURE 7.6 Gibbs' reflective cycle. *(Gibbs, 1998; Bassot 2013, citing Gibbs)*

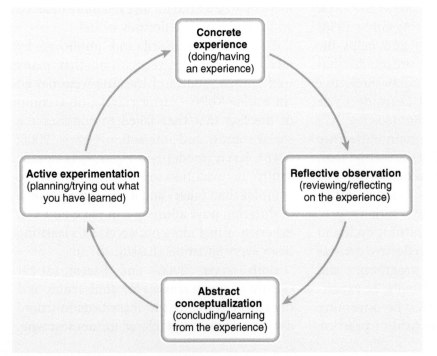

FIGURE 7.7 ■ Kolb's learning cycle. *(Kolb, 1984)*

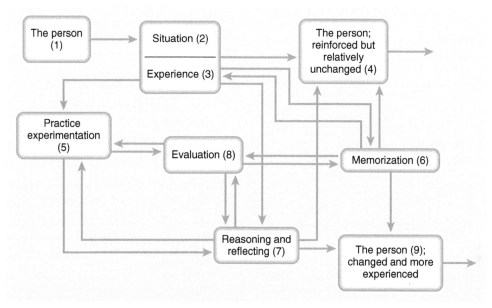

FIGURE 7.8 ■ Jarvis' reflective cycle. *(Jarvis, 2006 and 2010)*

The main reasons offered by Jarvis, and further succinctly explained by Bassot for nonlearning, are paraphrased as follows:

Presumption – the practitioner practices based upon presumptions gained through previous knowledge and experience; is rather automatic; besides, it is not possible for the practitioner to continually think through all that they do all of the time.

Nonconsideration – no response to a learning opportunity for a variety of reasons ranging from a lack of resources through to a lack of insight or understanding of the need to take advantage of the learning opportunity.

Rejection – a conscious rejection of aspects of the learning opportunity that may be for similar reasons to those previously mentioned.

In other words, nonlearning may be a subconscious or conscious choice-matter and nonengagement in reflection or rejection of a learning opportunity, leading to the premature exit from the cycle by the prospective learner tracking from Box 1 to Box 4 without engaging in any of Boxes 5, 6, 7 or 8 (see Fig. 7.8). Jarvis (2006) criticizes his own work accepting that there may be different routes through the cycle and, importantly, does not in entirety accept his earlier categorizations of the routes through, which are available in Table 7.3.

As every academic discipline that focuses on the human being as a learner, has a contribution to make to the understanding of learning (Jarvis, 2009), it would be pertinent to offer such a contribution by suggesting another possible route a clinician may follow through Jarvis' learning cycle using the following contextualised example.

The practitioner may experience a patient with psychosocial needs expressed through a

## TABLE 7.3

### Categories, the Routes Through and Outcomes of Jarvis' (2006) Learning Cycle

(see also Fig. 7.8)

| Category of Learning | Learning Cycle Route | Outcome of the Learning Route |
|---|---|---|
| Nonlearning through presumption | Boxes 1–4 | Individuals presume upon the situation and do not learn from it |
| Nonlearning through nonconsideration | Boxes 1–4 | For a variety of reasons the individuals do not consider the situation and do not learn from it |
| Nonlearning through rejection | Boxes 1–4 | For a variety of reasons the individuals reject the opportunity to learn from the situation |
| Nonreflective preconscious learning | Boxes 1, 3, 6 and either 4 or 9 | Individuals experience situations albeit with low awareness, where they do not really consider them but that they have learned something |
| Nonreflective practice learning | Boxes 1, 3, 5, 8, 6 and either 4 or 9 | Individuals learn basic skills without thought |
| Nonreflective memorization learning | Boxes 1, 3, 6, 8 and either 4 or 9 | Individuals remember the information which they were given |
| Reflective learning through contemplation | Boxes 1, 3, 7, 8, 6 and 9 | Individuals reflect upon a situation and either accept or change it |
| Reflective learning through reflective practice | Boxes 1, 3, 5, 7, 5, 8, 6 and 9 | Individuals think about the situation and then act upon it, either conforming or innovating upon it |
| Reflective learning through experiential learning | Boxes 1, 3, 7, 5, 7, 8, 6 and 9 | Individuals think about the situation and agree or disagree with what they have experienced |

belief of perhaps never being able to undertake exercise activity or participate in a particular employment activity again. The causation of the expressed beliefs may be difficult to unravel during the initial therapeutic session, but it may be as a result of a plethora of possible single reasons or a combination of a range of reasons such as the presence of chronic or long-standing low back pain radiating into the buttock and having been exposed to many conflicting practitioner opinions or approaches to treatment and rehabilitation. The practitioner on the other hand, may informally have widely read around psychosocial issues and, for example, cognitive behavioural therapeutic approaches and adopted published strategies to deal with such an example of a complex patient. In addition, the practitioner may have felt that the frequency of such patients was increasing in the service they have recently become employed in and that perhaps formal training is required to ensure that they are practising within their scope of practice. On completion of such a formal course, the practitioner may, from a recollection of reading, have resultant subject knowledge and understanding and further experience may, on reflection and evaluation, emerge reinforced and relatively unchanged as little more has been learnt. It is therefore possible to still emerge from the cycle reinforced and relatively unchanged via Box 4 without necessarily exiting Jarvis' cycle prematurely. The key here is the choice for active engagement and reflection (Bassot, 2013) to move around the cycle and the previous example illustrates how the practitioner may not necessarily emerge changed and more experienced as in Box 9 (see Fig. 7.8).

Jarvis' model of reflection may suit the more experienced practitioner where, as Bassot explains (2013, citing Jarvis), the model builds on Kolb's Learning Cycle, but is significantly more complex and recognizes that practitioners may not necessarily learn from a situation for various reasons. Bassot explains that Jarvis highlights how learning from experience is not automatic, that engagement in reflection is a choice matter and if practitioners fail to choose to engage, they can exit Jarvis' cycle prematurely by simply tracking across the top of the cycle rather than moving round it. In other words, it is fine to exit the cycle reinforced and relatively unchanged, provided there has been a period of reflection and reasoning. For example, the experienced practitioner may attend a formal course on cognitive behavioural therapy (refer to Evans and Hickey, Chapter 5 as well as Chapter 9 of this text, for more on the subject of cognitive behaviour therapy) and find that many strategies learnt have already been adopted into practice, but they have been reinforced with reference to the literature and research accessed through the formal course attendance and, as

a result, may remain unchanged in some aspects of practice.

It is beyond the scope of this chapter to discuss all learning theories per se, as this is more suited to the expert theorist and researchers in the field, but as an autonomous professional practitioner, you will have been transformed as you moved through the teaching and learning system underpinned by pedagogical theories and methods, where the learner is dependent, through to andragogical methods and practices, where the learner is more independent or cooperative in their learning. The Jarvis model of refection may support the more autonomous, experienced, expert and advanced learner in their reflective practice.

To be fair to Kolb, the idea of experiential learning cycle being too simplistic has been superseded more recently. The original experiential learning cycle has been widely used and adapted in the design and conduct of a myriad of educational programmes and indeed, Kolb has been disturbed by the oversimplified interpretations and applications of it (Kolb, 2015). Kolb in recognition of the cycle of learning being more complex has extensively updated the theory of experiential learning, its modern application in education, adult development and the working environment. In doing so, he has built on the scholarly works and theories of others (eg, William James, John Dewey, Kurt Lewin, Jean Piaget and Lev Vygotsky) and reflected on 30 years of research, theoretical issues and practice from within the fields of knowledge of psychology, philosophy and physiology that followed his first edition of Experiential Learning. The reader is therefore referred to Kolb's recent text for updating.

## Theoretical Clinical Models

Theoretical clinical models can equally be considered for adoption, development, evolvement and adaption. One such model adopted by many of those in musculoskeletal spinal mechanical diagnosis and therapy practice was the McKenzie model, which was first published in 1981. The model was further developed to help structure, support and justify accurate clinical analysis and decision-making through the formulation of a visual aid algorithm (Kilby et al., 1990) (see Fig. 7.9). The model was further adapted to reflect changes in thought and opinion following research findings. These will be considered

more, following two clinical examples from practice to demonstrate how theory and practice are inextricably linked and how practitioners need to really critically think through theoretical models, practice, protocols, procedures and guidelines that underpin their understanding and apply in their decision-making.

For those readers who are not familiar with the work of the late Robin McKenzie and the postgraduate courses provided by the McKenzie Institute, you may need to bear with the author, as a clinical example of model application 'is considered,' with and without adequate clinical reasoning, involving anatomical structure and related function and

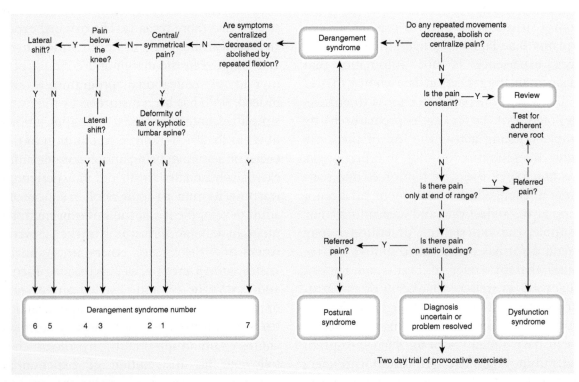

FIGURE 7.9 ■ The original McKenzie method of mechanical diagnosis and the therapy classification algorithm. *(Kilby, Stigant and Roberts, 1990)*

pathology is presented; together with a rationale for deviating from guidelines in practice.

To help those who are unfamiliar with the McKenzie method of mechanical diagnosis and therapy, the term derangement will be used. If a reducible derangement is an internal disc displacement with a competent annulus and an irreducible derangement is a displacement with an incompetent, or ruptured annular wall (McKenzie and May, 2003), it is understandable how some practitioners adopt the term discogenic derangement, rather than the preferred term of derangement syndrome within the mechanical diagnosis and therapy literature. The adoption of the term discogenic derangement is understandable when the same practitioners may be used to testing for, or differentiating between a peripheral joint derangement and non-derangement to determine management decisions. Irrespective, the term derangement in the context of this chapter is mainly referring to the intervertebral disc, in order to facilitate the understanding of additional secondary pathology.

## Clinical Scenario Example 1

On more than one occasion as a physiotherapist working with the McKenzie model of lumbar spinal mechanical diagnosis and therapy, in conjunction with others when employed in a primary care setting of an outpatient department and community service, some patients were observed to be not improving with persistent peripheralization of pain symptoms down the leg as a result of a derangement. The site and distribution of the peripheral pain symptoms serves to inform the practitioner of the status of a lumbar spinal intervertebral disc in terms of the affected spinal level, the direction of the protruding derangement with the outer annular wall intact (eg, more commonly postero-lateral, posterior or lateral) and the extent of the derangement (ie, whether it is a smaller or larger derangement with/without nerve root compression). In simple terms for non-physiotherapy readers, the protruding outer wall of the disc is a derangement, considered to be so, having developed a tear within the inner wall of the annulus. The protrusion can be minor where pressure is exerted against the innervated area of the posterior wall of the annulus producing pain locally and possibly referred to the buttock of the affected side, or it can be larger and protruding against other anatomical structures such as an adjacent nerve root. The problem with such pathology is that it does not occur in an anatomical and self-limiting pathological vacuum, as secondary pathological effects may take place and may give confusing signs and symptoms during examination. If the reader refers to Figures 7.9–7.11 (but preferably the text by McKenzie and May, 2003), it can be seen that if the practitioner determines from examination that a derangement is protruding onto a spinal nerve root, symptoms will be referred down the leg beyond the knee joint line and that through specific directed physiological positioning, movement, or loading, the derangement protrusion could be reduced and a sign of this amongst other possible abnormal neurological sign reversal, is when pain symptoms centralise. In other words, the pain symptoms have had their distribution reduced towards the centre of the body. From theory and practice, this may produce a greater intensity

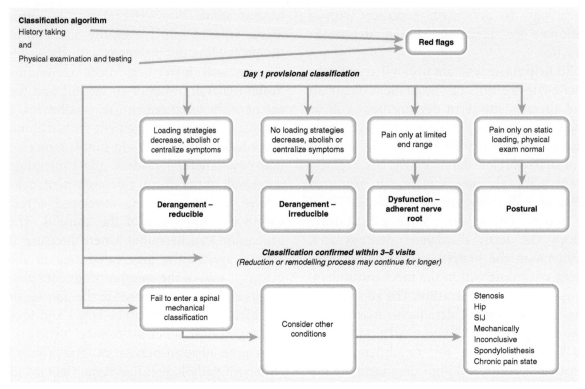

FIGURE 7.10 ■ McKenzie and May (2003, p. 426) adaption of the original McKenzie method of mechanical diagnosis and the therapy classification algorithm.

more proximally, as the distribution of symptoms reduce.

Practitioners need to remain critical in their reasoning skills and recognize when they may need to deviate from theoretical models, practice, protocols, procedures and guidelines that underpin their knowledge, understanding and clinical skills for decision-making.

Before proceeding with the McKenzie mechanical diagnosis and therapy clinical scenario example further, another brief example is provided below, where a model and guidelines may be critiqued or deviated from in practice, based on theoretical understanding rather than research.

In the management of acute soft-tissue injuries, the acronym PRICE (see Table 7.1) was recommended by original guidelines published by the Association of Chartered Physiotherapists in Sport Medicine in 1998 (Kerr et al., 1998), where the letter 'I' represented the need to apply ice. But for a duration of 20 to 30 minutes (Bleakley, 2010, citing Kerr Daley and Booth 1998) was represented. However, it is also recognized that Lewis' hunting response occurs causing vasodilatation within 3 to 8 minutes (Bleakley, 2010 citing Lewis). If the rationale for ice application is to induce a vasoconstriction response and therefore achieve haemostasis in the acute injury of superficial soft tissue,

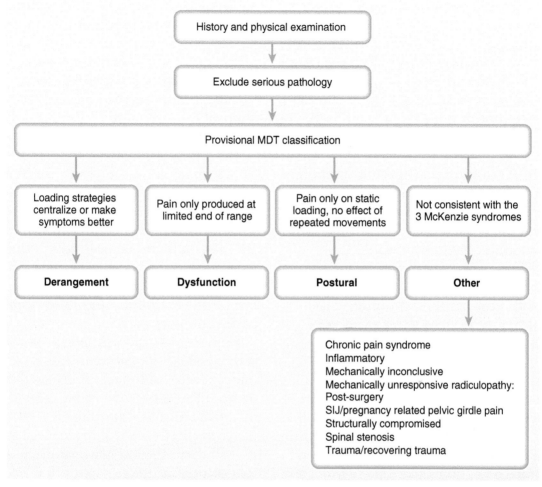

FIGURE 7.11 ■ The most recent developed McKenzie method of mechanical diagnosis and therapy classification algorithm. *(The McKenzie Institute International, in print)*

such as the lateral ligament complex of the ankle where there is subcutaneous haemorrhaging of the ligaments, it is suggested that the practitioner consider deviating from those earlier published guidelines and have a much shorter duration of ice application that induces vasoconstriction rather than the vasodilatation of Lewis' hunting response, which would potentially cause more harm than good.

Deviation from models of practice may be necessary in the real world of clinical practice as previously mentioned and the following serves to illustrate how the McKenzie model of mechanical diagnosis and therapy may need to be deviated from, either on a temporary or permanent basis depending on the findings.

Serving as an excellent example of the need to deviate from a model on a temporary basis is the problem experienced by the author on more than one occasion, where practitioners following the McKenzie diagnosis and therapy method either disregarded or had unwittingly not realized that secondary effects of the derangement were present and producing a nonresponse or worsening response when in fact, initially, the correct directional movement technique was employed. In simple terms, if the movement direction determined by the derangement is correct and a worsening response or nonresponse results, then there must be another component to consider such as those indicated next.

Examples of clinical reasons for peripheralization when the correct discogenic derangement diagnosis and disc derangement reduction movement technique is deployed include:

■ The derangement may be larger than anticipated and the derangement can be compressed to create peripheralization as the annulus bulges further towards pain sensitive nerve tissue. The suggested way to proceed is to unload and decompress, which may involve in the event of a posterior derangement, for example, a period of minutes to hours of prone lying; possibly in flexion and a gradual reduction of flexion towards extension as symptoms allow.

■ The relative space in the intervertebral foramina may be reduced by the disc derangement itself, by dural sleeve swelling produced by direct annular wall irritation of the nerve root, or by facet joint swelling. In the event of the latter two, a restful period of a number of hours (up to 24 hours) may be required to allow for the swelling to reduce and this is better obtained by encouraging elevation of the

lumbar area by prone lying rather than being supported by a lumbar roll in supine. This can be considered as specific back pain and deviation from nonspecific back pain guidelines can therefore be deviated from, where normal physical activities would be encouraged.

The previously mentioned scenarios serve as an example of applying anatomical, physiological and pathological clinical reasoning skills in combination and adapting a clinical model to suit how the patient presents and responds to derangement reduction movement. When therapists pugnaciously follow what may well be the correct movement direction in the presence of secondary presentations, as previously described, those same therapists may well induce or worsen such secondary problems by not reasoning through what additional problems may be present. The answer may be to temporarily wait, rather than deviate from the model and those who fail to reason through the presence of secondary effects of a derangement, do so at their peril, as the therapist could actually induce not only chronic pathology, but those psychosocial problems that may be found in low back pain patients.

The effectiveness of the McKenzie method on bio-behavioural factors such psychosocial and cognitive variables in patients with low back pain is argued to be contentious (Mbada, Ayanniyi and Ogunlade, 2015 citing Al-Obaidi et al., 2013 and Udermann et al., 2004). However, if McKenzie interventions can reduce the physiological perception of pain and possibly modify the cognitive and bio-behavioural factors influencing physical performances enabling realistic quantification and perception of pain associated with physical performances, as well as reducing related fear and disability beliefs (Al-Obaidi et al., 2013) through accurate mechanical diagnosis and therapy, it is argued the converse could apply in the event of any inaccuracies of clinical application and reasoning during the therapeutic episode. The need to constantly evaluate and re-evaluate practice throughout a therapeutic episode is therefore highly important in ensuring practitioners do not engender a long-term condition and possible yellow flags.

Management of acute to chronic conditions, including spinal and other common musculoskeletal (MSK) problems, can be a complex area of practice requiring equally complex approaches to their management. The approaches will be again considered later, but for now, the reader is referred to past McKenzie Institute literature (eg, McKenzie and May (2003) and future imminent updates) for greater development of clinical knowledge, understanding and reasoning skills in the application of the theoretical model and approach in mechanical diagnosis and therapy. However, for the purpose of this chapter, considering associated models of practice, the reader will be introduced to the rationale of the development and evolvement of the clinical McKenzie model that will lead to the suggestion of yet a further minor adaptation teaching and learning purposes at undergraduate, or early postgraduate stages of professional development.

In the comparison of Figures 7.9–7.11, it can be seen that the mechanical diagnosis and classification of a derangement was subclassified by numbers ranging from derangement 1 to 7 (D1–D7) in Figure 7.9, but have been removed in Figures 7.10 and 7.11. The rationale for the removal of the derange-ment subclassification numbers was based on research demonstrating poor reliability of the visual identification and presence of, for example, a lateral deformity (McKenzie Mechanical Diagnosis and Therapy Organisation, Undated). This is understandable if, for example, there is the additional presence of a marked protective paraspinal muscle spasm (the body's own natural splinting mechanism), or where adipose overlies the area making it difficult to visualize.

As a clinician using the McKenzie method of mechanical diagnosis and therapy, the numbering system became problematic when difficulty was experienced in notating or recording the diagnosis (having accurately classified the derangement and determined whether the derangement was reducible through the repeated movement testing protocol), because it was occasionally difficult to accurately recall the classification number. Consequently it was necessary to resort to a written description of the derangement rather than a number, together with the movement direction preference to reduce it. The adaption of the theoretical model and algorithm is therefore welcomed, not only based on research findings, but also for reasons explained from personal practice.

An academic argument has been constructed to support the adaptation of the McKenzie algorithm by triangulating to a greater or lesser proportionate amount, theory, research and practice. However, there is scope for a further adaptation of the most recent algorithm (see Fig. 7.11) based on the strength of the earlier (Fig. 7.9) and a weakness of the later algorithm (Fig. 7.10). For teaching and learning purposes, the earlier algorithm (Fig. 7.9) developed by Kilby, Stigant and Roberts (1990), includes the original derangement subclassifications espoused by McKenzie (1981), who equally advocated that a lateral component of a derangement must be reduced before the posterior component through lateral movement for the former and sagittal movement for the latter. This remains the case today and is fully clinically explained by McKenzie and May (2003). The algorithm of Kilby, Stigant and Roberts explicitly conveys the need to recognize the lateral component of a derangement, whereas it is implied by that illustrated by McKenzie and May (Fig. 7.10). If the full text of May and McKenzie (2003) is read alongside their adaptation of

the algorithm however, it is clear that the lateral component remains the priority component to reduce, prior to proceeding to move to reduce a posterior component. On the basis of making the priority loading strategy for each component explicit and in order to help reinforce the need to consider the lateral component first, there is perhaps scope for a minor adaptation that includes making the required loading strategy for derangement reduction clear (see Figure 12). However, this adaptation is perhaps of most use to those being introduced to the McKenzie method of Mechanical Diagnosis and

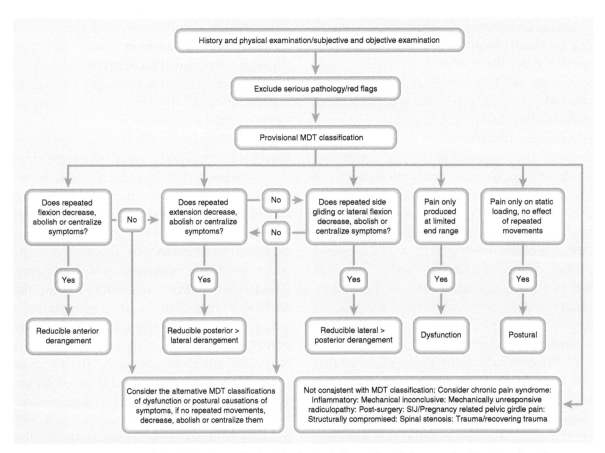

FIGURE 7.12 ■ Adaption of the McKenzie method of mechanical diagnosis and therapy classification algorithm.

Therapy such as those on undergraduate programmes rather than those attending specialist postgraduate clinical programmes offered by the McKenzie Institute.

It is beyond the scope of this chapter to discuss the minor adaptation further, but it is emphasized that it is only a suggested adaptation that may serve to visually remind undergraduate and neophyte therapists without having to recall text, in order to consider the three anterior, lateral and posterior derangements and the respective movement loading strategies of flexion, lateral and extension.

It is also beyond the scope of this chapter to offer other areas where a review and simplification of a less logical numbering system of clinical tests may be appropriate, but perhaps the numbering system of the current neural dynamic testing equally may be worth updating, as they can be equally difficult to recall for note and record keeping purposes, but may be considered a little dubious and especially where there is a move to reduce abbreviations, acronyms and hieroglyphics in clinical records, in order to avoid ambiguity for medico-legal reasons. However, and later, the clinical flag system framework will be considered for potential further development and operationalization within the context of biopsychosocial practice.

## THE CLINICAL FLAG SYSTEM

The Clinical Flag System has already been covered in a previous Chapter (see Selfe and Greenhalgh, Chapter 3) and this section serves to augment the work of these authors, rather than duplicate. As physiotherapists increasingly become frontline practitioners in the private and public sectors of health services, they need to be increasingly aware of and prepared for the application of the Clinical Flag System in practice. Although physiotherapists may remain vigilant throughout a patient's treatment episode in practice, the safety net of another practitioner, such as a general practitioner conducting medical and other screening examinations, may, in the near future no longer be a precursory requirement for accessing a public sector physiotherapy service in England in parallel with other parts of the UK, such as Scotland, or other parts of the world, such as Australia. In other words, the physiotherapist may be the first practitioner to find evidence of other pathology, conditions or other factors that may render the patient inconducive to physiotherapy and rehabilitation.

### The Clinical Flag System: It May Not Be a Red Flag, but Do Not Induce a Yellow Flag

It is clear from practice and the literature that individual Red Flags are insufficiently sensitive in isolation to act upon above that of raising suspicion of serious pathology. Anecdotally, one of the commonest false Red Flags reported is night pain and, although in combination with other Red Flags it would raise suspicion, it could be regarded as a false positive when alone. It is perhaps understandable why the updated hierarchical list of Red Flags includes severe night pain that precludes sleep (Greenhalgh and Selfe, 2010), rather than night pain per se alone. However, pain is, after all, subjective and is whatever a patient says it is and many spinal pain patients may subjectively have variable pain-induced sleep disturbance. It is therefore useful to try and consider another example of night pain in order to illustrate the presence of this false positive. Before doing so, it would be beneficial for the reader to know and recognize the difference between mechanical and chemical induced pain mechanisms. As it is beyond the scope of this chapter to adequately explain these anatomically, physiologically and pathologically at the micro and macro tissue levels (ie, cellular through to organ level of tissue), the following will serve as a useful tool for understanding another reason for night pain, which will help link the earlier clinical models of practice previously discussed and in other chapters within this book. After presenting the next clinical scenario example, a useful tool in practice in the education of your patients and carers will be offered and, although it is difficult to recall which tutor used the example to explain and demonstrate the difference between mechanical and chemical pain during a formal clinical postgraduate course, it continues to be used by many to do so.

When considering the McKenzie model for mechanical diagnosis and therapy, one of the mechanical diagnoses is the posture syndrome with '…pain only on static loading, physical examination normal…', it must be remembered that a patient could have a combination of dysfunction and posture problems. However, when there is a posture problem or what can also be known as repetitive postural strain, paraspinal tissues will present with other signs. As a therapist, and it does not matter whether the repetitive postural stress is cervical, thoracic or lumbar, it is important to identify repetitive postural strains for reasons across the biopsychosocial spectrum. If it is not identified and addressed

(or worse, repeatedly missed or misinterpreted by consecutive therapists or service providers), it can induce anxiety and psychosocial responses of fear of, for example, not being believed about their symptoms or some other pathology being missed. The same patient may report that it is worse at night and so it is worth considering why this may be, through the following case scenario.

### Clinical Scenario Example 2

Susan is a full-time 47-year-old school teacher who has teenage children and a husband who works long hours. Both her and her husband commute for an hour each way to and from their place of work. Susan's role in her place of employment involves a mix of face-to-face teaching, meetings, marking, preparatory and subsequent work for long periods on a personal computer, she is often driving to and from work and comanaging the home and family.

Susan may have some mild to moderate dysfunctional restriction of cervical and thoracic spinal range of movement (ROM) and this is a separate issue to address. Indeed, the repetitive postural strains may have contributed to the development of the dysfunctional restriction and it is for the therapist to clinically reason through why that may be the case. In the meantime, Susan is complaining of paraspinal pain of the cervical and midthoracic spine. Other than some restriction of cervicothoracic ROM, there is little else other than tender, thickened paraspinal muscles. In the absence of trauma, it is likely that the muscles are thickened with inflammatory responses. It is possible to traumatically strain these muscles, but had Susan done so, the therapist would hopefully have identified this possibility during the subjective examination and history taking. The therapist rarely undertakes a single test or examination technique to determine a mechanical, or any other clinical diagnosis, as a collection of tests are normally required to do so. Likewise, a collection of subjective and objective examination techniques are required to form the mechanical diagnosis of postural syndrome, or repetitive postural straining. Subjectively, if there are risk indications and, objectively, there is palpable tender thickening, the examination is not normal. So as a clinician, a therapist would have to reason through why there are thickened and tender paraspinal muscle fibres in the absence of trauma.

In order to understand why paraspinal muscles may be thickened and tender through repetitive postural strain, try the following technique, provided you do not have any contraindications to doing so. With your dominant hand, passively hyperextend the interphalangeal and metacarpal joints of the nondominant hand to a point you clearly feel pain. This pain is mechanical in nature and is a normal defence mechanism to alert that end range tension of the tissues has been achieved. Maintain the end of range tension for a minute or so and make an observation of the colour of the palmar aspect of the hand and fingers. Irrespective of ethnicity and skin colour, you will observe blanching of the skin, which indicates that the arterial and venous blood supply has been temporarily diminished or interrupted as a result. On a cellular level there is no exchange of nutrition and oxygen for their respective waste products and the latter are building up within the tissues at this cellular level, as the nutrition and oxygen is metabolized. As you hold your hand at the end of range tension you may find your mechanical pain relatively fades, but ensure you maintain holding your hand in this position at the end of passive range for a whole minute. After at least a minute, let go and simultaneously try and speedily flex your fingers as you do! You should, on release of the end of range tension, experience sudden pain across the palmar aspect of the metatarsophalangeal joints and fingers. You have just experienced chemical pain; observe the skin colour and appearance as you simultaneously palpate the skin with the dorsum of the dominant hand. You should observe and palpate the cardinal signs of inflammation, albeit on a temporary basis. That is redness or *rubor*, swelling or *tumor*, and an increase in skin temperature or *calor* and in this case, this is yet another defence mechanism, a neurovascular system reflex to prevent tissue damage at the cellular level. The waste products of nutrition and oxygen are noxious to the body; cells would die without an adequate blood supply to transport the nutrition and oxygen to the cells and tissues and the subsequent waste products away. In an attempt to neutralize and eradicate the waste products that are released from the cells into the extracellular space, hypervasodilatation occurs with extracellular fluid increasing to dilute the noxious products, followed by a return to the vascular system transporting them away for the body to dispose of. Had this reflex response not taken place, cellular and collateral cellular damage could occur. If blood supply is completely lost through trauma or disease, the tissues become ischaemic and die.

Now consider a constantly contracted postural maintaining muscle intrinsically reducing its own blood supply, and then imagine this being sustained for long periods followed by muscle relaxation by lying down or sitting back and adopting a different posture. The physiological responses are likely to be as previously described, but because the tissues have not been placed at the end of range tension, mechanical pain would not be experienced. Furthermore, while lying down, or possibly not until going to sleep in a bed, chemical pain may be experienced. In this scenario, and if this is repeated chronically on a daily basis, the inflammatory response would lead to paraspinal muscular thickening and it is often bilateral. However, with mobile technology items containing screen displays and long periods of looking down at these, or where PC operators are working with a screen to one side, the symptomatic and palpable findings may be unilateral. It is worth noting that as patients correct their postural habits and the paraspinal thickening reduces, a residual fibrotic feel to the muscles may be palpated as the chronic inflammatory response leads to the development of scar tissue that can reduce and remodel to an insignificant and, indeed, impalpable level over time.

The previous example serves to warn against making assumptions that serious pathology exists in the presence of an isolated Red Flag such as night pain and as Selfe and Greenhalgh (Chapter 3) explain if in any doubt, always seek a colleague to discuss your suspicions with. In addition, try to consider and exhaust all the biological reasons and causations for pain before labelling a patient with a Yellow Flag, or worse, inducing unnecessary anxiety which will further induce psychosocial problems. Greenhalgh and Selfe (Chapter 3) warn not to forget the 'bio', which

should serve as a warning to practitioners, professionals, service providers and all other stakeholders with an interest in the biopsychosocial health of the individual and society at large.

## The Clinical Flag System: From Red, Orange, Yellow, Blue and Black Flags to the Green Flag

In order to avoid repetition, the reader should refer to the refer to Chapter 3 (Selfe and Greenhalgh) and add any other Chapters that may refer to the Clinical Flag System in any large part.

The clinical coloured flag system is excellent as a model for raising clinician awareness and as a screening tool for guidance in clinical practice, giving direction for decision-making and serving to simplify and classify what can be a complexity of potential and actual findings during examination and assessment of the patient. Similarly, the previously referred to models, such as the redundant numbering system for derangement syndrome in the McKenzie method of mechanical diagnosis and the current numbering system for neural dynamic or tension testing, appear to be an attempt to simplify and classify a mechanical diagnosis following examination by site, direction and the extent of derangement in the former and examination technique to help determine the neural dynamic diagnosis and treatment intervention for the latter. Some therapists in previous years may have experienced a greater problem recalling the numbers of the numbering systems and their respective definitions rather than the definitions or classifications themselves. The same could apply to the colours of the clinical flag system, where the clinician has to recall the flag colour as well as the definition and as flag colours are added, recalling the respective flag colour and definition can equally become problematic. It is for this reason that this chapter embraces the biopsychosocial model, which is integrated into the World Health Organization's (WHO, 2013) International Classification of Functioning, Disability and Health framework (ICF).

If the practitioner should find themselves having difficulty recalling the clinical flag system colours and definitions, the biopsychosocial model by virtue of its name prompts the practitioner to consider the patient more holistically across the biopsychosocial spectrum.

The biopsychosocial model was conceptualized, during the 1960s and 1970s by Engel (Adler, 2009; Alonso, 2003; Engel, 1981) and initially introduced to health professional education in North America during the 1970s (Ross, 2007), but it was not until the turn of the twenty-first century that the model was recognized and began to be adopted across the health and medical professions in the UK.

If psychological stress can lead to disease, such as cancer and death, which is widely accepted within the literature, there is a duty of care to ensure we fully address the bio of MSK problems, its causations, contributing factors and safe criteria-based habilitation or rehabilitation and reintegration into a higher level of functional activity, in order to avoid therapist or service provision/nonprovider inducement of psychosocial problems.

It remains to operationalise the Clinical Flag System through the Biopsychosocial Model and on screening for serious medical and psychiatric pathology and psychosocial barriers to rehabilitation; the practitioner would need to decide whether other referrals are required to address any positive findings before proceeding to intervene with treatment and management of the physical problems the patient presents with. Through this screening process, examination and assessment, the practitioner should recognise being able to safely proceed with physical interventions. At the risk of introducing yet another coloured flag, it would be worth introducing a coloured flag that indicates it is safe to proceed with physical intervention. A Green Flag has been introduced in the following algorithms that have been designed for the undergraduate and early graduate practitioner to engage with for their own professional biopsychosocial practice and clinical flag system application development. Figure 7.13 is to be considered in conjunction with Figures 7.1B and 7.4 in order to determine where strengths and weaknesses in practitioner knowledge and skills may exist with regards to the application of the clinical flag system and the biopsychosocial model and to determine whether they exist and where, in addition to how the learning needs are going to be met and/or what other support is required in practice.

Figure 7.14 serves to guide the undergraduate and neophyte practitioner through the clinical flag system screening process in the context of application of the biopsychosocial model and to determine whether it is safe and pertinent to progress towards physical intervention, which is denoted by a Green Flag. If, however, alternative or coreferrals are appropriate in the presence of a Red, Orange, Yellow, Blue or Black Flag for alternative intervention or comanagement, this is made explicit through engaging with the algorithm.

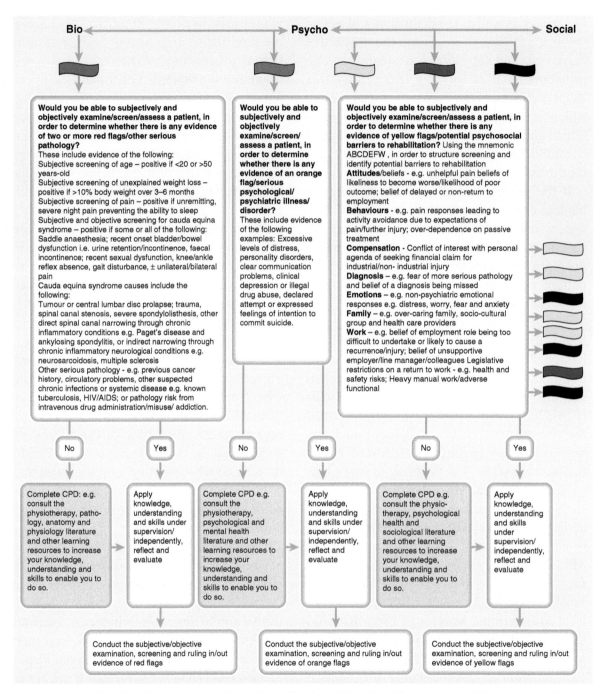

FIGURE 7.13 ■ Algorithm for your preparedness for application of the clinical flag system and biopsychosocial analysis of patients.

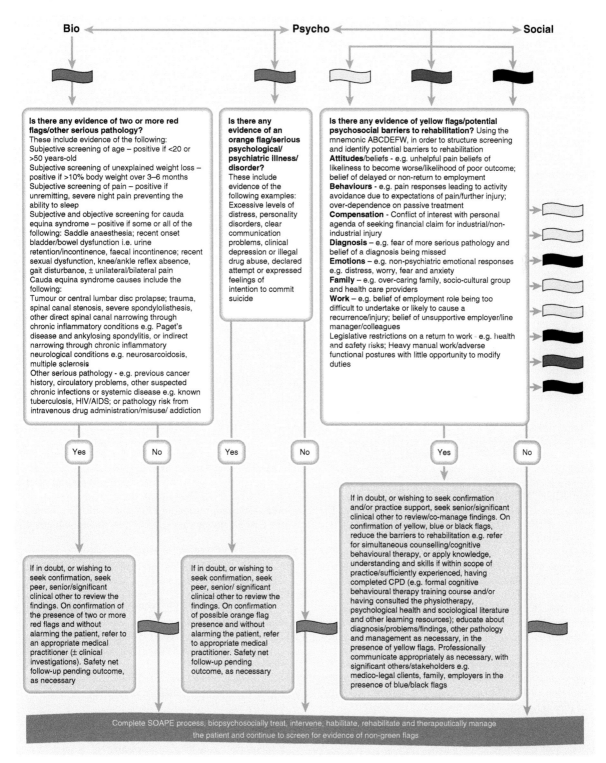

FIGURE 7.14 ■ Clinical flag system algorithm for determining whether it is safe and pertinent to progress towards physical intervention and whether additional or coreferrals are appropriate for alternative or comanagement.

Using the algorithms, determining whether you are either prepared or are supported to work safely and methodically in practice, determines whether a Green Flag indicates to proceed with physical intervention.

## References

Adler, R.H., 2009. Engel's biopsychosocial model is still relevant today. J. Psychosom. Res. 67, 607–611.

Al-Obaidi, S.M., Al-Sayegh, N.M., Nakhi, H.B., Skaria, N., 2013. Effectiveness of McKenzie Intervention in Chronic Low Back Pain: A Comparison Based on the Centralisation Phenomenon Utilizing Selected Bio-behavioural and Physical Measures. In: International Journal of Physical Medicine and Rehabilitation, vol. 1, No. 4. pp. 1–8. Available online at: <http://www.omicsonline.org/effectiveness-of-mckenzie-intervention-in-chronic-low-back-pain-a-comparison-based-on-the-centralization-phenomenon-utilizing-selected%20bio-behavioral-and-physical-measures-jpmr.1000128.pdf> (accessed 04.22.16).

Alonso, Y., 2003. The biopsychosocial model in medical research: the evolution of the health concept over the last two decades. Patient Educ. Couns. 53, 239–244.

Bassot, B., 2013. The Reflective Journal. Palgrave Macmillan, Basingstoke, p. 35, 58, 28, 48.

Baxter, R.E., 2003. Pocket Guide to Musculoskeletal Assessment, second ed. Elsevier, Philadelphia.

Bleakley, C.M., 2010. Acute Management of Soft-tissue Injuries: Protection, Rest, Ice, Compression & Elevation Guidelines. ACPSM, London.

Bleakley, C.M., Glasgow, P., MacAuley, D.C., 2012. PRICE needs updating, should we call the POLICE? Br. J. Sports Med. 46 (4), 220–221.

Chamberlain, A., (Unpublished). The Planning and Management of Work-based Continuing Professional Development in NHS Physiotherapy Departments: Focusing on the In-service Education Model.

Chamberlain, A., Munro, W., Rickard, A., 2013. Muscle Imbalance. In: Porter, S. (Ed.), Tidy's Physiotherapy, fifteenth ed. Churchill Livingstone Elsevier, Edinburgh, p. 164.

Chartered Physiotherapy of Physiotherapy, 1994. Continuing Education Information Paper No. 3, Continuing Professional Development Strategy. Chartered Society of Physiotherapy, London, pp. 1–7.

Chartered Physiotherapy of Physiotherapy, 2001. Developing a Portfolio: A Guide for CSP Members. Chartered Society of Physiotherapy, London, p. 73.

Chartered Society of Physiotherapy, (2015), The CPD Cycle. available at <http://www.csp.org.uk/documents/cpd-cycle> (accessed 22/1015).

Engel, G.L., 1981. The Clinical Application of the Biopsychosocial Model. J. Med. Philos. 6, 101–123.

Gibbs, G., 1988. Learning by Doing: A Guide to Teaching and Learning Methods. Further Education Unit, Oxford Polytechnic, Oxford.

Gibbs, G., 1998. Learning by Doing: A Guide to Teaching and Learning Methods. Further Education Unit, Oxford Polytechnic, Oxford.

Greenhalgh, S., Selfe, J., 2010. Red Flags II: A Guide to Solving Serious Pathology of the Spine. Churchill Livingstone Elsevier, Edinburgh, p. xx.

Griffin, C., 1995. Curriculum and Course Design – Study Guide. University of Surrey, Unit 0-10, p. 5.8.

Hengeveld, E., Banks, K. (Eds.), 2005. Maitland's Peripheral Manipulation, fourth ed. Elsevier Butterworth-Heinemann, Philadelphia.

Jarvis, P., 1985. The Sociology of Adult and Continuing Education. Croom Helm, London, p. 50.

Jarvis, P., 1987. Adult Learning in the Social Context. Croom Helm, London.

Jarvis, P., 2006. (ebook 2010). Towards a Comprehensive Theory of Human Learning. Routledge, Abingdon, p. 23.

Jarvis, P., 2009. Contemporary Theories of Learning: Learning Theorists in Their Own Words. Routledge, London, p. 4.

Jarvis, P., Holford, J., Griffin, C., 2003. The Theory and Practice of Learning. Kogan-Page, London, p. 71.

Kerr, K.M., Daley, L., Booth, L., 1998. for the Association of Chartered Physiotherapists in Sports and Exercise Medicine (ACPSM), Guidelines for the Management of Soft-Tissue (Musculoskeletal) Injury With Protection, Rest, Ice, Compression and Elevation (PRICE) During the First 72 Hours. Chartered Society of Physiotherapy, London.

Kilby, J., Stigant, M., Roberts, A., 1990. The reliability of back pain assessment by physiotherapists, using a McKenzie algorithm. Physiotherapy 76 (9), 579–583.

Kolb, D., 2015. Experiential Learning: Experience as the Source of Learning and Development. Prentice Hall Book, New Jersey. page reference required, pp. 50–64.

Kolb, D.A., 1984. Experiential Learning: Experience as the Source of Learning and Development, first ed. Prentice Hall, New Jersey.

Maitland, G.D., Hengeveld, E., Banks, K., English, K. (Eds.), 2005. Maitland's Vertebral Manipulation, seventh ed. Butterworth-Heinemann, Philadelphia.

Mbada, C.E., Ayanniyi, O., Ogunlade, S.A., 2015. Comparative Efficacy of Three Active Treatment Modules on Psychosocial Variables in Patients with Long-term

Mechanical Low Back Pain: A Randomised Controlled Trial. In: Archives of Physiotherapy, vol. 5, No. 10. pp. 1–9. Available online at: <https://archivesphysiotherapy.biomedcentral.com/articles/10.1186/s40945-015-0010-0> (accessed 04.22.16).

McKeown, C., Summers, E., 2008. Collins English Dictionary. Harper Collins, Glasgow, pp. 196, 208.

McKenzie, R., 1981. The Lumbar Spine: Mechanical Diagnosis and Therapy. Spinal Publications New Zealand, Waikanae. Book page reference required.

McKenzie, R., May, S., 2003. The Lumbar Spine Mechanical Diagnosis and Therapy, vols. 1-2. Spinal Publications New Zealand, Waikanae, pp. 426, 701.

McKenzie Institute International, (in print). Mechanical Diagnosis and Therapy Educational Material Part A-D Manuals. The McKenzie Institute International, Raumati Beach, New Zealand.

McKenzie Mechanical Diagnosis and Therapy Organisation, (Undated). Mechanical Diagnosis and Therapy: Classification. Available online at: <http://www.mckenziemdt.org/forms/ClassificationChanges.pdf> (accessed 09.22.15).

O'Sullivan, J., 1996. The benefits of structured learning in the workplace. Frontline 2 (18), 14–15.

Oxford Dictionaries, (2016), Accessed online 03/3/16 at <http://www.oxforddictionaries.com>.

Panjabi, M.M., 1992a. The stabilising system of the spine, part I. Function, dysfunction, adaptation and enhancement. J. Spinal Disord. 5 (4), 383–389.

Panjabi, M.M., 1992b. The stabilising system of the spine, part II. Neutral zone and instability hypothesis. J. Spinal Disord. 5 (4), 390–397.

Ross, J., 2007. Occupational Therapy and Vocational Rehabilitation. Wiley, Chichester, pp. 61–62.

Sanghvi, S., 2013. Cardiac rehabilitation. In: Porter, S. (Ed.), Tidy's Physiotherapy, fifteenth ed. Churchill Livingstone Elsevier, Edinburgh, pp. 147–168.

Selye, H., 1951. General-adaptation-syndrome. Annu. Rev. Med. 2, 327–342.

World Health Organization, 2013. How to Use the ICF: A Practical Manual for Using the International Classification of Functioning, Disability and Health (ICF). Exposure Draft for Comment. WHO, Geneva, p. 5.

# THE PSYCHOLOGY OF THE ATHLETE – THE PHYSIOTHERAPIST'S PERSPECTIVE

ANDREW MITCHELL

## CHAPTER CONTENTS

## BACKGROUND

I am a chartered physiotherapist with a master's degree in sport and exercise science. I have worked in five different professional sports clubs and been the head physiotherapist at four football clubs, namely Burnley, Bolton Wanderers, Wigan Athletic and Chel-tenham Town. The exposure I received to the latest treatments and rehabilitation techniques was therefore an outcome of touring the world whilst working in professional sport.

Within the professional domain, I have rehabilitated a multitude of injured athletes back to competing at a professional standard,

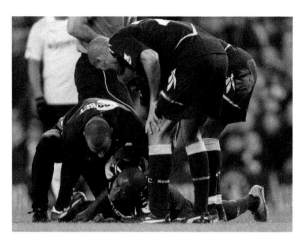

FIGURE 8.1 ■ Physiotherapist Andy Mitchell administering medical care to Fabrice Muamba who suffered a cardiac arrest during an FA Cup football match at White Hart Lane in March 2012.

many of whom have been premiership footballers with international experience. My experience in the field of physiotherapy extends to academia as well, where I have lectured on physiotherapy to undergraduate and postgraduate students at York St John and the University of Salford, UK.

Therefore this chapter, which draws on both personal experience and desk based research, reflects a meeting point between my training and expertise in professional and academic settings. Its overall aim is to provide an overview of the potential psychological responses a professional or amateur sports person may experience and to present certain tools you can use as a chartered physiotherapist to care for them.

## INTRODUCTION

This chapter describes the psychological responses of athletes to injury and the ways in which a physiotherapist can employ psy-

chological strategies to help the athlete through the process. The possible psychological precursors to injury opens up this discussion which is aptly followed by an explanation of the responses of athletes in the three critical stages of the injury process; (1) the onset of the initial injury, (2) the rehabilitation phase and (3) the return to competition (RTC) phase. The subsequent section highlights the importance of goal setting and how this can be utilized to the advantage of the athlete during the previously named stages. With a focus on social support, the third section first examines what athletes can expect from their physiotherapist and concludes with further expansion on the types of social support that are required in the specific stages of recovery. The closing section gives an overview of other psychological strategies that can be used and the manner in which the whole process can be monitored with several psychological tools that are being used clinically.

## PSYCHOLOGICAL PRECURSORS AND ATHLETIC RESPONSES TO INJURY

### Psychological Precursors to Athletic Injury

An awareness of the psychological precursors to athletic injury can help the physiotherapist better understand the athlete in their care. Injuries are deemed to be freak unexplainable incidents resulting from either a tackle that comes from a blind side or from an innocuous tendon rupture which occurs despite no history of symptoms. However, for most athletes a plethora of psychological reasons have been suggested as having the capacity to increase the likelihood of the onset of injuries.

These reasons are split into three main categories and appear to indicate that athletes who are frequently injured have certain personality characteristics, a history of stressors and poor coping resources (Johnson, 2006).

What these reasons seem to suggest, in essence, is that they are inextricably linked and interconnected. Physiotherapists need to be aware that athletes who are more susceptible to injury tend to have low self-confidence and self-esteem. They perceive situations as stressful and lack hardiness within their makeup compared with athletes that appear less at risk and more resilient (Williams and Andersen, 1998). Athletes may exhibit higher levels of competitive anxiety and sense that the locus of control in sporting situations is outside of their influence.

A history of stressors in the athlete's past is also present in these high-risk athletes (Johnson, 2007). These could be large historical events such as bereavements, failures and relationship problems or even more short-term daily hassles. The short-term daily hassles could include irritations over performance, finances, daily responsibilities and difficult relationships with coaches and peers. Although previous athletic injury is a key factor that falls within the category of previous stressors, it can cause fear, apprehension and hesitancy during training and competition (Johnson, 2006). An athlete's coping resources enables them to appropriately appraise and keep situations in perspective. The presence of a support network of people around them has been shown to buffer stress, reduce fear and self-blame and keep a level of control in their sporting activity. Athletes with a poor coping system and minimal support network have been shown to exhibit heightened stress and to have a higher risk of being subject to injury (Ivarsson and Johnson, 2010).

The athletes that experience those previously listed factors have been shown to appraise situations as stressful and threatening. This leads to an increased distractibility, increased levels of muscle tension and a narrowing of their field of vision or attention span (Monsma et al., 2009). These variables may increase the vulnerability to injury by disrupting the athlete's coordination, movement and ability to detect important environmental cues (Maddison and Prapavessis, 2005). Consequently the physiotherapist needs to be aware of all of these potential underlying factors when working with athletes during the recovery process. Inevitably the personality, individual history of stressors and coping resources of the athlete will influence how they respond to injury, rehabilitation and RTC (Walker et al., 2007).

## Responses to the Initial Onset of Injury

The overriding feelings at the onset of injury are made up of shock, disbelief and helplessness through a complete lack of control (Evans et al., 2012; Johnston and Carroll, 1998). Often the physical harm to the body and the shock of incapacitation deeply affect the athlete, because the injury to the athlete's body may change as injured body parts become swollen, bruised and cause pain. Surgery may result in scars, muscle wastage and the need to use aids such as crutches, slings, braces or boots. These physical adaptions can heighten this negative emotional response, especially if the injury is severe. Arguably the same process occurs on a shorter more minor scale with less severe injuries as the physical changes and incapacitation can be outlived within days.

During this initial incapacitation at the onset of injury, clear communication is vital as verbal insensitivity from medical staff, peers and coaches about factors such as the diagnosis and prognosis can have dramatic psychological effects on the athlete (Bianco and Eklund, 2001). Sometimes cementing the fate and diagnoses can even be, in some cases, emotionally disabling for the athlete. Similarly a lack of an accurate diagnosis can fuel the feelings of helplessness, frustration and, undoubtedly, a sinking feeling of depression. Changes to the routine of being away from the team and the lack of stimulation from exercise can lead to boredom and the feeling of isolation. Athletes frequently cite the inability to drive, cook, and complete activities of daily living (ADL) as being the main causes behind the negative emotions they experience at the onset of injury as they lose their independence and become ever more isolated (Mitchell et al., 2014).

### Responses to the Rehabilitation Phase

Once the initial onset phase has subsided and the athlete enters the rehabilitation process, they generally become much more settled. Regaining a certain degree of independence and being able to exercise manifests itself in physical and mental signs of progression (Carson and Polman, 2008; Podlog et al., 2015).

Despite this general uplift in emotions and wellbeing, many athletes can plateau during this rehabilitation phase and display negative emotional responses. A repetition of exercises, the same uninspiring gym accompanied with a lack of progress or even rehabilitation

setbacks, such as pain and repeated swelling, can be a recipe for possible unrest (Rees et al., 2010). As a consequence, athletes will report feeling bored, frustrated and suffer a drop in motivation levels. Classically this combination reduces self-confidence and adherence to the rehabilitation plan (Bianco et al., 1999). This is heightened in long-term injuries by a seemingly inevitable loss of fitness and skills, and occasionally a weight gain as a result of relative inactivity. Moreover athletes feel isolated from their peers, fans, and especially time strapped coaches who tend to focus on the team and the next game or event. A lack of contact and communication between both of these key parties widens the gap increasing the guilt and lack of identity felt by the athlete. Athletes feel guilty for not being able to help and support their peers during events as they cannot perform. This is further explained by how often athletes report losing their sense of identity as a sports person feeling useless and worthless to their peers or the coaches during this rehabilitation phase (Evans et al., 2012; Podlog and Dionigi, 2010).

### Responses to the Return to Competition Phase

The RTC phase is a notorious period for a whole host of emotional responses felt by the athlete. Physically and psychologically the athlete may be expected to go from being injured to performing again. This transition from being cared for and labelled as injured to actually putting the kit on, competing in front of thousands and being judged on every move is a difficult transition. Understandably this intensifies their anxiety, their feelings of stress and often their lack of control during this key transitional period (Clement et al., 2015; Glazer 2009). They automatically question the robustness of the injury, their fitness and skill levels and tactical decision-making. They will ask themselves, can I still do it? Will my body hold out and has the competitive standard gone up since I last played (Podlog et al., 2011)?

Furthermore, athletes feel a tremendous amount of vulnerability over the fear of reinjury. This is a common feeling that athletes describe as leading to heightened levels of anxiety and stress. Completing the position or action that led to the injury could therefore be very unsettling. Athletes become hesitant, lose confidence and sometimes hold back from giving 100% because of this fear of reinjury (Wadey et al., 2014).

External pressures from coaches and peers as well as the influence of the 'sport ethic' are other important factors to consider in the RTC phase. The sporting culture comprises the notion that athletes should play in pain and play while carrying injuries or they will be viewed as soft or letting the team down (Podlog and Eklund, 2005). For these reasons they may lose their sense of control over when to RTC, as the decision may in some cases appear to be made by other parties like the coach or the physiotherapist. In light of this, during this delicate decision of RTC, the consideration of all parties, such as the medical personnel, coaches and most importantly the athlete, are critical. A strategic approach to open communication and goal setting needs to be established so the athlete can openly voice their ideas and feelings regarding rehabilitation and their RTC. This keeps the locus of control with the athlete, where there is an element of input from the other key parties (Arvinen-Barrow et al., 2014; Podlog and Eklund, 2007a).

Conversely to the perfectly planned RTC decisions are the ones that are rushed and pressured. In such circumstances, the athlete may still be experiencing pain, swelling and minor setbacks. If the whole RTC process has been poorly organized there will be a lack of communication and trust. This will lead to athlete distress, anxiety and a feeling of being out of control about the prospect of returning to competitive action (Podlog and Eklund, 2009).

## GOAL SETTING AND CREATING THE RIGHT ENVIRONMENT

### Introduction to Goal Setting

Goal setting is the most widely used technique by physiotherapists in the rehabilitation process of athletes (Arvinen-Barrow et al., 2010). It is the area physiotherapists feel they know most about with regards to its application and potential benefits. Simply put, it is the process of setting targets or aims for the athlete to work towards. If set appropriately, goals can increase adherence, motivation, confidence and the athlete's feeling of self-worth (Evans and Hardy, 2002a). Physical goals can be utilized to increase the manner of the athlete's physical characteristics, ranging from flexibility, strength, proprioception, skill acquisition and power, among others (Bizzini et al., 2012).

### Time Scales and Types of Goals That Can Be Used

The physiotherapist, with a sound understanding of the types of goals and factors surrounding each goal, can really utilize them for the benefit of the athlete. With the rehabilitation process being described as an unpredictable matrix of rapid progression and disappointing setbacks, it is paramount that goals are flexible and can be adjusted when required (Gilbourne and Taylor, 1998). Failure to do this will debilitate the athlete's response and confidence instead of facilitating them. Ideally goals should be joint decisions made between all parties; often at the onset, and in the rehabilitation phase, this is restricted to the athlete and the physiotherapist. Once the athlete enters the RTC phase input from the coach can also be extremely beneficial. At all times keeping the athlete at the centre of the process is paramount as it will fuel their sense of autonomy, value and self-esteem (Arvinen-Barrow et al., 2014; Hamson-Utley et al., 2008).

For long-term injuries of 3 months or more, goals are often set into short-, intermediate- and long-term categories. Short-term goals are normally 7 to 10 days or could even be within the space of a couple of days. These are frequently readjusted and improved upon to mount towards the intermediate-term goals, which may be set every 6 to 12 weeks. Long-term goals naturally come to be poignant towards the latter stages and can make up the RTC criteria or performance based specifics that the athlete may want to achieve (Podlog and Eklund, 2009). It is therefore highly recommended that the time scales of goals are kept flexible in order to adapt them for the specific athlete in need.

Further clarity can be given to goals as they are set to be either performance or outcome based. These types of goals aim to achieve specific scores for time, distance, weight or repetition. Conversely they could be set as process driven goals. These aim to achieve a certain skill, movement or technique; for example, accomplishing heel strike while walking, or the execution of a specific turn or technique with a ball (Evans et al., 2000). Setting holistic goals for the rest of the athlete's body to improve fitness capabilities that they may feel weak in are also valuable. This will drive their sense of accomplishment, satisfaction and achievement. Finally, lifestyle type goals like completing studies, coaching certificates or starting a business all have proven to be significantly beneficial in stimulating a positive vibe for the recovering athlete (Podlog et al., 2011). Once again the time scales of goals should be very flexible, but the principles discussed are important and can be applied to athletes according to their specific individual needs.

With the physiotherapist having this underpinning knowledge to set them, let us look in more detail at the potential positive, and in some cases, if set inappropriately, negative effects goal setting can have.

## Positive and Negative Effects of Goal Setting

The psychological benefits of goal setting are well published and should not be ignored (Hamson-Utley et al., 2008). Reemphasis of this to the physiotherapist can in turn be really beneficial for the recovering athlete, if implemented correctly. Appropriate goal setting can, as a result, foster communication, trust and rapport between both parties involved. Ideally setting goals in such a way that the athlete is at the centre of the decision-making process increases their sense of control and autonomy and reduces their anxiety. They verbally report a sense of direction, a mental route map for progress and a focus towards their goals (Clement et al., 2013; Vergeer, 2006). This will manifest itself through increased adherence, motivation and commitment to the treatment and rehabilitation exercises. The exclusion of the athlete in the decision making process and setting unrealistic goals will often prove to be counterproductive and result in decreased adherence, confidence and motivation (Brewer et al., 2000). Poorly planned goals that lack physiotherapist and athlete interaction will inevitably debilitate the latter on their route to recovery (Podlog and Eklund, 2007b).

## A Clinical Example of Goal Setting With an Elite Athlete (Professional Footballer) Recovering From an Anterior Cruciate Ligament Rupture Injury

The physical characteristics of the elite athlete being considered for this case study can be presented in the following manner. The professional footballer is 25 years in age, 190 cm in height and weighs 80 kg. Having been a full-time professional since the age of 16, he competes at premiership and international levels. Although he is right foot dominant, he occupies the centre back position. The athlete in question has had no previous history of major injury or trauma. Having twisted the right knee on landing (flexion, valgus, external rotation mechanism of knee injury), he has suffered an isolated anterior cruciate ligament (ACL) rupture, which was reconstructed with a bone-patella-tendon-bone graft from the ipsilateral knee 10 days post injury.

Given that this athlete is recovering from ACL reconstructive surgery and has no post-surgical complications, a whole host of goals can be set around the specifics of the injury. These could include goals that target reducing the pain or swelling, goals centred on how many repetitions of flexion they can do

| TABLE 8.1 |
|---|
| **An Example of Short-, Intermediate- and Long-Term Goals for an Elite Athlete (Professional Footballer) Recovering From an ACL Rupture** |

**ACL Day 1 Post Surgery, Short-Term Goals (0–10 Days)**

1   Achieve 90-degree knee flexion

2   Normal gait pattern on stairs with crutches

3   Complete 10 minutes on a static cycle with no resistance

4   Sign up for a coaching course or external commitment outside of the club/work environment

5   Complete two light upper body sessions with team mates

**ACL Day 10 Post Surgery, Intermediate-Term Goals (6–12 Weeks)**

1   Achieve 120-degree knee flexion

2   Normal gait pattern to start low level running drills

3   Can now complete all cycle sessions unlimited

4   Feedback information to coaches, peers or medics on progress of external learning

5   Can now complete all team upper body sessions unlimited

**ACL 9 Months Post Surgery, RTC Long-Term Goals (6–12 Months)**

1   Full prone knee bend (by being able to kneel comfortably)

2   Complete bleep, sprint and agility fitness running tests

3   Complete fitness sessions with sports scientists/conditioners or physiotherapist on the grass and in the gym

4   Complete external learning activity and conduct sessions on the topic, etc.

5   Complete all team lower limb strength/fitness sessions unlimited

or what range of extension they have achieved. All of these are perfectly valid and clinically useful, but often the professional athlete under daily care will already be working towards these goals regardless. They will form their daily drudgery of rehabilitation, their daily treatment and will not carry the sense of achievement and special identity that a goal should have. Achieving a goal needs to be acknowledged and considered as something special so that it in turn gives the athlete a sense of fulfillment, increasing their confidence and well (Clement et al., 2013).

### Short-Term Goals

Table 8.1 provides some alternative goals that were set for this case study and have been frequently requested by players in the sporting environment. Goal number one is an outcome type of goal aiming to achieve 90 degrees of flexion. Goal number two is more of a process driven goal requiring the injured player to carry out the process and skill of being able to walk normally up the stairs. By completing this it will also help in the recovery of their ADL. They will be able to move better at home as they become more confident in starting to regain their independence. The cycling in goal number three will produce not only the underlying physiological benefits of range of movement and muscle strengthening, but often, and more importantly, psychological benefits. This should be carried out in the team gym or a public gym where teammates can work alongside the recovering athlete as this positive interaction will reduce the feeling of being isolated. Furthermore, it offers the case study in question some team involvement, as often coaches passing through provide encouragement, support and positive interaction.

Goal number four is a lifestyle type goal, allowing the case study to complete a coaching course would broaden their experiences, allow them to meet new people and face fresh challenges giving them something new to share at home or at work. Finally, although goal number five has very little association with the knee, its implications are highly relevant from the psychological perspective. The completion of the upper body sessions will give the case study the exercise feel-good factor they all experience after an exercise session and permit the athlete to continue to interact with their team mates. This positive social interaction will increase their sense of wellbeing, self-worth and reduce isolationism as it is carried out within the normal team schedules.

In this case study, daily interaction between the physiotherapist and the elite athlete to continually discuss and work towards the classic ACL rehabilitation goals is essential. These goals of range, pain and swelling in this short-term phase should never be overlooked or underestimated, as they are imperative for the knee to successfully heal. However, from a psychological perspective, the player actively selecting and engaging in the goals listed in Table 8.1 will provide a holistic plan with varying strands they can work towards. Too many goals will become unmanageable and the focus will be lost. Too few will not provide the wide array of physical and psychological benefits that have been explained. Ideally between four and six will prove to be a feasible number for the case study to work towards, focus on and ultimately gain a sense of achievement from once they are accomplished.

## Intermediate-Term Goals

Intermediate-term goals for an elite athlete similar to the one being discussed in this case study could be set on day 1 with the aim of achieving them at roughly 12 weeks post surgery.

The first goal stays in alignment with the short-term goal number one as the flexion is increased now to 120 degrees. This is often achieved before 12 weeks increasing their sense of accomplishment and a desire to keep improving. The word 'running' stimulates any sportsperson. This has been left flexible as it could be done on the antigravity running machine (alterG), a treadmill, on the grass or even in the pool depending on how competent the player has become. This wide scope and flexibility means the goal will be achieved through some method of running and will not cause player disappointment and frustration by failure to achieve it.

In the intermediate-term goals, numbers three and five include unlimited cycling and upper body sessions, which will stress and highlight to the case study their independence as they will do these with the rest of the squad. The professional athlete that trains daily can be integrated with their peers for these sessions. They can buddy up with other injured players, work with their teammates and even work under the supervision of other members of the multidisciplinary team (MDT) such as a strength and conditioning coach or sports scientist for these sessions, see Fig. 8.2. The physiotherapist with medical knowledge will know the exact parameters the injured body part can work under. This can be shared and relayed to the strength and conditioning coach so that they are com-

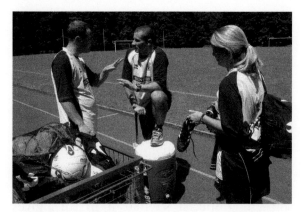

FIGURE 8.2 ▪ Members of the multidisciplinary team (MDT) discussing how to integrate an injured athlete into the appropriate team sessions.

pletely aware of the injury-specific limitations that the recovering athlete has and how they can be incorporated into team sessions. Athletes love and clamor for such team involvement. If this is discussed and carefully planned by all parties, it can have a very positive psychological and physical effect on the case study in question. Hopefully by now, goal number four, chosen as part of their lifestyle goal, is well underway so that they can provide positive feedback of their new education and experience to the physiotherapist, peers or, better still, to engaging coaches.

## Long-Term Goals

The long-term goals are inextricably linked to the RTC criteria for this elite level footballer. These can justifiably be set on injury specifics like achieving full knee hyperextension, flexion, proprioception, and isokinetic strength and hop scores, for example. From personal experience it could be said that these are very useful but are very specific physiotherapist-related goals. These classic physiotherapy type goals need to be achieved and accomplished if the athlete suffering from an ACL injury is going to have a safe RTC. From a physiotherapeutic perspective these clinically relevant goals should not be overlooked. Close attention should be paid to precise detail as it is vital that they are accomplished.

However, they give primary satisfaction to the physiotherapist and often secondary satisfaction to the athlete. To make them more functional, Table 8.1 has suggested functional goals athletes would choose, aspire to and focus on for their safe return. The theme from day 1 is continued throughout all of the goals. The goal of range of movement progresses from 90 degrees, to 120 degrees, to now full kneeling down completing the full range of knee flexion. The second goal, which initially involved stair walking, is improved to a form of running at the 12 week stage. This is then further progressed to be unlimited running on the traditional running tests used for an elite level footballer. The cycling fitness sessions are translated into functional fitness sessions where players have to reproduce preinjury statistics on key aspects such as sprints, match day running distances and heart rates. By this stage the case study, who often has a lot of time on their hands, should also have completed goal four, the lifestyle goal, and thereby educated themselves. This goal driven process offers a feeling of positivity to the player's rehabilitation process. If the player is successful in these four goals, fulfilling goal number five will be a natural progression as they can be classed as similar to their peers in the squad strengthening and fitness sessions. This is another point of integration and method in encouraging the transition from being injured to being fit and normal again.

## Goal Setting – A Summary

Goals, as previously explored, can be presented through different media, in either the written or verbal formats. They in essence need to be functional, interesting and challenging for the athlete. As a result seemingly perfect physiotherapeutic designed goals like firing a multifidus at a certain level or improving balance by 1 second will not necessarily stimulate or motivate athletes in the same way as the ones we have discussed in this clinical example. Similarly setting too many goals and changing them too often will reduce their importance and lessen the athlete's focus and drive towards reaching their milestones.

With a view of setting goals in a feasible and pragmatic manner, they can be organized in conjunction with other team members or other recovering athletes. Although fostering a sense of camaraderie, it will surely raise performance and improve outcomes. Goals can be made public, when appropriate, on the treatment room or gym wall (Podlog and Eklund, 2006). They can also be signed for which can all aid to increase their sense of importance. Occasionally having standard goals that peers have previously achieved can help peer modelling. Peers will offer their empathy and encouragement as they see their supportive role as beneficial in helping the recovering athlete. In brief, goals are vital for athletes and should be employed as often as possible. What is more, making them functional, and interesting whilst placing the athlete at the centre of the process is a means of heightening the success rate in the rehabilitation journey.

## The Key Characteristics and Attributes of a Physiotherapist Working With Athletes

An eminent physiotherapist working with athletes tends to demonstrate the following characteristics and attributes: on one hand they need to be positive, enthusiastic, understanding and caring, and show high levels of motivation, on the other hand, they need an up-to-date skill base, have the capacity to set goals, maintain perspective and be a source of support at all times (Francis et al., 2000). The physiotherapist needs to make the athlete feel safe, special and feel like they are a high priority (Tracey, 2008).

A sense of trust and rapport can be developed quickly, especially if the physiotherapist projects an atmosphere of equality and empowerment in the decision-making and recovery process. The sports physiotherapist should never compromise professionalism as they are regularly pressurized by players, coaches, agents and sometimes even teammates to return the athlete. At all times an appropriate attitude, dress code and choice of language help to constitute the persona of a successful physiotherapist working with athletes. Furthermore, although being consistently professional, it is vital that the physiotherapist is able to recognize which attributes they need to emphasize in a given situation (Arvinen-Barrow et al., 2014; Tracey, 2008).

These situations vary considerably as the sports physiotherapist could often find themselves working and making decisions in a variety of settings ranging from the pitch side, the gym and even hotel rooms converted into treatment rooms whilst on tour (Jevon and Johnston, 2003). At the pitch side or when the initial injury occurs it is vital

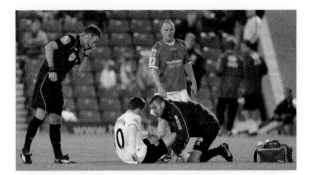

FIGURE 8.3 ▪ The physiotherapist has to maintain a standard of care despite working in challenging environments in the sporting world.

that the physiotherapist is organized and remains calm, see Fig. 8.3. In such situations, which are beyond one's control, athletes typically experience confusion and uncertainty (Mitchell et al., 2014). Undeterred by the crowded pitch side or the congested medical room, the physiotherapist needs to be composed and methodical in their approach to assisting the injured athlete. Once removed from the arena the physiotherapist can commence their assessment after emptying the medical room of coaches and peers. One should take care never to lose sight of one's role as a chartered physiotherapist. The creation of a quiet environment to conduct your traditional subjective and objective assessment is paramount for the physiotherapist to insist on. This will enable the physiotherapist to make an accurate diagnosis, administer appropriate treatments and ensure high physiotherapeutic standards throughout.

When touring with teams or covering camps, athletes may require treatment and rehabilitation in unfamiliar surroundings; in the event where physiotherapists set up an *ad hoc* treatment room or open-air facility and use poorly equipped gyms for rehabilitation.

Every situation is unique but it is necessary that the physiotherapist be armed with a range of preplanned rehabilitation sessions for that specific athlete. Utilizing sports like rowing, cycling, swimming and boxing, and having a vast catalogue of exercises for rehabilitation can reduce the athlete's boredom and prevent or minimize frustration from setting in. Being flexible and thoughtful in the approach adopted by the physiotherapist means the athlete's time is always well spent and purposeful for their needs. Athletes unable to complete tasks or take part in rehabilitation sessions are ultimate disappointments for them, but the successful physiotherapist with ingenuity and ideas can overcome this scenario and keep them involved.

It is inevitable that athletes experience highs and lows during the recovery process and it is vital that the physiotherapist maintains a state of relative equilibrium. Sometimes it may even be the role of the physiotherapist to deliver bad news, which can be uncomfortable and unsettling. Occasionally athletes seek alternative care and may not agree with the advice being offered by the physiotherapist. These situations can occur with the highly motivated athlete and as a physiotherapist it is crucial to maintain professionalism despite potentially personal and clinical differences about the best care pathway. Hopefully working with the athlete and investing time in them as a patient and a person will permit you, as the physiotherapist, the most appropriate way to communicate information to the individual (Podlog and Eklund, 2007a). As with all patients, delivering the information in a thoughtful, simple and honest manner is all within your professional scope and practice as a chartered physiotherapist.

During the unfortunate incident of a career-ending injury, the transition experience may be worse for the athlete because, unlike in the injury process, there is no return. Consequently those with unfulfilled ambitions forced into an abrupt sporting end may feel anger, loss, helplessness and frustration. It can lead to many negative effects such as isolation, depression, addiction and in rare cases even suicide (Stoltenburg et al., 2011). For the amateur athlete the end of the one off weekly sporting venture can potentially be accepted more easily than the elite level performer that has devoted their life and sole ambition to their sport. This sudden lack of routine, focus and constant absorption in their sport is taken away from them. For the elite who have often foregone education, hobbies, family life and travelling because of being consumed by their sporting activity from a young age, the sport is all they have experienced and known. It can therefore leave them psychologically poorly equipped for coping with life after sport, which can occur in the twenties or thirties for many sports people (Smith and McManus, 2008).

In such rare scenarios one key priority of the physiotherapist is to provide the best medical care pathway for the injured athlete. This includes care for the foreseeable future and long-term advice on how to manage the injury with a view to achieving the best quality of life after sport. Throughout the injury process and in this career-ending stage, the physiotherapist should encourage a passion in the athlete for other endeavors like education, hobbies and social circles inside and outside of the sporting environment

(Stoltenburg et al., 2011). Social support is vital during this end point, mobilizing relationships with peers that have been through the process, coaches and teammates can all help the athlete cope with the transition. Support services from professional bodies and organizations from within the specific sport should also be sought to help the athlete accept the change and transition ahead (Drawer and Fuller, 2002). Encouraging the athlete to plan for retirement early in their career is important and can actually be harvested during the injury process of a long-term injury. Appropriate injury care, social support, goal setting and offering ideas of a plan B for when retirement occurs are all part of the psychological interventions the physiotherapist could offer the athlete in a career ending scenario.

## SOCIAL SUPPORT FOR ATHLETES

### What Athletes Expect From Their Physiotherapist

Injured athletes spend a lot of time in the presence of physiotherapists. Physiotherapists physically provide treatment, a variety of rehabilitation techniques and, often, engage in time-consuming activities like travelling with and transporting athletes around. As this encapsulates a lot of time, it should come as no surprise that injured athletes view the physiotherapist's role as increasingly critical in their recovery (Arvinen-Barrow et al., 2007). Athletes expect the physiotherapist to be an educator, to simplify and teach them about the specifics of their injury. They expect them to be able to clarify medical terms, set goals and provide an uncomplicated route map they can relate to (Podlog and Dionigi,

2010). Athletes consider such communication from the physiotherapists to be vital. They want to be informed, listened to, understood and empowered in the recovery process they are enduring. Athletes want physiotherapists to understand their needs, fears, desires and even more holistically how this injury may affect their lives on a wider scale. If the physiotherapist can meet such expectations of the athlete then a trusting rapport between the two parties can be fostered by regular, clear and honest communication (Tracey, 2008).

On a more day-to-day basis athletes expect the physiotherapist to be open, trustworthy and likeable. Athletes respond to physiotherapists who listen, motivate them and make them feel safe in their presence (Walker et al., 2007). Athletes claim that successful physiotherapists, in addition to having all these traits, often depict deeper psychological skills. Physiotherapists who are positive and have a sense of leadership and a purpose are viewed more favourably by the athlete. They hope the physiotherapist can sense the intricacies of the balance between work and rest for each individual case (Clement et al., 2012). They are able to add variety and fun whilst keeping the focus on the underlying goals and objectives (Arvinen-Barrow et al., 2007). Athletes warm to the physiotherapist who shares their of desire to return quickly and safely back to competition (Bianco, 2001). They like physiotherapists who have up-to-date techniques, and are knowledge bound by a positive energy to return the athlete safely back to competition (Francis et al., 2000).

### Types of Social Support

Research surrounding the role of social support has shown to have significant beneficial psychological effects in health care and especially sports medicine. Providing athletes with social support during the recovery process has been shown to reduce distress and increase their motivation and adherence levels. By influencing these three factors alone it will undoubtedly increase the likelihood of positive outcomes post injury (Mitchell et al., 2014; Rees et al., 2010).

Social support can be provided intentionally and in some instances even unintentionally by a wide spectrum of people that the injured athlete comes into contact with. Physiotherapists, coaches, peers, family members, surgeons, supporters, agents, to name a few, will all interact with the injured athlete. These complex relationships and interactions will form the basis of the social support surrounding the athlete (Podlog and Eklund, 2007a). As can be seen in Table 8.2, social support has been categorized as either taking the form of emotional, informational or tangible. Emotional social support is when the person in contact with the athlete assumes

### TABLE 8.2

**Types of Social Support and Examples the Athlete May Require During the Recovery Process**

| Types of Social Support | STAGE OF THE RECOVERY PROCESS | | |
|---|---|---|---|
| | **Initial Onset** | **Rehabilitation** | **Return to Competition** |
| Emotional | Family members, peers and the physiotherapist may engage in: listening, comforting, compassion, empathy, understanding and sharing | A physiotherapist may: be positive and enthusiastic, set up peer modelling for emotional support and to reduce isolation, provide a positive atmosphere in the treatment and rehabilitation setting | Physiotherapist, peers and coaches may engage in: building confidence, positive reassurance, reducing competition anxiety, encouragement, reducing fears of reinjury or poor performance |
| Informational | The physiotherapist may: clarify medical terms and resolve unwanted myths, answer questions<br><br>Educate the athlete: about the injury, the types of treatment and rehabilitation that is required, provide a sense of perspective, set short-term goals and an injury route map the athlete can relate to | Effective communication about the efficacy of treatment and rehabilitation; ideas and methods to overcome the potential lack of progress and/or rehabilitation setbacks<br><br>Appropriate goal setting | Medical clearance, education about the test results and goals moving forward<br><br>Coaches may provide: sports specific technical information, performance analysis, help to plan realistic performance expectations |
| Tangible | Assistance with activities of daily living (ADLs), transportation, transfers around the work place or to appointments | Potentially utilizing different environments to reduce boredom; willingness to provide a variety of exercises and rehabilitation sessions | Organizing fitness tests, 1–1 sessions, practice sessions with peers |

the role of listening, understanding and caring as they provide empathy. Informational social support occurs as the other person in the relationship (often the physiotherapist) provides education, answers specific questions and sets goals, for example. Tangible social support is the physical help received by the athlete with activities like preparing food, driving and ADLs. In the later stages tangible social support may come in the form of the sessions and practices organized by the coach or physiotherapist to help the injured athlete in their quest to return (Bianco and Eklund, 2001).

Social support for all human beings, especially for athletes, is in higher demand during crisis points, which, as suggested by research, are often at the onset of the injury, during the rehabilitation setbacks and finally at the critical RTC phase (Mitchell et al., 2014). With this in mind, the discussion of this section will now move on to social support in these three key areas and highlight concurrently the traditional types of social support that are specifically required during a particular phase of the recovery process.

## The Initial Onset of Injury

At the initial onset of an injury, athletes experience dramatic physical and psychological changes within a short space of time. Physically they will be in pain, have swollen limbs, scars and bruises and may even require surgery, often putting them into complete immobilization. Losing their place in the team as a result of the injury will affect them psychologically; they will feel isolated as their sense of self-esteem and confidence is shattered. Because of these abrupt changes, it is vital that they get the right type, and amount

of, social support (Podlog and Eklund, 2004).

On leaving the pitch or arena where the injury occurred, players report the events that happen following either in slow motion or too fast, leaving no room for clarity or comprehension. After the initial incident athletes often face endless questions from medics, surgeons, physiotherapists, players, coaches and family members. They sometimes are bombarded with information from scan results, hospital appointments and other tests. With the athlete being medically untrained this can be a very unsettling period. The uncertainty, the what ifs and the medical dialogue involving unknown terms and decisions mean that, naturally, the athlete will require appropriate social support (Horvath et al., 2007).

Initially family members take on the role of offering emotional social support as the armor most sportspeople wear in their sporting setting is removed once they are home in familiar surroundings. Family members will need to be able to listen, comfort and allow the athlete to vent their frustrations and fears. Similarly in the professional setting the physiotherapist will need to empathize, show comfort and affection during this initial crisis point (Bianco, 2001; Carson and Polman, 2008).

From Table 8.2 it is clear that informational social support is key to the physiotherapist's skill set during this initial stage. In the midst of the appointments, scans and examinations they need to provide perspective and accurate information to the athlete. They need to be able to answer questions, allay fears and provide a route map for the injury so the athlete can easily understand and relate to it.

The physiotherapist needs to be professional and trusting during this time. They are ideally situated to unravel and simplify the athlete's concerns, which is a vital social skill in supporting the injured athlete (Bianco and Eklund, 2001).

Accompanying this, the physiotherapist, in this initial onset of injury phase, will set some short-term goals for the athlete to focus on. They will provide some role models in the form of well-educated peers and generally make the athlete feel safe and trusting in the care they receive (Mitchell et al., 2014). Often the athlete's family members who also need some subtle social support tend to go unnoticed. Their emotional response to their dearest family member being injured can often manifest itself in a similar way to the athlete's emotions. From personal experience, it could be said that family members are no different from the athlete and need educating about the injury and how it will unfold. They need to be listened to, have their fears calmed and gain trust in the care pathway the physiotherapist has laid out for their loved one. Further emotional social support is sometimes needed for the coaches who feel a loss, report feeling depressed and frustrated by the loss of a key player. Table 8.2 suggests how tangible social support, such as transport to treatment sessions; help with ADLs and assistance in the work place should not be overlooked either. Creating this safe and caring environment at work and at home is essential for the type of social support athletes require during this initial stage (Clement et al., 2012).

Once in the work place, the coach has a small but very important role in the social support an injured athlete receives during this stage. Although general reassurance from the coach about the long-term outlook is advisable, it should be reiterated that simple words reassuring the athlete that they will be supported through the process can be priceless when delivered by the coach. Moreover, coaches informing players that an injury will not affect their long-term place and future is invaluable for the player's overall sense of wellbeing. Similarly, during this time, peers, especially those who have suffered similar emotions and changes, can provide empathy. They can act as a confidante and role model the athlete can look to as someone who overcame adversity. This source of perspective, encouragement and inspiration is close to hand and should be encouraged. The physiotherapist is suitably placed to encourage these relationships between injured athletes and their peers (Podlog et al., 2011).

## The Rehabilitation Phase

Once in the rehabilitation phase, athletes commonly show strong motivation and are extremely focused as their self-confidence is mirrored by their progress. However, this progressive phase can have setbacks which can be psychologically testing for multiple reasons. As a sense of boredom at the continual drudgery of monotonous exercises may set in, the lack of progress and setbacks may make the athlete frustrated and demotivated. Besides the separation from the rest of the team and sometimes even the financial costs of rehabilitation, not having the ability to compete can weigh heavily on the injured athlete causing psychological stress (Evans et al., 2012).

Another point Table 8.2 highlights is how the climate of the rehabilitation room can prove to be a valuable source of social support during this time. A positive atmosphere and vibe in the treatment room and gym can be very productive and powerful during the rehabilitation process (Magyar and Duda, 2000). Ideally it gains its supportive, positive and inspiring nature from how it has been designed and the people that work in it. Furthermore having a rehabilitation buddy can be extremely beneficial to injured athletes. It not only allows them to share troubles and achievements, but also to form an alliance and a bond as they motivate one another. This would help to reduce their feeling of isolation as they have somebody to work with, to pick them up and to encourage them, other than the physiotherapist who chiefly has this role (Clement et al., 2013; Gould et al., 1997).

During this phase the physiotherapist principally supplies social support, as all of the key attributes they have will be utilized. The close interaction between both parties gives the physiotherapist a prime position to see what is physically and psychologically feasible for a specific athlete at a given point in time. For example, sometimes for the injured athlete being around their peers and fellow athletes may be a positive influence. With this in mind encouraging further team sessions and involvement can translate into a form of positive social support.

Conversely continual frustrations and negative social comparisons may require the physiotherapist to suggest the athlete withdraw from team sessions (Podlog and Eklund, 2007a). A rest from rehabilitation, a different working environment and fresh people to work with may provide the athlete with a different form of social support (Arvinen-Barrow et al., 2010); an environment they feel

more comfortable with, where they feel it is more positive and energizing. Consideration can be given to whether the athlete would benefit from speaking to peer models away from their normal working environment, as they may provide an independent arm of social support unaware of the pressures and hassles of the environment they normally exist in (Podlog and Dionigi, 2010).

## The Return to Competition Phase

During this complex phase the athlete will naturally experience a whole host of emotional responses that may range from fear of reinjury and failure, to worry over not hitting preinjury performance standards, to hesitancy and a lack of self-confidence (Ardern et al., 2012). Players may feel hugely uncertain about their fitness level and technical skills, and the ability of their injured body part to withstand competitive demands. This all tends to manifest itself in a competitive anxiety, lack of confidence and fear.

Once the player has entered this phase, the role of the physiotherapist and the coach is critical, as indicated in Table 8.2. The physiotherapist, along with other members of the medical team, must provide the athlete with a medical clearance for the injury in question (Ardern et al., 2013; Bianco et al., 1999). This is made possible once they safely complete relevant fitness and injury tests. The athlete should achieve certain criteria to be given the medical all-clear. Accomplishing these requires the physiotherapist to provide all forms of social support to the athlete: tangible support by organizing the correct sessions and tests, informational support by educating the player about the testing and future direction for the injury and finally emotional social support to encourage and positively reinforce the athlete throughout this process. The collective ingredients of these types of social support will help to build confidence and self-esteem and provide the reassurance the athlete needs to go on to successfully compete again (Podlog et al., 2015; Vergeer and Hogg, 1999).

Arguably one of the most important individuals to provide social support in this RTC phase is the coach. Coaches that distance themselves, alienate athletes and rarely interact with them will only enhance the athlete's negative emotions already mentioned. Limited communication and interplay does not build trust between the coach and the athlete. Coaches choosing not to discuss and set realistic expectations for the returning athlete will only increase the pressure the athlete feels and heighten their negative emotions (Podlog and Eklund, 2007b).

A successful coach during this phase takes an active role. They should view themselves as facilitating the athlete's return to play. They are a vital cog in the decision making process, but should not be claiming the role of chief decision maker. Ideally they can provide emotional social support by providing feedback, encouragement and a sense of perspective on expectation levels. When an athlete is out for several months with a long-term injury, returning immediately at preinjury levels is impossible. Their speed of return varies from case to case but often takes several months and a sense of perspective about this being relayed to the athlete by the coach can certainly help to alleviate pressure (Podlog and Eklund, 2006). Informational social support from the coach can take the form of technique tips and game analysis that only

the coach is in a position to provide. The coach can ease the athlete's fears and help them through this phase by informing them of positional specifics and tactical information. Finally, tangible social support such as organizing one on one sessions, practice exercises or matches can be extremely positive in building the player–coach relationship and alleviating the negative emotions athletes experience during this phase (Podlog and Eklund, 2007a).

Similar to the coach, peers and senior athletes in the sporting environment can help provide the social support mentioned in Table 8.2. Failure by the coach or the teammates to deliver such support leaves the physiotherapist to offer as much of it as they feel comfortable doing. Recognizing one's own personal limitations in this situation is what the physiotherapist should consider as the main aim in returning the athlete to competition safely and successfully. Conversely negative coaches or peers can have a debilitating effect on how the athlete reacts during this phase. Precisely, as stated in the initial onset of injury phase, it falls to the remit of the physiotherapist to regulate and monitor these interactions for the benefit of their patient, the athlete.

## FURTHER INTERVENTION, PSYCHOLOGICAL ASSESSMENT, TIPS AND WHEN TO REFER ON

### Imagery

Imagery is defined as cognitively reproducing or visualizing an object, scene or sensation as though it were occurring in an overt physical reality (Driediger et al., 2006). From an injury perspective, it is clear how an athlete can use imagery to visualize a skill or even more simply imagining an injured body part healing. However, there has been reluctance by some sports physiotherapists to use imagery in the athlete's rehabilitation process. This may result partly from hesitancy over why it should be used and how it can be employed successfully (Green and Bonura, 2007). When adopted, it can be utilized in a very specific and organized fashion with set time periods for imagery per day, or alternatively subtly woven into the athlete's daily care (Johnson, 2000). If executed correctly imagery has been shown to decrease pain levels, increase strength, speed recovery and improve the athlete's confidence and adherence (Vergeer, 2006). Because of the uncomplicated method of its application, imagery can be encouraged and incorporated into all stages of the athlete's recovery process.

## Initial Onset of Injury

During this stage when the athlete will be experiencing pain, swelling and uncertainty about the injury, healing imagery can be extremely useful. Providing the athlete with simple images, ie, videos, pictures or anatomical models of what has happened and more importantly of the process of repair allows them to visualize this process (Schwab Reese et al., 2012). The provision of education by the physiotherapist using simple terms and images will enable the athlete to comprehend, understand and encourage the repair process. Emphasis and focus on this moving forward can be calming and self-rewarding for the athlete. Visualizing pain and what is physiologically happening if pain is present can emphasize the need to avoid and reduce it.

Accompanying this visualization, the slow stretching type of sensation often envisaged as the tissue starts to heal and regain flexibility can enhance the athlete's understanding of how to use this sensation to their advantage. Educating and training the athlete to differentiate between these two sensations is a vital skill as they seek to reduce pain and enhance the healing process in the injured body part (Vergeer, 2006).

## The Rehabilitation Phase

The imagery skills taught initially can be incorporated and encouraged through all stages of the rehabilitation process. Traditionally the rehabilitation phase is considered to be progressive and energetic as the athlete can use imagery to visualize achieving goals, learning new exercises and relearning sport-specific skills (Schwab Reese et al., 2012). The athlete can be trained to use imagery to visualize achieving a future goal or the specific execution of an action for the injured body part, all of which should be encouraged. Attentively focusing on physical cues and details has been shown to increase self-confidence, speed recovery and increase the athlete's adherence to rehabilitation. The advantage of utilizing goals and promoting peer modelling often allows injured athletes to visibly see the necessary requirements being performed by their peers. Visually affirming what they are focusing on and trying to achieve this will naturally embed positive images in their subconscious mind (Monsma et al., 2009).

## The Return to Competition Phase

Ideally through the two stages already discussed the athlete has been visualizing the route map they are travelling along. The final section of this rehabilitation journey is the RTC phase. As a result of raised anxiety in this phase imagery can be extremely useful. The fear of reinjury and underperforming should be counterbalanced by more facilitative images. DVDs of successful past performances or the athlete performing challenging end stage rehabilitation should be encouraged and provided (Green and Bonura, 2007). The athlete should be encouraged by the physiotherapist to picture positive experiences and images of successful past performances. This will foster confidence and raise their level of self-esteem as they picture themselves competing successfully against and with their peers (Podlog and Eklund, 2009). It will contribute to their sense of control and comfort as they use imagery to visualize their injured body part meeting the required standards to compete again. Positive reinforcement during this stage from the physiotherapist, the athlete's peers and more importantly the coach can help their psychological wellbeing (Podlog and Dionigi, 2010).

### Psychological Tools That Can Be Used to Assess Athletes

To date there have been over 300 psychological tests published related to sport and exercise. Questionnaires designed for sports medicine practitioners measure anything from the athlete's stress, adherence, motivation, confidence, mood state, to even readiness to return to sport. The main aim in this instance of using such a tool is to gain reliable information about a specific factor in the athlete's recovery process. The chosen questionnaire needs to be user friendly and accessible so that ideally athletes can complete it within minutes. Minimal disruption to the

athlete's routine means you can gain multiple sets of data which can help to spot subtle pertinent differences (Sachs et al, 2007).

Honest and regular use of the questionnaires by athletes could demonstrate slight differences that may be lost in day-to-day communication. Detection of vital trends such as a loss of confidence, drop in energy levels or adherence can be identified accurately through the correct use of such inventories. After this, issues can be openly discussed and the appropriate strategies put in place to aid in the recovery of those psychological aspects the athlete may be suffering from. Therefore the use of regular, quick and easy questionnaires can be extremely beneficial to the physiotherapist and athletes as opposed to laborious and irregular data collection through inappropriate methods (Sachs et al., 2007).

Three simple questionnaires to consider which assess mood, readiness to return to sport and reinjury anxiety are worth further consideration by physiotherapists working with athletes. Initially McNair et al. (1971) created the profile of mood states, but Dean et al. (1990) reduced the 65-point questionnaire into a six-point assessment. The brief assessment of the mood questionnaire uses a six-point scale to assess anxiety, sadness/depression, confusion, anger, vigor/energy and fatigue. By adding all of the negative scores and then subtracting by the positive score (vigor) the amount of total mood disturbance can be revealed. A low score may mean the athlete is in a positive mood state, whereas a high score may suggest that they have a negative mood state. The athlete can be asked to evaluate their mood over the previous 24 hours, 7 days or a much longer period leading up to the time of the assessment (Dean et al., 1990).

Walker et al. (2010) devised a 28-item reinjury anxiety inventory (RIAI) which can be used to assess reinjury anxiety in rehabilitation and competition. It reflects the athlete's confidence, fear of reinjury and their overall anxiety about their rehabilitation or the prospect of competing. Finally, the injury-psychological readiness to return to sport (I-PRRS) is a six-item questionnaire assessing all the key concerns athletes have about their readiness to return to competition. It addresses their overall confidence in their skills and injured body part, their pain awareness, their hesitancy and concentration levels. Each component is scored out of 100 and divided by 10, ideally scores between 50 and 60 may suggest that the athlete feels they are ready to compete. Scores below 50 should be treated with concern as psychologically it may indicate the athlete does not feel they are quite ready to compete again (Glazer, 2009).

These three questionnaires are ideal for the athlete because of the ease with which they can be completed and the direct information and feedback they can provide. For the chosen tool to be used wisely it should be presented to the athlete regularly throughout their recovery process. The information, like all medical information, needs to be carefully reviewed as it can present subtle trends and problems that can be successfully addressed through the psychological strategies suggested. These strategies can be added to the honest and frank discussions between the athlete and physiotherapist that need to regularly occur throughout the whole recovery process. Failure to have open communication will inevitably produce problems in this complicated process of caring for the injured athlete. Like all tests the physiotherapist and the athlete should realize that these tools are a part of the whole process of care. The results of the tools used should not be treated in isolation. Instead, they should be considered in conjunction with other psychological and physical factors that the physiotherapist and athlete are reviewing regularly.

### Other Tips and Considerations

The discussion so far has provided a comprehensive account of the psychology of the injured athlete from the physiotherapist's perspective. The sections that follow provide further tips that can complement and build on those previously mentioned fundamentals.

Athletes, especially team sportspeople, respond to rehabilitation exercises that contain variety and are functional to the sport they compete in (Arvinen-Barrow et al., 2007). Ideally stimulating the injured athlete, while using a ball or a racquet depending on their sport, will help to keep it fun as they will always push themselves harder in sports-specific rehabilitation exercises. This notion of sports-specific rehabilitation does not need to be exclusive to the end stage, as imagination and close attention to the pathology can employ these methods early on (Gould et al., 1997). A change of the rehabilitation scenery with the use of a variety of settings and the creation of a reward system within the routine can aid in the athlete's motivation. Rewarding athletes on completing tasks may allow them to pick certain aspects of the follow sessions or grant them periods of down time, which are useful ploys. It encourages the athlete's feelings of empowerment and helps to maintain motivation during months and months of daily rehabilitation in long-term injuries (Clement et al., 2013).

The ingenuity and variety of the rehabilitation always need to be closely linked to the athlete's goals. Keeping them athletically active with clearly defined goals will help to maintain their adherence to the long-term plan (Naylor, 2007). After the injury, pursuing nonsporting goals, like learning a new skill, a hobby or spending time with family can aid in their coping process, especially in the case of the elite athlete. Often the elite athlete has disposal time, unlike the working amateur sportsperson, so channelling this time into positive outcomes is beneficial (Carson and Polman, 2008; Podlog et al., 2014).

Similarly encouraging athletes to keep a blog, write a diary or chart their feelings and progress is a good way to foster self-efficacy and confidence (Evans and Hardy, 2002b; Schwab Reese et al., 2012). Athletes now often keep a video diary allowing them to share their accomplishments with peers, which encourages peer support and interest. The physiotherapist should encourage all of these ways to engage with the athlete. Athletes feeling a sense of worth will take a positive interest in their own rehabilitation, inevitably leading to positive outcomes (Podlog et al., 2011).

Finally communicating to the coach about their role in the recovery process should not be underestimated, see Fig. 8.4. Coaches need to be educated about the injury process, psychological implications and the transition back into competition (Podlog and Dionigi, 2010). The physiotherapist should express to the coach how they need to maintain regular

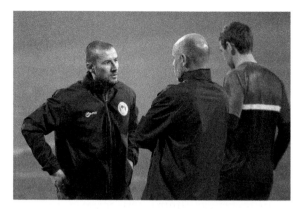

FIGURE 8.4 ■ The physiotherapist should work closely with the coach to educate them and encourage their role in the recovery process of the injured athlete.

communication with all injured athletes. Athletes need the coach to be providing encouragement and support through their rehabilitation process and technical assistance when starting the RTC phase. Clarifying with coaches how some athletes can take up to 6 months to regain full confidence in their injury and performance is vital to set realistic expectations and clear goals that everybody can work towards (Podlog and Eklund, 2006).

Commonplace in hospital settings are regular MDT meetings, during which patients and their needs are reviewed. These should be adopted in the care of the athlete whenever possible to discuss care pathways and management. Also meetings incorporating the athlete help to create open communication, clearer goals and expected outcomes everybody can agree on (Francis et al., 2000; Gilbourne and Richardson, 2005; Podlog, 2006).

### Referring on and the Rationale

The close relationship and time spent between the physiotherapist and the athlete naturally places the physiotherapist in a prime position to detect abnormal responses and behaviours in the athlete. Many athletes will certainly feel isolated, depressed and anxious about their injury and pending rehabilitation. The physiotherapist needs to be aware of the host of behaviours athletes may exhibit and be especially conscious of more deep-rooted problems that may manifest during this period (Mitchell et al., 2014).

Athletes being overly withdrawn, restless or lethargic all need to be observed closely by the physiotherapist. Injury can cause a loss of identity resulting in athletes feeling cheated, worthless and even in rare cases suicidal (Walker et al., 2007). Consequently, observing for substance abuse, lack of sleep and strange eating habits all need to be carefully considered by the physiotherapist. Similarly, exercise addiction, eating disorders and a poor attention span are abnormal behaviours which are not normally associated with athletes and should raise alarm bells for the physiotherapist (Arvinen-Barrow et al., 2010).

If the physiotherapist working with injured athletes suspects behaviour they feel unskilled to care for, referral should be made to other members of the MDT (Arvinen-Barrow et al., 2014). Sensitivity in handling this information and these patients means it should only be discussed with the correct members of the MDT. Ideally the athlete's GP, sports doctor or lead physiotherapist will have the appropriate procedures in place to refer on to specialists. The named senior practitioners will hopefully have encountered this rare type of patient before and have experience in how to manage them. As with all patients that have complex needs, sensitivity is paramount during communication to promote the correct referral pathway and best serve the athlete's clinical requirements.

## CONCLUSION

This chapter has described the psychological responses of athletes to injury and the ways in which a physiotherapist can use psychological strategies to help the athlete through the process of recovery. After acknowledging the variety of responses that athletes may demonstrate one can start to employ beneficial psychological strategies to aid the athlete. The benefits of setting appropriate goals and creating a positive environment for the athlete were reiterated in the former half of the discussion. It was also noted that a positive effect on the athlete could be enhanced further by providing the right social support, by meeting the athlete's expectations and by possessing certain characteristics as a physiotherapist. Drawing on experience and evidence, the use of imagery was then suggested as a useful method in the different stages of the recovery process. The closing remarks of this chapter emphasized that the attentive physiotherapist will observe many psychological responses and should be well placed to detect abnormal responses that require the athlete to be referred on for specialist psychological care. Overall, this chapter provides a basis of potential psychological strategies the chartered physiotherapist could employ whilst managing an injured athlete.

### References

Ardern, C.L., Taylor, N.F., Feller, J.A., Webster, K.E., 2012. Fear of re-injury in people who have returned to sport following anterior cruciate ligament reconstruction surgery. J. Sci. Med. Sport 15 (6), 488–495.

Ardern, C.L., Taylor, N.F., Feller, J.A., Webster, K.E., 2013. A systematic review of the psychological factors associated with returning to sport following injury. Br. J. Sports Med. 47 (17), 1120–1126.

Arvinen-Barrow, M., Hemmings, B., Weigand, D., Becker, C., Booth, L., 2007. Views of chartered physiotherapists on the psychological content of their practice: A follow-up survey in the UK. J. Sport Rehabil. 16 (2), 111–121.

Arvinen-Barrow, M., Massey, W.V., Hemmings, B., 2014. Role of sport medicine professionals in addressing psychosocial aspects of sport-injury rehabilitation: professional athletes' views. J. Athl. Train. 49 (6), 764–772.

Arvinen-Barrow, M., Penny, G., Hemmings, B., Corr, S., 2010. UK chartered physiotherapists' personal experiences in using psychological interventions with injured athletes: An interpretative phenomenological analysis. Psychol. Sport Exerc. 11 (1), 58–66.

Bianco, T., 2001. Social support and recovery from sport injury: elite skiers share their experiences. Res. Q. Exerc. Sport 72 (4), 376–388.

Bianco, T., Eklund, R.C., 2001. Conceptual considerations for social support research in sport and exercise settings: The case of sport injury. J. Sport Exerc. Psychol. 23 (2), 85–107.

Bianco, T., Malo, S., Orlick, T., 1999. Sport injury and illness: elite skiers describe their experiences. Res. Q. Exerc. Sport 70 (2), 157–169.

Bizzini, M., Hancock, D., Impellizzeri, F., 2012. Suggestions from the field for return to sports participation following anterior cruciate ligament reconstruction: soccer. J. Orthop. Sports Phys. Ther. 42 (4), 304–331.

Brewer, B.W., Van Raalte, J.L., Petitpas, A.J., Sklar, J.H., Pohlman, M.H., Krushell, R.J., et al., 2000. Preliminary psychometric evaluation of a measure of adherence to clinic-based sport injury rehabilitation. Phys. Ther. Sport 1 (3), 68–74.

Carson, F., Polman, R.C.J., 2008. ACL injury rehabilitation: A psychological case study of a professional rugby union player. J. Clin. Sport Psychol. 2 (1), 71–90.

Clement, D., Arvinen-Barrow, M., Fetty, T., 2015. Psychosocial responses during different phases of sport-injury rehabilitation: A qualitative study. J. Athl. Train. 50 (1), 95–104.

Clement, D., Granquist, M.D., Arvinen-Barrow, M., 2013. Psychosocial aspects of athletic injuries as perceived by athletic trainers. J. Athl. Train. 48 (4), 512–521.

Clement, D., Hamson-Utley, J., Arvinen-Barrow, M., Kamphoff, C., Zakrajsek, R.A., Martin, S.B., 2012. College athletes' expectations about injury rehabilitation with an athletic trainer. Int. J. Athl. Ther. Train. 17 (4), 18–27.

Dean, J.E., Whelan, J.P., Meyers, A.W., 1990. An incredibly quick way to assess mood states: The incredibly short POMS. *Paper presented at the annual meeting of the Association for the Advancement of Applied Sport Psychology*, San Antonio, TX. p.177 in Sachs, M.L., Sitler, M.R., and Schwille, G. (2007) Assessing and Monitoring Injuries and Psychological Characteristics in Intercollegiate Athletes: A Counseling Prediction Model. In:

Pargman, D. (Ed.), Psychological Bases of Sport Injuries. FiT Publishing, West Virginia University, pp. 131–147.

Drawer, S., Fuller, C.W., 2002. Perceptions of retired professional soccer players about the provision of support services before and after retirement. Br. J. Sports Med. 36 (1), 33–38.

Driediger, M., Hall, C., Callow, N., 2006. Imagery use by injured athletes: A qualitative analysis. J. Sports Sci. 24 (5), 261–272.

Evans, L., Hardy, L., 2002a. Injury rehabilitation: a goal-setting intervention study. / Effet de l'intervention de la psychologie dans le processus de reeducation physique. Res. Q. Exerc. Sport 73 (3), 310–319.

Evans, L., Hardy, L., 2002b. Injury rehabilitation: a qualitative follow-up study. / Reeducation physique: etude qualitative du suivi medical. Res. Q. Exerc. Sport 73 (3), 320–329.

Evans, L., Hardy, L., Fleming, S., 2000. Intervention strategies with injured athletes: An action research study. Sport Psychol. 14 (2), 188–206.

Evans, L., Wadey, R., Hanton, S., Mitchell, I., 2012. Stressors experienced by injured athletes. J. Sports Sci. 30 (9), 917–927.

Francis, S.R., Andersen, M.B., Maley, P., 2000. Physiotherapists' and male professional athletes' views on psychological skills for rehabilitation. J. Sci. Med. Sport 3 (1), 17–29.

Gilbourne, D., Richardson, D., 2005. A practitioner-focused approach to the provision of psychological support in soccer: Adopting action research themes and processes. J. Sports Sci. 23 (6), 651–658.

Gilbourne, D., Taylor, A., 1998. From theory to practice: the integration of goal perspective theory and life development approaches within an injury-specific goal-setting program. J. Appl. Sport Psychol. 10, 124–139.

Glazer, D.D., 2009. Development and preliminary validation of the Injury-Psychological Readiness to Return to Sport (I-PRRS) scale. J. Athl. Train. 44 (2), 185–189.

Gould, D., Udry, E., Bridges, D., Beck, L., 1997. Coping with season-ending injuries. Sport Psychol. 11 (4), 379–399.

Green, L.B., Bonura, K.B., 2007. The use of imagery in the rehabilitation of injured athletes. In: Pargman, D. (Ed.), Psychological Bases of Sport Injuries. FiT Publishing, West Virginia University, pp. 131–147.

Hamson-Utley, J., Martin, S., Walters, J., 2008. Athletic trainers' and physical therapists' perceptions of the effectiveness of psychological skills within sport injury rehabilitation programs. J. Athl. Train. 43 (3), 258–264.

Horvath, S., Birrer, D., Meyer, S., Moesch, K., Seiler, R., 2007. Physiotherapy following a sport injury: stability of psychological variables during rehabilitation. Int. J. Sport Exerc. Psychol. 5 (4), 370–386.

Ivarsson, A., Johnson, U., 2010. Psychological factors as predictors of injuries among senior soccer players. A prospective study. J. Sports Sci. Med. 9, 347–352.

Jevon, S.M., Johnston, L.H., 2003. The perceived knowledge and attitudes of governing body chartered physiotherapists towards the psychological aspects of rehabilitation. Phys. Ther. Sport 4 (2), 74–81.

Johnson, U., 2000. Short-term psychological intervention: a study of long-term-injured competitive athletes. J. Sport Rehabil. 9 (3), 207–218.

Johnson, U., 2006. Sport Injury, Psychology and Intervention: An overview of empirical findings. From: <http://www.idrottsforum.org>.

Johnson, U., 2007. Psychosocial antecedents to sport injury prevention: a case study of competitive soccer players at risk. In: Pargman, D. (Ed.), Psychological Bases of Sport Injuries. FiT Publishing, West Virginia University, pp. 39–49.

Johnston, L.H., Carroll, D., 1998. The context of emotional responses to athletic injury: a qualitative analysis. J. Sport Rehabil. 7 (3), 206–220.

Maddison, R., Prapavessis, H., 2005. A psychological approach to the prediction and prevention of athletic injury. J. Sport Exerc. Psychol. 27, 289–310.

Magyar, T.M., Duda, J.L., 2000. Confidence restoration following athletic injury. Sport Psychol. 14 (4), 372–390.

McNair, D.M., Lorr, M., Droppleman, L.F., 1971. Manual: Profile of Mood States. Educational and Industrial Testing Service, San Diego, CA.

Mitchell, I., Evans, L., Rees, T., Hardy, L., 2014. Stressors, social support, and tests of the buffering hypothesis: Effects on psychological responses of injured athletes. Br. J. Health Psychol. 19 (3), 486–508.

Monsma, E., Mensch, J., Farroll, J., 2009. Keeping your head in the game: Sport-specific imagery and anxiety among injured athletes. J. Athl. Train. 44 (4), 410–417.

Naylor, A., 2007. The Key to Committed Rehabilitation. Athl. Ther. Today 12 (3), 14–16.

Podlog, L., 2006. Returning to sport following injury; Key considerations for coaches and health practitioners. Sport Health 4 (24), 14–17.

Podlog, L., Dimmock, J., Miller, J., 2011. A review of return to sport concerns following injury rehabilitation: practitioner strategies for enhancing recovery outcomes. Phys. Ther. Sport 12 (1), 36–42.

Podlog, L., Dionigi, R., 2010. Coach strategies for addressing psychosocial challenges during the return to sport from injury. J. Sports Sci. 28 (11), 1197–1208.

Podlog, L., Eklund, R.C., 2004. Assisting injured athletes with the return to sport transition. Clin. J. Sport Med. 14 (5), 257–259.

Podlog, L., Eklund, R.C., 2005. Return to sport after serious injury: a retrospective examination of motivation and psychological outcomes. J. Sport Rehabil. 14 (1), 20–34.

Podlog, L., Eklund, R.C., 2006. A longitudinal investigation of competitive athletes' return to sport following serious injury. J. Appl. Sport Psychol. 18 (1), 44–68.

Podlog, L., Eklund, R.C., 2007a. Professional coaches' perspectives on the return to sport following serious injury. J. Appl. Sport Psychol. 19 (2), 207–225.

Podlog, L., Eklund, R.C., 2007b. The psychosocial aspects of a return to sport following serious injury: A review of the literature from a self-determination perspective. Psychol. Sport Exerc. 8 (4), 535–566.

Podlog, L., Eklund, R.C., 2009. High-level athletes' perceptions of success in returning to sport following injury. Psychol. Sport Exerc. 10 (5), 535–544.

Podlog, L., Hannon, J.C., Banham, S.M., Wadey, R., 2015. Psychological readiness to return to competitive sport following injury: a qualitative study. Sport Psychol. 29 (1), 1–14.

Podlog, L., Heil, J., Schulte, S., 2014. Psychosocial factors in sports injury rehabilitation and return to play. Phys. Med. Rehabil. Clin. N. Am. 25 (4), 915–930.

Rees, T., Mitchell, I., Evans, L., Hard, L., 2010. Stressors, social support and psychological responses to sport injury in high- and low-performance standard participants. Psychol. Sport Exerc. 11 (6), 505–512.

Sachs, M.L., Sitler, M.R., Schwille, G., 2007. Assessing and monitoring injuries and psychological characteristics in intercollegiate athletes: a counseling prediction model. In: Pargman, D. (Ed.), Psychological Bases of Sport Injuries. FiT Publishing, West Virginia University, pp. 131–147.

Schwab Reese, L.M., Pittsinger, R., Yang, J., 2012. Effectiveness of psychological intervention following sport injury. J. Sport Health Sci. 1, 71–79.

Smith, J.L., McManus, A., 2008. A review on transitional implications for retiring elite athletes: what happens when the spotlight dims? Open Sports Sci. J. (1), 45–49.

Stoltenburg, A.L., Kamphoff, C.S., Lindstrom Bremer, K., 2011. Transitioning out of sport: the psychosocial effects of collegiate athletes' career ending-injuries. Athletic Insight Journal 3 (2), 115–133.

Tracey, J., 2008. Inside the clinic: health professionals' role in their clients' psychological rehabilitation. J. Sport Rehabil. 17 (4), 413–431.

Vergeer, I., 2006. Exploring the mental representation of athletic injury: A longitudinal case study. Psychol. Sport Exerc. 7 (1), 99–114.

Vergeer, I., Hogg, J.M., 1999. Coaches' decision policies about the participation of injured athletes in competition. Sport Psychol. 13 (1), 42–56.

Wadey, R., Podlog, L., Hall, M., Hamson-Utley, J., Hicks-Little, C., Hammer, C., 2014. Reinjury anxiety, coping, and return-to-sport outcomes: a multiple mediation analysis. Rehabil. Psychol. 59 (3), 256–266.

Walker, N., Thatcher, J., Lavallee, D., 2007. Psychological responses to injury in competitive sport: a critical review. J. R. Soc. Promot. Health 127 (4), 174–180.

Walker, N., Thatcher, J., Lavallee, D., 2010. A preliminary development of the Re-Injury Anxiety Inventory (RIAI). Phys. Ther. Sport 11, 23–29.

Williams, J.M., Andersen, M.B., 1998. Psychosocial antecedents of sport injury: review and critique of the stress and injury model. J. Appl. Sport Psychol. 10 (1), 5–25.

# 9

# USING COUNSELLING AND PSYCHOLOGICAL STRATEGIES WITHIN PHYSIOTHERAPY

LOUISE HENSTOCK ■ HELEN CARRUTHERS

## CHAPTER CONTENTS

## INTRODUCTION

Recognition of the relationship between the physiotherapist and patient is crucial when attempting to achieve optimal patient outcomes. This partnership must be nurtured to create an environment where patients feel comfortable to share often very personal details to allow for a full assessment, and to acknowledge and engage in effective treatment. As such it is important for physiotherapists to consider techniques and strategies that can be used to enhance and nurture engagement in therapy.

This chapter will introduce psychosocial strategies that could be used to this end and the evidence base surrounding them. This area is often not considered a part of the traditional tools and strategies used within physiotherapy, but it is argued that by considering such areas the effectiveness of treatment may be enhanced. It does not aim to provide all of the information needed to use these approaches, but rather to guide and stimulate interest in topics for further study and education.

## WHY DO WE NEED TO USE PSYCHOLOGICAL STRATEGIES?

Communicating meaningfully with patients and family members who are struggling to manage their emotions and mood can be challenging for physiotherapists. Patients attending physiotherapy will be in some degree of distress about their symptoms and prognosis, but this may extend to significant anxiety, depression and/or grief that will

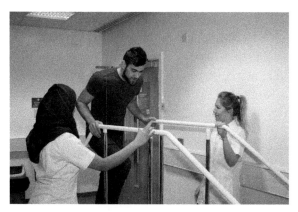

FIGURE 9.1 ■ Therapists should make the most of their interactions with patients.

affect their ability to engage in therapy. Skills gained when using psychological strategies may offer appropriate tools to communicate and engage in these situations to create effective therapeutic alliances.

The aim of using psychological approaches is to ultimately improve the therapeutic relationship and allow the patient to engage in treatments and strategies to improve their health. As physiotherapists, our aim is not to be the sole provider of psychological strategies and to replace other members of the interprofessional team, but to use such strategies to supplement our assessment and management skills in physical therapy. They allow recognition of problems that affect assessment and management and deliver treatment in a way that motivates the patient and produces optimal engagement and effectiveness. As physiotherapists we are a part of the wider interprofessional team and there are other members who are trained specifically to provide more in-depth care if required.

When discussing the effect of a relationship between a health care professional and patient, 'therapeutic alliance' is a term that is often used. A therapeutic alliance is the bond that is created between two parties in a care- or treatment-giving relationship, and the subsequent collaboration and agreement on treatment goals. It is a fundamental element within patient-centred care as explored by Mead and Bower (2000), and must be considered when attempting to create an environment to allow power sharing between the patient and therapist.

Therapeutic alliance has been described and evaluated in different health professional–patient dyads, it has been found to improve patient outcomes and is a long-standing acknowledged dimension of the counsellor–client relationship. Rogers (1967), when introducing patient-centred therapy, explored the empathy, congruence and unconditional positive regard that is necessary and sufficient to create positive change in clients. Physiotherapists and health care professionals could use such strategies to engage with patients and improve therapeutic alliance. The extent of therapeutic alliance between a physician and patient was positively associated with adherence and treatment satisfaction and patient quality of life (Bennett et al., 2011), and a strong relationship exists between therapeutic alliance and self-efficacy with regards to patients following a treatment plan (Fuertes et al., 2007).

There is no reason that the therapeutic alliance should not be applied to the physiotherapist–patient relationship without equally positive results. In fact Hall et al. (2010) discovered that it creates improved patient treatment adherence, physical function and treatment satisfaction and reduces depressive symptoms. In addition, enhanced

therapeutic alliance training for physiotherapists was found to have an effect on the pain
intensity experienced by patients in a double-
blind randomized controlled trial (Fuentes
et al., 2014). If nurturing positive therapeutic
alliances has such positive effects, the effectiveness of physiotherapists will be enhanced
by using strategies to promote them.

## INTERPERSONAL SKILLS
## NECESSARY TO ENHANCE
## THERAPEUTIC ALLIANCES

After acknowledging the importance of nurturing the relationship between the physiotherapist and patient, we must now consider
the interpersonal skills that are important in
developing it. Kidd et al. (2011) explored the
perceived elements of patient-centred care
during physiotherapist treatment. Clear communication, confidence, the understanding
of people, the nature of professional relationships and the transparency of progress and
outcome were emerging themes of importance to patients. Such themes are associated
with the personal qualities of the therapist
and Taber et al. (2011) suggested that it was
personality similarity between the professional and patient that was associated with
enhanced working alliances.

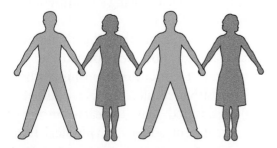

FIGURE 9.2 ■ Patients and therapists should work as a
alliance.

This would suggest that a therapist who is
able to create effective relationships with patients
has an innate quality, but is it enough to accept
that one is just good at this or should we explore
the important aspects so we can engage patients
when struggling to relate to them?

Patient-centred communication is important in creating effective therapeutic alliances,
such as provision of emotional support and
allowing patient involvement in the consultation process (Pinto et al., 2012). Not ignoring
emotional issues that patients may explore
and asking questions with a focus on emotional issues was another finding that emerged
from a related systematic review (Pinto et al.,
2012). Factors that have been found to impede
a therapeutic alliance include discrepancies
between health care professionals and patients
about abilities and family discord (Sherer
et al., 2007). In cases when professionals are
struggling to relate to patients, acknowledging and reflecting on interpersonal skills is
important to ensure that efforts are made to
create effective relationships and engage
patients to the best of our ability.

If communication is important to ensure
patient-centred care is perceived by the
patient, then we must truly listen and attend
to what is being said. Attending involves
becoming focused on the patient and attempting to be fully aware of what they are trying
to communicate. It will involve paying attention not just to what is being said, but also to
our thoughts and reactions to it. Burnard
(2005) discussed three zones when considering attention:

■ *Zone 1* – act of listening to the patient and
  attending to linguistic, paralinguistic and
  nonverbal aspects

- *Zone 2* – act of paying attention to the therapist's own thought processes and being aware of what the patient is saying in the background
- *Zone 3* – therapist is theorizing and interpreting what is happening to the patient.

To effectively communicate with patients in a therapeutic relationship, physiotherapists need to use all three zones. They must listen to and hear what is being said to them, they also need to start to interpret what is happening and its meaning for physical treatment and management. When emotional issues are being discussed, caution needs to be used when interpreting meanings, as some may be fantasy; so checking back to the patient may be useful. Awareness of linguistics is useful when identifying a patient's opinion and includes the words and figures of speech. For example, a person could communicate ambivalence towards their self-efficacy by using the phrase *'I don't know if I can do …'* or *'c'est la vie'*. Paralinguistic aspects such as timing, volume and tone, alongside nonverbal cues are useful to be aware of, as they will also indicate and give insight to the opinion and thoughts of the communicator. Attending to these aspects will enable the physiotherapist to uncover and interpret opinions and allow the relationship to be improved by using psychological strategies. When communicating back to the patient, attention to the words used is equally important and further exploration of neurolinguistic programming may be useful.

## NEUROLINGUISTIC PROGRAMMING

Communication between the therapist and client is of the upmost importance, and attention to the language we use, and the way in which we use it is vital. Neurolinguistic programming is the study of the dynamics between the brain (neuro) and language (linguistics) and how these two aspects interact to affect behaviour (programming).

A system of interpersonal communication and behavioural change intervention was developed by Bandler and colleagues in the 1970s (Dilts, 2011). They studied language patterns used by therapists who excelled in their chosen fields and named this neurolinguistic programming (NLP). The NLP approach to therapy aims to enhance the effectiveness of communication.

According to Dilts and DeLozier (2000), NLP can be viewed as a technology, a methodology and as epistemology. As a technology, NLP consists of frameworks, tools and techniques that can be applied in a clinical arena to strengthen communication and the setting of clear achievable goals. The foundations of the technology are a set of rules known as 'NLP presuppositions' and these are the beliefs that govern NLP. These presuppositions are a guide to how we may not always be able to control what goes on around us; however, we can always control how we respond to it.

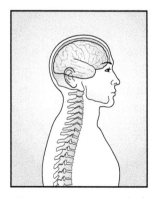

FIGURE 9.3 ■ Can we reprogramme the brain?

■ **The map and territory** – acknowledged as the single most important presupposition in the whole of NLP (originally developed by Alfred Korzybski). The 'map' is a representation of how we organize our experiences in the world and that this is different than the 'territory' – what is actually happening around us. Good communicators realize that we need to remind ourselves to be responsive to what is actually occurring and not just our preconceived perceptions.

■ **The meaning of communication is the elicited response** – people will respond to what they think you mean, regardless of whether that is an accurate or inaccurate representation of what you had intended. Good communicators will be constantly aware of other people's responses and adjust their communication (both verbally and nonverbally) accordingly in order to get their achieved outcome.

■ **You cannot not communicate** – despite people imagining they can avoid communication by saying nothing, nonverbal communication illustrates the thoughts and feelings inside of you. We are constantly communicating not just by what we say but by what we do not say. On this basis a good communicator will realize that there is more to be gained by verbalizing rather than by staying aloof.

■ **There is no such thing as failure, only feedback** – every result will give you information. Instead of something being wrong, we can view this as a learning experience and are therefore prepared to try again.

■ **Everyone has all the resources they need** – people will already have the knowledge of how their problem occurred and therefore already have the capacity to be able to deal with it. Often people may not have considered that their skills in another arena can by utilized elsewhere to solve their own problem. Equally people may know how to find the skills they do not have elsewhere.

■ **The person with the greatest number of choices is likely to get the best outcome** – if you imagine the problem only has one solution then the likelihood is that you will not achieve it. Whereas someone who is open to the possibility of several solutions or outcomes is much more likely achieve success.

■ **If you want something different, you must do something different** – there is a solution to every problem if you can be prepared to keep looking for it.

■ **Every behaviour has its appropriate context** – behaviour that was exhibited alongside previous events or experiences can limit your current potential. Think not about past feelings, thoughts or emotions but look for new ways to adapt to new behaviours that are most beneficial for the experiences now.

■ **Mind and body are inseparable** – it was previously thought that mind and body were separate entities. Now it is recognized that your thoughts and emotions affect your body and *vice versa*.

■ **If one person can learn to do something, anyone else can learn to do it** – this is about modelling behaviour. Recognizing that if one person can achieve something, looking at the way in which they did and replicating it will also bring similar results.

■ **Change makes change** – this is acknowledging that if your behaviour changes it will have an effect on those around you.

■ **Action develops understanding** – you do not really fully understand something until you personally do it.

■ **Every behaviour has a positive intention** – this presupposition can be often misinterpreted and controversial. It alludes to the fact that the person exhibiting the behaviour is looking for a positive intention.

NLP has now been used by practitioners for over 30 years. NLP can be used in everyday practice by physiotherapists in their assessment and management of patients. NLP centres on maximizing our communication and as physiotherapists we should possess advanced communication skills. This enables us to ensure patients are active participants in their care and for us to truly reflect on our practice. It is a widely contested area of practice and there is a need for up-to-date research to substantiate its claims (Wake et al., 2013).

## PSYCHOTHERAPY AND COUNSELLING

As discussed previously, this chapter is not intended to cover all aspects of psychotherapy and counselling, or to train you as counsellors. Instead this section is aimed at giving you a background to the different approaches of counselling, to provide insight into the therapy and to stimulate interest. We are part of an interprofessional team and we must utilize the expertise of all members. It is hoped that this section of the chapter will encourage you to discuss possible therapies with the multiprofessional team and patients, and potentially guide future study.

There are many different approaches to guiding people through emotional distress, each with its own view on human nature and emotional drive. These range from the analytical view point, where clients are analysed to discover maladaptive thoughts from their past, to postmodern theory, which accepts the client's views whether rational or not. Some of the different approaches are detailed further in Table 9.1.

Most of these approaches would not be relevant to the role of a physiotherapist, but some could be adopted to improve the therapeutic alliance and allow for the physiotherapist to be able to discuss emotional issues affecting patients. It may also encourage the patient to acknowledge their problems, facilitate positive movement and reassure them in seeking further help from a counsellor. Approaches that could be useful to physiotherapists are explored further in this chapter.

## THE PATIENT-CENTRED APPROACH

Patient-centred therapy was derived from ideas introduced by Dr Carl Rogers, an American psychologist. His view of human nature was that everyone had the potential for growth if the conditions and environment, as perceived by the client, were sufficient (Rogers, 1957a). These six necessary and sufficient conditions are described in Box 9.1. This approach places more trust in clients to lead therapy, encourages them to make positive changes and gives them the freedom to make correct choices (Corey, 1996).

Rogers extended his ideas wider than counselling and psychotherapy, and could see the application to other fields such as health, education and politics. He stated that such conditions are relevant in helping relationships and are not restricted to that between counsellor and client (Rogers, 1957b). As physiotherapists, we could use the counsellor 'ways of being' advocated by Rogers to provide a more truly patient-centred approach. These are congruence, unconditional positive regard

TABLE 9.1

## Comparison of Different Psychotherapy and Counselling Approaches

| | Approach | Key Figures | View of Human Nature | Aims of Treatment | Role of Therapist and Methods Used |
|---|---|---|---|---|---|
| *Analytical* | Psychoanalytical | Sigmund Freud (1856–1939) | ■ Life goals are to avoid pain and gain pleasure<br>■ Behaviour is affected by irrational forces and instinctual drives<br>■ Personality determined by three systems; Id (ruled by biology and survival), ego (regulates between instincts and the external world) and superego (judicial system that strives for perfection)<br>■ Anxiety is the tension that is needed to motivate; caused by a conflict of these three systems) | To make the unconscious conscious and allow clients to love, work and play | ■ The therapist is a blank personality to allow projection of relationship with others and to foster feelings associated with significant others<br>■ An analytical framework of psychotherapy where nothing is taken at face value<br>■ Interpretation of the unconscious from analysis, dream analysis, interpretation of resistance and transference (from projection) |
| | Adlerian therapy | Alfred Adler (1870–1837) | ■ There is some agreement with Freud's theory, but says that behaviour is guided by social relatedness and is purposeful rather than unconscious<br>■ It is human nature to strive for superiority and mastery<br>■ Explores the effect of birth order in the family | To explore and acknowledge mistaken goals and assumptions; to develop a sense of belonging | ■ To offer encouragement to the client by being open and guiding in the relationship<br>■ Exploring the client's dynamics including their place in the family and early recollections<br>■ To encourage the client to understand themselves; reorientation to being more useful |

| Humanistic | Existential therapy | Viktor Frankl (1905–1997) | ■ It is never fixed but constantly reshaping<br>■ There is a potential for freedom but the responsibility of this can cause tension<br>■ Being a person is concerned with making sense of life, understanding values and the awareness of death | To recognize insecurity; to encourage coping and allow the client to be authentic in recognizing when they are deceiving themselves | ■ To understand the view of the client and help them to understand<br>■ To be a 'mirror' reflecting back their image and behaviour<br>■ Focus on freedom |
|---|---|---|---|---|---|
| | Patient-centred therapy | Carl Rogers (1909–1987) | ■ People are trustworthy and have potential for growth in the right conditions<br>■ Everybody is able to find meaning to life | The focus is not to analyse the problem but to enable growth | ■ To create the necessary conditions for growth which are: unconditional positive regard, congruence and empathetic understanding<br>■ To focus on the way of being rather than techniques |
| | Gestalt therapy | Fritz Perls (1893–1970) and Laura Perls (1905–1990) | ■ People are capable of remodelling and discovering more about themselves<br>■ Everybody is capable of understanding what is happening internally and externally<br>■ People need to be able to deal with problems themselves | To achieve awareness and encourage greater choice; to promote self-regulation and reliance | ■ Confrontational style focusing on experiencing rather than talking<br>■ Presents experiments and shares observations |

*Continued*

**TABLE 9.1** *cont*

## Comparison of Different Psychotherapy and Counselling Approaches

| | Approach | Key Figures | View of Human Nature | Aims of Treatment | Role of Therapist and Methods Used |
|---|---|---|---|---|---|
| **Cognitive and Behavioural Therapies** | Reality therapy | William Glasser (1925–2013) | ■ All we do is behave and everything is chosen<br>■ People choose behaviours as a way of coping with frustrations<br>■ Problems mainly caused by a lack of satisfying relationships with others | To encourage effective choices when dealing with others and allow clients to become connected | ■ The therapist and client need a connection<br>■ Not to evaluate but to challenge self-evaluation<br>■ Emphasize choice and instill hope |
| | Cognitive Behavioural Therapy – Refer to Chapter 5 | | | | |
| | Solutions focused therapy | Insoo Kim Berg (1934–2007) Steve De Shazer (1940–2005) | ■ No view on human nature and cautious of assumptions | To help clients to talk about solutions rather than problems, focusing on the present and future rather than past | ■ To accept the client's reality without disputing its accuracy<br>■ The therapist is an expert in change, but the client is an expert in their life<br>■ Uses small, realistic and achievable changes |
| **Systems** | Feminism | Jean Baker Miller (1927–2006) Carolyn Zerbe Enns Olivia Espin Laura Brown | ■ Psychotherapy is bound to culture<br>■ Social arrangements are rooted in gender<br>■ Gender roles that we are socialized to accept lead to tension | To empower others to live according to internal drives rather than societal norms | ■ To change client and society as a shared journey<br>■ Uses self-help books, power analysis, assertiveness training, social action |
| | Family systems | Murray Bowen (1913–1990) | ■ Although individuals have freedom of choice, we discover ourselves and our meaning of life in a family system<br>■ Development of one individual within a family is interconnected to that of others in the family | To enable understanding of the functioning of the family unit to identify problems and find solutions | ■ Collaborative relationship between clients and therapist<br>■ Group and individual sessions<br>■ Actively listening and connecting with each member of the family |

## BOX 9.1
### SIX NECESSARY AND SUFFICIENT CONDITIONS FOR THERAPEUTIC CHANGE

1. Two persons in psychological contact
2. The first, whom we shall refer to as the client, is in a state in incongruence, vulnerability or anxiety
3. The second person, whom we shall term the therapist, is congruent and integrated in the relationship
4. The therapist experiences unconditional positive regard for the client
5. The therapist experiences an empathic understanding of the client's internal frame of reference and endeavours to communicate this experience to the client
6. The therapist's empathic understanding and unconditional positive regard is communicated to the client to a minimal degree

*(Rogers, 1957)*

## BOX 9.2
### A THERAPIST'S 'WAYS OF BEING' TO PROMOTE EMOTIONAL GROWTH

#### CONGRUENCE

Congruence could also be termed as genuineness, honesty or realness. The therapist is real in the relationship without playing roles, or being untruthful in their reaction or expression of feelings. It means not pretending to be something that they are not. Any negative feelings are not suppressed but only shared if it is felt to be therapeutically relevant. By behaving this way, the therapist becomes a 'model' for behaviour and encourages the other person to become congruent in their own behaviour and to recognize incongruence. The therapist will need to engage in self-reflection and have an awareness of their feelings to behave in this way, using clinical supervision or reflective partners may be helpful.

#### UNCONDITIONAL POSITIVE REGARD

Unconditional positive regard refers to deep and genuine caring for the other person. It is not necessarily about liking the person, but acceptance of them as they are. This is important in allowing the other person to feel free to express themselves honestly and without a fear of loss of regard. Pretending that such feelings can be easily seen through affects the congruence displayed by the therapist. It is accepting the person's right to have their emotions and reactions.

#### EMPATHETIC UNDERSTANDING

Empathetic understanding is the understanding of the other person's experiences, feelings and behaviours. By sensing underlying feelings and reflecting on them, it may encourage the other person to feel more intensely and recognize incongruence. It is challenging for the therapist not to project their feelings and to remain with their emotions, so again the use of reflection is important.

and empathetic understanding, discussed in more detail in Box 9.2. The 'conditions' of patient-centred therapy are directly relevant to three of the five dimensions of patient-centred care stated by Mead and Bower (2000). They are as follows: 'patient as a person', 'sharing power and responsibility' and 'the doctor as a person'.

Using the counselling skills as a physiotherapist will not provide counselling to the patient. There are trained psychotherapists and counsellors who have the skills necessary for such therapy. It will, however, allow patients to express themselves honestly, in a helping relationship, and may allow them to consider such therapy in the future. It will provide people in crisis with an opportunity to express themselves and to ground them in keeping calm while in turmoil, think more clearly and make better decisions (Burnard, 2005).

No investigation has looked into the effect of the counselling skills discussed in this section on physiotherapy. Basler et al. (2007) found no evidence of counselling sessions in conjunction with physiotherapy to have an effect on physical activity or functional activity of range of movement. In the counselling sessions studied in this trial, no mention was made of counselling style other than that it was based on the transtheoretical model of change. Therefore it is impossible to use when evaluating the utilization of the 'ways of being' in the patient-centred approach advocated by Rogers.

Using the counselling skills or the 'conditions' from Box 9.2 will provide the physiotherapist with a set of skills that could be used to explore the emotions affecting the patient. It will allow the patient to feel comfortable when sharing their feelings and provide for a better understanding and relationship between the physiotherapist and patient. It will therefore positively affect the therapeutic alliance and could be used effectively when enhancing the patient–physiotherapist relationship.

## MOTIVATIONAL INTERVIEWING

Defined as a 'directive, client-centred counselling style for eliciting behaviour change' by Rollnick and Miller (1995), motivational interviewing is a strategy that could easily be adopted by physiotherapists when discussing behaviour changes or treatment adherence. It involves exploring ambivalence to change and assisting the patient to resolve it. The strategy is a development from the patient-centred approach in that it focuses on the patient's own motivations to change (Hettema et al., 2005), however it is more focused and goal directed (Rollnick and Miller, 1995). The spirit of motivational interviewing is explored further in Box 9.3.

When using this strategy the therapist encourages and reinforces the patient's own motivation and argument to change, having faith that they will move in a positive direction (Hettema et al., 2005). The patient voices this argument rather than the therapist as it is thought to strengthen their commitment to change (Miller and Rose, 2009). The relationship between the patient and therapist is

> **BOX 9.3**
> **THE SPIRIT OF MOTIVATIONAL INTERVIEWING**
>
> ■ Motivation to change is elicited from the client and is not imposed
> ■ It is the client's task, not the counsellor's, to articulate and resolve his or her ambivalence
> ■ Direct persuasion is not an effective method for resolving ambivalence
> ■ The counselling style is generally a quiet and eliciting one
> ■ The counsellor is direct in helping the client examine and resolve ambivalence
> ■ Readiness to change is not a client trait but a fluctuating product of interpersonal interaction
> ■ The therapeutic relationship is more like a partnership or companionship than one with expert/recipient roles
>
> *(Rollnick and Miller, 1995)*

important to be conscious of, as it should be supportive and use the conditions used in the patient-centred approach (Box 9.2). Any resistances to change should be explored and any discrepancies in their discussions highlighted to help resolve ambivalence, but it must be the patient's own motivation to change rather than be enforced by the therapist (Rollnick and Miller, 1995).

Motivational interviewing has a growing evidence base in a variety of settings and is generating interest in more medical settings. It has been found to have small to medium positive effects in improving health outcomes (Hettema et al., 2005), and across a variety of problem domains (Lundahl et al., 2010). In meta-analyses motivational interviewing has been shown to significantly increase weight loss in overweight patients (Armstrong et al., 2011) and to have modest improvement in physical activity for people with chronic health conditions (O'Halloran et al., 2014). When exploring the results of the trials further, O'Halloran et al. (2014) discovered that the effect size was larger when the level of participation with motivational interviewing was higher, suggesting it may be more effective when used more consistently. With evidence that motivational interviewing can improve healthy behaviour, it must be considered an effective strategy for physiotherapists to adopt while discussing lifestyle changes with patients.

When exploring the effectiveness of motivational interviewing in medical care settings, Lundahl et al. (2013) discovered that motivational interviewing provides a moderate advantage over other interventions. Moreover, this systematic review suggested that this intervention is deliverable by different types of health care professionals. Physiotherapists could effectively provide motivational interviewing when discussing behaviour change with patients, and in light of the emerging evidence, they should be.

## MINDFULNESS

Mindfulness can be described as 'nonevaluative, present-focused awareness of physical and psychological experiences' (Kabat-Zinn, 2013). It cultivates the presence of thinking to that particular moment in time, fostering clear thoughts and disengaging from strong attachments to any negative emotions or beliefs. Mindfulness has the goal of promoting engagement and strengthening internal resources for both prevention and improvement from ill health by developing a better sense of wellbeing and emotional balance. It has been suggested that this technique has the ability to modulate a person's experience of pain and therefore their capacity to cope with disability and chronic disease (Ludwig and Kabat-Zinn, 2008).

There are different interventions that are based around mindfulness training such as mindfulness-based stress reduction (MBSR), mindfulness-based cognitive therapy (MBCT) and mindfulness-based functional therapy (MBFT). Many of these interventions involve an 8-week programme including guided breathing, gentle stretching and exercise, group dialogue and mindful communication exercises.

Mindfulness is an ancient concept that has origins in Eastern meditation practices, such as Buddhism. It has been more widely used in the last 40 years as a clinical intervention in the Western world. Empirical evidence has started to support the use of mindfulness in the treatment of certain disorders (Baer, 2003). These may include: reduction of stress, reduction in analgesia, decreased perception of pain/increased ability to tolerate pain, improved adherence to medical treatments, increased motivation for lifestyle changes and potential adaptations in the immune, nervous and endocrine systems (Ludwig and Kabat-Zinn, 2008).

In one of the first studies assessing the effects of MBSR on patients with chronic pain, Kabat-Zinn (1982) suggested that through the application of traditional mindfulness practice (often including sitting motionless for extended periods of time in relaxed postures), allows for the ability to observe pain sensations nonjudgmentally. It is postulated that this extended exposure to chronic pain, using mindfulness and observing no consequences, could lead to desensitization and therefore affect the decreased emotional response to the pain.

Current usage of invading technology such as smart phones and an increase in economic pressure and demands in productivity have given rise to the concept of 'continuous partial attention'. These factors are thought to influence the general health of the population and can diminish the client–therapist relationship significantly. Mindfulness may hold the key to combating some of these generational changes and returning the focus to improving both physical and psychological function. Although the current body of literature has significant methodological flaws, there are interesting suggestions that mindfulness could be used to combat a number of health problems (Dufour et al., 2014). Further high-quality randomized controlled trials of mindfulness in medicine and therapeutic intervention are needed (Baer, 2003).

## ACCEPTANCE AND COMMITMENT THERAPY

Acceptance and commitment theory has been described as the third wave of cognitive behaviour therapy. The fundamental principle of acceptance commitment therapy (ACT) is to construct a meaningful and full life whilst being in acceptance of the idea that pain may be an inevitable part of it. Symptom reduction is not a goal that ACT focuses on; rather it is achieved as a consequence through behaviour change. Most Western approaches to therapy are contrary to this with the basis of many being centred on symptom relief. The word 'symptom' is closely associated with pathology and so by focusing on symptom relief, this thought process can actually create

a clinical condition rather than abolish one. ACT is acknowledgement of a commitment to try and transform our affiliation with our thoughts, feelings and emotions. By accepting that 'symptoms' may not be harmful or constant events, but merely transitory, we can concentrate our attention on other aspects of life and feeling fulfilled (Flaxman et al., 2010). ACT has been used for a wide range of problems, including chronic illness, depression and work-related problems.

In ACT the emphasis is on two main principles: (1) when personal experiences that are out of your control occur, you learn to accept them and (2) making a commitment and taking action towards a valued life (Harris, 2006). There are six core areas that ACT centres around and these combine to produce what is described as 'psychological flexibility' (Hayes et al., 1999).

- **Acceptance** – the willingness to accept our feelings and sensations. To acknowledge that our thoughts and worries will change over time and have the ability to dismiss any resistance we have towards them. To accept that we can make room for these emotions and not feel the need to dispel them, but to learn how to allow them to come and go without a struggle.
- **Cognitive defusion** – attempts to modify the thoughts and language that we are immersed in. Often we can be caught in the literal meaning of those thoughts and language and they can have an enormous effect on our behaviour. Cognitive defusion means that we are able to disengage from those aspects of thought and language and recognize them with detachment; hence they have a lesser effect and

influence. This is in contrast to CBT where cognitive defusion would involve evaluation of those thoughts.

- **Contact with present moment** – the ability to identify internal and external influences and to engage fully with a positive attitude in whatever is occurring at the present moment. Allow thoughts and feelings to come and go but keep focus on what is happening in the here-and-now. Using mindfulness (as described previously) as a method to achieve contact with the present moment rather than be focused on thoughts and feelings.
- **Values** – being able to identify what is most important to you, what significant values you hold and what direction you would like your life to take. Often anxiety can accompany taking a new direction in life and embracing your core values. This is something that needs to be accepted with willingness in order to allow yourself to do something you value.
- **The observing self** – the process by which you allow any negative thoughts and feelings to pass through you without being defined by them. By not allowing yourself to be defined by any negative thoughts and feelings, you are able to establish that they are not as threatening and disabling as they initially may have seemed. In this way you

are able to engage in a more meaningful life and not use experiential avoidance to steer away from situations.

- **Committed action** – setting goals and continuing to behave in a committed way in order to achieve those goals. This is not just a promise or an agreement to achieve the goals set, but effective action to ensure they are accomplished, and the continuation of setting further goals.

Through the utilization of ACT, therapists can further develop their skills of compassion, understanding and reflection, and ultimately become a better communicator with a deeper therapeutic alliance. This can enrich the experience of physiotherapy and instead of directing efforts on trying to eliminate unwanted symptoms or feelings, learning to accept and deal with them through focusing on the positive aspects of patient-centred goals, with symptom reduction, can be a pleasant byproduct of ACT.

## CASE STUDIES

It was envisaged that it may be hard to see how such strategies could be used in everyday physiotherapy practice. Therefore some case studies are explored next where such techniques could be utilized effectively.

---

### CASE STUDY 1

#### The Use of Counselling Skills

A middle-aged man was referred to the respiratory physiotherapy out-patient clinic with suspected chronic hyperventilation syndrome (HVS). He attended clinic and during his assessment he became upset and started to cry. He was reluctant to share the reasons for being upset but was keen to continue with the assessment and discuss potential breathing exercises. During the examination it was noted that

*Continued*

## The Use of Counselling Skills

his lung function tests were normal, but that he had a dysfunctional breathing pattern consistent with HVS. His subjective symptoms were also consistent with this. Breathing retraining occurred and a follow-up appointment was organized for the following week. The physiotherapist reflected on the session and was unhappy with the way they reacted when the man started to cry as she tried to deflect his emotional distress and move on with the treatment. Subsequently she thought of the counselling skills she had used in the past pertaining to the patient-centred approach of counselling. She reflected that exploring the reasons for the man's distress is vital, as this anxiety was directly influencing his HVS.

In session two, the physiotherapist demonstrated unconditional positive regard to the patient and attempted to probe the reasons for his distress in the previous session. He admitted that he was struggling to find work as he could not read and was relying on his wife and children to help him in day-to-day life when reading was required. The man became upset again and the physiotherapist used empathetic and congruent responses to allow him to explore his feelings of guilt, anxiety, low self-worth and reliance on his family. He acknowledged that when he began to feel anxious about his life, this was when his symptoms of HVS appeared to get worse. Further breathing retraining occurred and another appointment was made for the following week. The physiotherapist asked the patient to note when he was feeling his symptoms and what was happening to his breathing.

In the following two physiotherapy sessions, the patient's knowledge of his breathing pattern progressed and his symptoms started to reduce. He still experienced episodes of dizziness associated with his overbreathing, but he recognized why this was occurring and used breathing control to rectify the problem. After a discussion with the physiotherapist about his worries, he started to discuss them more openly with his family who then became supportive in helping him start to learn how to read. However, during the fifth appointment, he was visibly distressed at the start of the session and needed the physiotherapist to use counselling skills to allow him to discuss his feelings again. He discussed a family argument which had increased his worries and he was struggling to cope with this. At this point the physiotherapist explained her role as a physiotherapist and her limits when using counselling skills and suggested that further counselling from a trained professional may help to reduce his anxiety levels. The patient was initially very reluctant but agreed to think about it.

During the final physiotherapy session the patient's breathing pattern was much improved and he had more control over his breathing. He still had episodes of light headedness and tingling lips, but he recognized that this would occur at times when he was particularly worried. He agreed that further input was required to help him manage his anxiety levels and was planning to see his general practitioner.

## The Use of Acceptance and Commitment Therapy

Jenny is a 35-year-old school teacher who suffered for several years with low back pain (LBP). She had seen several physiotherapists and had surgery all to no avail. During the musculoskeletal assessment, Jenny discussed the strategies she had used previously to try and avoid or alleviate her pain. These had included avoiding activity, taking pain medication, sleeping during the day, taking sick leave from work, avoiding certain social events and eating chocolate. Jenny identified that, although some of these strategies had helped her in the short term, none had had any long-term significant effect. She was also able to identify that in fact some of these previous approaches had exacerbated the LBP and had a detrimental effect on her quality of life, eg, she now has significant weight gain and her social life has been affected.

In session two Jenny discussed what her concerns were about the LBP and how it made her feel. She highlighted her fears about 'damage' and progressing disability and the effect this may have on her life. Alongside the progression of her musculoskeletal assessment, the focus of this session was to interact with her thoughts with the aim being that their effect be lost. There are several ways to do this – using visual imagery and words out of context until they become less distressing. Jenny was given the task to go away and practice these 'thought' exercises with the aim not to get rid of them, but to be able to step back and put them into context for what they were – just thoughts. This is known as *cognitive diffusion* within acceptance and commitment theory.

Session three focused on *acceptance* – Jenny was told to come to therapy and focus on her LBP. She described it and discussed her sensations in response to it. She concentrated on breathing exercises whilst remaining focused on her feelings surrounding the LBP. Jenny reported a feeling of tranquillity surrounding this and the aim was to allow those feelings to be present, not to eliminate them, but to let them come and go without anxiety surrounding them – to accept them.

Over the next couple of sessions mindfulness exercises were used to engage with all five senses and Jenny learnt to participate fully with whatever was occurring at that moment rather than being distracted by her own thoughts about her LBP. This is known as *contact with the present moment*. She also had to access her transcendent self, again through mindfulness, to be aware that the thoughts and feelings she was having were just that, thoughts and feelings, and that those things constantly change and do not define who you are. This is known as the *observing self*. This is to realize that thoughts are not harmful, nor defining.

In the last session Jenny was asked to identify what was significant and meaningful to her in her life. This is known as *identifying values*. Once she had identified what was important to her and decided she was willing to make room for the feelings she had about the LBP in order to pursue her values it was important to start making goals. This is called *committed action*. Jenny continued to practice the skills and exercises she had learned during previous sessions and started to achieve some of the goals she had set. She reported that overall her LBP had significantly reduced – this is not the goal of acceptance and commitment therapy, but merely a positive side effect.

CASE STUDY 3

### The Use of Motivational Interviewing Strategies

A physiotherapy team delivering an education and exercise class for people with osteoarthritis in the hips and/or knees recognized a recurring problem with attendees failing to keep up with physical activity after discharge from the class. One person in the team was reading about motivational interviewing and was keen to use some of the strategies he had read about. As a team, they discussed how they could change the way in which they communicated with patients about physical activity and continuance with exercise, and recognized they rarely discussed patients' beliefs about exercise. Consequently they met and discussed how they could change their practice to integrate motivational interviewing.

It was decided that small focus groups of four to five patients would be added to the end of each session. In these groups, one physiotherapist would lead a discussion about exercise and increasing the patients' physical activity. The physiotherapist would explore and 'roll with any ambivalence' demonstrated by the patients and make suggestions about physical activity. They directed the conversation, as it was trying to elicit the patients' beliefs about physical activity, but they did not direct what changes should occur, just allowed the patients to discuss what changes were possible for them.

This addition to the class was evaluated well by the patients as they discussed it was a good way for them to really think about how they could improve their physical activity. However, it was recognized by the team that goal setting in relation to the patients' readiness for change was needed. A further individual session was offered to patients upon completion of the exercise class, to discuss how they plan to continue with increasing their physical activity. In this session, the physiotherapist again used the spirit of motivational interviewing to guide their short- and long-term goals in relation to changing their behaviour.

## CONCLUSION

For physiotherapy to be effective and to engage the patient in the process of rehabilitation, attention must be paid to the relationship between the patient and physiotherapist. The therapeutic alliance should be considered and evaluated in the relationship in order to provide patient-centred care. In some situations, patients may need enhanced psychological support using counselling or psychotherapy and structured therapy but this is beyond the scope of physiotherapy. Despite this, physiotherapists can be trained in using counselling skills to enable conversations about emotional distress and to provide support in keeping with the patient–physiotherapist relationship. When support-ing a patient in adhering to a suggested treatment plan or improving their health and behaviour, physiotherapists can use other strategies such as motivational interviewing, acceptance and commitment therapy and mindfulness. This chapter has hopefully given some information with regards to what these strategies entail as far as stimulating interest for further research and training.

### References

Armstrong, M., Mottershead, T., Ronksley, P., Sigal, R., Campbell, T., Hemmelgarn, B., 2011. Motivational interviewing to improve weight loss in overweight and/ or obese patients: a systematic review and meta-analysis of randomized controlled trials. Obes. Rev. 12 (9), 709–723.

Baer, R.A., 2003. Mindfulness training as a clinical intervention: A conceptual and empirical review. Clin. Psychol. Sci. Prac. 10 (2), 125–143.

Basler, H.D., Bertalanffy, H., Quint, S., Wilke, A., Wolf, U., 2007. TTM-based counselling in physiotherapy does not contribute to an increase of adherence to activity recommendations in older adults with chronic low back pain—A randomised controlled trial. Eur. J. Pain 11 (1), 31–37.

Bennett, J.K., Fuertes, J.N., Keitel, M., Phillips, R., 2011. The role of patient attachment and working alliance on patient adherence, satisfaction, and health-related quality of life in lupus treatment. Patient Educ. Couns. 85 (1), 53–59.

Burnard, P., 2005. Counselling skills for health professionals. . Nelson Thornes.

Corey, G., 1996. Theory and practice of counseling and psychotherapy. Brooks/Cole Publishing Company, Pacific Grove.

Dilts, R.B., 2011. What is NLP. Retrieved from <http://www.nlpu.com/NewDesign/NLPU_WhatIsNLP.html>.

Dilts, R.B., DeLozier, J., 2000. Encyclopaedia of Systematic NLP and NLP New Coding. Meta Publications, California.

Dufour, S.P., Graham, S., Friesen, J., Rosenblat, M., Rous, C., Richardson, J., 2014. Physiotherapists supporting self-management through health coaching: a mixed methods program evaluation. Physiother. Theory Pract. 31 (1), 29–38.

Flaxman, P.E., Blackledge, J.T., Bond, F.W., 2010. Acceptance and commitment therapy: Distinctive features. Routledge.

Fuentes, J., Armijo-Olivo, S., Funabashi, M., Miciak, M., Dick, B., Warren, S., et al., 2014. Enhanced therapeutic alliance modulates pain intensity and muscle pain sensitivity in patients with chronic low back pain: An experimental controlled study. Phys. Ther. 94 (4), 477–489.

Fuertes, J.N., Mislowack, A., Bennett, J., Paul, L., Gilbert, T.C., Fontan, G., et al., 2007. The physician–patient working alliance. Patient Educ. Couns. 66 (1), 29–36.

Hall, A.M., Ferreira, P.H., Maher, C.G., Latimer, J., Ferreira, M.L., 2010. The influence of the therapist-patient relationship on treatment outcome in physical rehabilitation: a systematic review. Phys. Ther. 90, 1099–1110.

Harris, R., 2006. Embracing your demons: an overview of acceptance and commitment therapy. Psychotherapy in Australia 12 (4), 70.

Hayes, S.C., Strosahl, K.D., Wilson, K.G., 1999. Acceptance and commitment therapy: An experiential approach to behavior change. Guilford Press, New York.

Hettema, J., Steele, J., Miller, W.R., 2005. Motivational interviewing. Annu. Rev. Clin. Psychol. 1, 91–111.

Kabat-Zinn, J., 1982. An outpatient program in behavioral medicine for chronic pain patients based on the practice of mindfulness meditation: Theoretical considerations and preliminary results. Gen. Hosp. Psychiatry 4 (1), 33–47.

Kabat-Zinn, J., 2013. Full catastrophe living, revised edition: how to cope with stress, pain and illness using mindfulness meditation. Hachette, London.

Kidd, M.O., Bond, C.H., Bell, M.L., 2011. Patients' perspectives of patient-centredness as important in musculoskeletal physiotherapy interactions: a qualitative study. Physiotherapy 97 (2), 154–162.

Ludwig, D.S., Kabat-Zinn, J., 2008. Mindfulness in medicine. JAMA 300 (11), 1350–1352.

Lundahl, B., Moleni, T., Burke, B.L., Butters, R., Tollefson, D., Butler, C., et al., 2013. Motivational interviewing in medical care settings: a systematic review and meta-analysis of randomized controlled trials. Patient Educ. Couns. 93 (2), 157–168.

Lundahl, B.W., Kunz, C., Brownell, C., Tollefson, D., Burke, B.L., 2010. A meta-analysis of motivational interviewing: Twenty-five years of empirical studies. Research on Social Work Practice. 000 (0), 1–25.

Mead, N., Bower, P., 2000. Patient-centredness: a conceptual framework and review of the empirical literature. Soc. Sci. Med. 51 (7), 1087–1110.

Miller, W.R., Rose, G.S., 2009. Toward a theory of motivational interviewing. Am. Psychol. 64 (6), 527.

O'Halloran, P.D., Blackstock, F., Shields, N., Holland, A., Iles, R., Kingsley, M., et al., 2014. Motivational interviewing to increase physical activity in people with chronic health conditions: a systematic review and meta-analysis. Clin. Rehabil. doi:10.1177/0269215514536210.

Pinto, R.Z., Ferreira, M.L., Oliveira, V.C., Franco, M.R., Adams, R., Maher, C.G., et al., 2012. Patient-centred communication is associated with positive therapeutic alliance: a systematic review. J Physiother. 58 (2), 77–87.

Rogers, C., 1967. On Becoming a Person: A Therapist's View of Psychotherapy. Constable, London.

Rogers, C.R., 1957a. The necessary and sufficient conditions of therapeutic personality change. J. Consult. Psychol. 21 (2), 95.

Rogers, C.R., 1957b. On becoming a person. S. Doniger.

Rollnick, S., Miller, W.R., 1995. What is motivational interviewing? Behav. Cogn. Psychother. 23 (04), 325–334.

Sherer, M., Evans, C.C., Leverenz, J., Stouter, J., Irby Jr., J.W., Eun Lee, J., et al., 2007. Therapeutic alliance in post-acute brain injury rehabilitation: predictors of strength of alliance and impact of alliance on outcome. Brain Inj. 21 (7), 663–672.

Taber, B.J., Leibert, T.W., Agaskar, V.R., 2011. Relationships among client–therapist personality congruence, working alliance, and therapeutic outcome. Psychotherapy (Chic.) 48 (4), 376.

Wake, L., Gray, R., Bourke, F., 2013. The clinical effectiveness of neurolinguistic programming: a critical appraisal. Routledge.

# MAKING EVIDENCE-BASED DECISIONS AND MEASURING EFFECTIVENESS IN PSYCHOLOGICALLY INFORMED PRACTICE

LOUISE HENSTOCK ■ HELEN CARRUTHERS ■ CHRISTINE PARKER

## CHAPTER CONTENTS

## INTRODUCTION

Evidence based practice is about:

'..using evidence wisely and integrating evidence appropriately with individual patients. It is a skilled activity concerned with combining the best available evidence with clinical experience to turn the evidence into useful information for a specific patient, in particular circumstances.'

**Hammond, 2004**

As physiotherapists we must ensure that we are working in the best interests of our patients and providing effective treatments and strategies. To do that, deciding on the best evidence based strategy and measuring our effectiveness in using the chosen strategy are vital. The aim of this chapter is to discuss the challenges in identifying the most appropriate approach to use in a psychologically informed physiotherapy practice and measuring its effectiveness, in order to justify decision making.

Of course there is a key challenge for evaluation, as 'psychologically informed practice' is not a separate treatment technique or

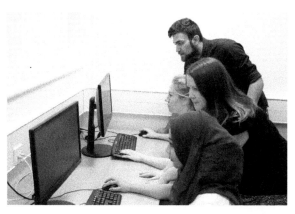

FIGURE 10.1 ■ Make sure that your evidence is high quality – your patients deserve the best.

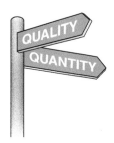

FIGURE 10.2 ■ Quantitative research is not automatically the best quality – have the researchers and you as the clinician used the right tool for the right job?

approach; we may choose psychological strategies that are evidence based but we are unlikely to use them in isolation. Psychologically informed practice in contemporary physiotherapy will involve the integration of a range of physical, psychological and social aspects in order to reach functional goals. So unless you are doing some research comparing clinical outcomes, before and after introducing psychological strategies, or maybe introducing psychological strategies with one group of patients and comparing outcomes with a control group, then it will be difficult to draw any direct conclusions around the effectiveness of your psychologically informed practice. Instead you may need to consider drawing inferences from the use of a broader range of outcome measurements. This will be considered later in the chapter.

## DECIDING ON THE MOST APPROPRIATE APPROACH TO ADOPT

Modern health care demands that decisions be made on effective care and treatments be based on the best available evidence. Making decisions on the most suitable psychosocial strategy to use can be difficult as research questions in psychologically informed practice are unlikely to be answered by those methodologies higher up on the hierarchy of evidence, namely meta-analyses and randomized controlled trials (RCTs) (Fig. 10.3). Physiotherapists will require skills in reviewing a range of evidence sources to reach decisions. We will now consider how you might appraise this evidence, in relation to psychologically informed practice decisions. These methodologies include quantitative, qualitative and mixed methods.

### Using Quantitative Evidence

The effectiveness of using psychological strategies can be measured using quantitative methods. Using inductive reasoning would allow effectiveness to be proven and measured for specific populations. Decisions could then be made about whether it would be effective for your population. The strength of this approach is that it minimizes error and bias when measuring effectiveness; giving more definitive results (Lewis and Warlow, 2004). The problems in these approaches may revolve around the specificity of the treatment or approach tested, and the ability to

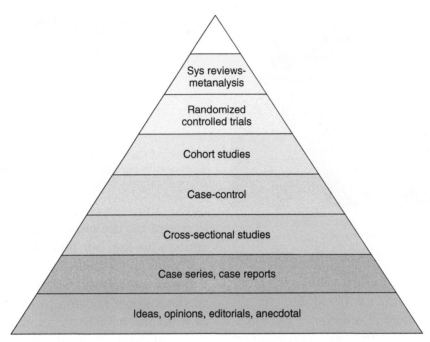

FIGURE 10.3 ■ Remember the hierarchy of research evidence.

measure effectiveness of techniques across a variety of outcomes and domains, ie, quality of life, mental health, adherence.

### Levels of Quality

RCTs aim to reduce extraneous variables that could affect the outcome measurements. Because of this, methods will use strict inclusion and exclusion criteria with specific interventions to minimize bias. The very specific population used in trials may not be representative of the population as a whole (Clay, 2010) and when investigating psychologically informed practice, being specific in relation to the interventions the participants received may be difficult as a result of the patient-centred approach of most techniques. Blinding of participants is virtually impossible to achieve because of the nature of the intervention and the need to gain informed

consent for participation in the trial, which could affect the judgement of researchers or the behaviour of participants (Lewis and Warlow, 2004). Although methodologically sound RCTs may more strongly demonstrate effectiveness in psychologically informed practice, they may well be subject to bias.

Quasiexperimental or nonrandomized designs could be used to measure effectiveness when randomization is not possible (Harris et al., 2006), and could be used when evaluating psychologically informed strategies. However, there are limitations in such trials which must be remembered when using the results to make decisions. Controlled clinical trials allow for comparisons between control and intervention groups but the lack of randomization may create meaningful differences between the groups and affect the results. Cohort studies using one group could measure the effects of person-specific strategies but the lack of a control group reduces the chance that the results are directly attributed to the intervention. However, if two groups are used (one being a control group) this could show meaningful differences between the groups.

This discussion highlights some of the challenges in conducting quantitative research in this area. However, quantitative research will strengthen the evidence base so long as you consider whether the research is relevant to your practice and population; and whether the results are useful and trustworthy depending on the methods utilized. To complement quantitative results, other methodologies may offer insight into the problem, usefulness of the intervention and the types of effects observed.

## Using Qualitative Evidence

Qualitative methodologies are well suited to address research questions about patient experiences in order to improve psychosocial outcomes, or in exploring the theoretical framework when using such techniques. Qualitative research can be used to address research questions related to why improvement occurs or detecting obstacles to treatment (Pope et al., 2002), and so could be ideally suited when physiotherapists are exploring whether a technique is suitable to use in a certain population. Qualitative research can also be used to tackle complex problems that arise with psychosocial issues (Curry et al., 2009), they can give more insight into the views of patients (Al-Busaidi, 2008) and shed light on the relevancy of certain techniques to tackle multifaceted psychosocial problems. Although quantitative research is

difficult to implement in practice because of strict inclusion and exclusion criteria, qualitative data can explore barriers to implementing strategies in practice (Pope et al., 2002) providing a richer picture to inform your decisions. With these benefits, qualitative data comprise an appropriate choice when considering using psychosocial techniques.

Qualitative methods are deductive rather than inductive (Curry et al., 2009) and involve deductions from multiple factors investigated, rather than proving effectiveness per se, in order to create new understanding. Different methodologies are used to create new information in a variety of ways and the choice is driven by the research question or the existential viewpoint of the researcher. Grounded theory methods may be used if the researcher wants to create a new theory concerning their psychologically informed practice and will involve moving between theory, data collection and analysis fluidly to generate new ideas and thoughts (Hall et al., 2013). Phenomenology methods involve understanding the meanings and experiences of others (Lopez and Willis, 2004), and in this context will explore the experiences of using psychologically informed strategies from the patient's and/or practitioner's viewpoints. Ethnography methodology involves exploring a group and their structure and function (Al-Busaidi, 2008), and could potentially explore the use of psychologically informed practice for specific populations. Case study designs were the most frequently used designs in the review by Weiner et al. (2011) and involve an in-depth and all-encompassing exploration of one or a small number of individuals. This methodology could be used to investigate psychologically informed practice, but generalizability will be limited and such consideration must be made when using the data.

Despite the variety and benefits of qualitative methods in aspects of psychologically informed practice, the use of qualitative research does remain controversial with doubts over the strength of the evidence it produces (Rahman and Majunder, 2013). Qualitative research produces rich and detailed data from a purposively selected sample that is extremely valid if the research is conducted well, but may have limited generalizability to different populations. Another challenge is in recognizing good-quality qualitative research: the problems in reporting qualitative research limit the reader's ability to appraise articles. In a systematic review and analysis of qualitative trials reported over a 10-year period, Weiner et al. (2011) discovered that half of the articles failed to describe key details of the study methods. Qualitative data are rich and detailed and a significant number of words are required to explore the methods and results. The strict word limits in many journals restrict the detailed explanation of methodology in trials. As such, it will limit decision making when we cannot recognize whether the results are robust.

## Using Mixed Methods Evidence

Mixed methodology would appear to be a sensible solution that would utilize the benefits of quantitative and qualitative research whilst minimizing the problems. A methodology that is rooted in the pragmatic philosophical paradigm provides insight into real world practice and the consequences of interventions (Creswell and Piano Clark, 2009). Using mixed methods will provide a more comprehensive representation of effectiveness than either method alone (Wisdom, 2012). There are different ways of conducting mixed methods, mainly concerned with how the sampling, data collection and analysis of each element are conducted, ie, concurrently or not. This will affect the way in which the data from a qualitative or quantitative element are used to inform the design or analysis of the other (Halcomb and Hickman, 2015), and could enhance the validity of the findings. In psychologically informed practice such methodology could analyse the feasibility of using psychosocial techniques and investigate effectiveness.

Alongside the problems previously discussed surrounding publications of qualitative studies, similar problems surround the publication of mixed method trials. In a review, Wisdom et al. (2012) discovered that key methodological components were often missing which was attributed to word count limitations and journal reviewers' lack of familiarity with the methodologies. To attempt to rectify this issue, trials could be reported in a segregated model with the methods reported in separate articles or chapters (Halcombe and Hickman, 2015) but this will restrict how the reporting of two arms of the trial affected one another. Furthermore when assessing the quality of the trials, the methods of demonstrating rigour in mixed method designs is still poorly defined (Halcomb and Hickman, 2015) and even though the design enhances validity, trials should still demonstrate rigour (Lavelle et al., 2013). With an unclear definition of rigour it is hard to critique trials and decide if the results and conclusions of mixed method studies are trustworthy.

## Making Evidence Informed Decisions About Psychologically Informed Practice

The potential problems concerning the different methodologies affect how we use the results to make decisions. However, by using a variety of trials and different methodologies, a more holistic view of psychologically informed practice and applicable interventions in physiotherapy can be considered. When making evidence-based decisions in this area, physiotherapists will need to explore areas and sources outside of the traditional 'physical therapy' domain and consider the applicability of a variety of research to their clinical practice.

When searching for literature about psychologically informed practice, research across a variety of professions may need to be accessed using other databases alongside those of medical practice, such as the PsycINFO database. If using sources outside of physiotherapy you will need to consider whether the strategies used are within, or outside of, your scope of practice. Such strategies and practice may be very pertinent to physiotherapy practice and, if so, clear justification is necessary when liaising with patients, colleagues and commissioners.

Critical quality appraisal is needed when any professional is using the evidence to inform practice. There are a variety of tools available to assist critical appraisal, but the correct tool for the methodology should be used to more effectively identify the qualities and trustworthiness of the results. This will allow balanced decisions to be made in relation to the underpinning evidence base, especially if results of different trials are conflicting. In addition, although there may

be a lack of rigorous evidence in relation to the specific population you treat, trials investigating the effects of interventions in related or nonspecific populations may exist. However, if doing so, you should be aware of how your population differs from the population studied and if these differences may affect the applicability of the results. If not, it could be possible to use such studies as long as the issue is raised when justifying your psychologically informed practice.

Some of the psychological strategies that you are looking at may not have a strong empirical evidence base, but a lack of evidence does not necessarily mean a lack of effectiveness. You may need to take a pragmatic approach in some cases and consider broader evidence. We cited Hammond (2002) at the start of this chapter, where he says that evidence based practice includes *'combining the best available evidence with clinical experience to turn the evidence into useful information for a specific patient, in particular circumstances.'* Your own experience and that of your peers, guidance from senior staff, opinion pieces and case reports in professional journals and other publications can all be factored in, so long as you take a critical and analytical approach to assessing this information. Where the evidence is conflicting or lacking, you should consider the degree of risk involved in applying a new strategy. This is discussed in more detail later in this chapter.

When implementing new practice, clinical effectiveness must be considered to measure the effect on patients. For this reason, the next section of this chapter explores potential ways to evaluate psychologically informed practice.

## EVALUATION AND MEASUREMENT OF PSYCHOLOGICALLY INFORMED PRACTICE

Ensuring excellence in the delivery of care, regardless of clinical setting, is paramount to any clinician. With time and cost effectiveness as added pressures, there is an ever increasing focus on 'measuring' the quality and delivery of what we do. As part of the Chartered Society of Physiotherapy's (CSP) Quality Assurance Standards, using outcome measures which are valid and standardized is an explicit requirement.

But, please consider what Einstein said ............

> 'Not everything that can be counted counts and not everything that counts can be counted'.
>
> *Albert Einstein*

So why do we use outcome measures when looking at psychologically informed practice? Health care providers have a duty to engage in evidence based practice, in which using outcome measures allows for

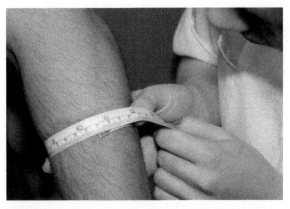

FIGURE 10.4 ■ Outcome measures – yes of course they are important.

the physiotherapist to provide credible and reliable justification for the employed intervention. Psychological outcome measures can monitor a range of both subjective and objective markers that we may be interested in as physiotherapists, thus giving us the potential of collecting either qualitative or quantitative data. These data can be utilized in many different ways. It may allow us to measure the effect of pathology on an individual, establish baseline measurements for evaluating change, assess the effect of an intervention or the effect a service may be providing. Outcome measures also have implications for use in clinical trials, audit and quality assurance.

As evidence based practitioners, we should be aware of the instrument or tool that we select to capture our outcomes. There are several considerations to make in order to achieve best practice with the instrument/ tool chosen. Firstly, is the reliability of the outcome measurement tool – will the results it produces be repeatable, will it yield the same (or similar) results despite when, where or who administers it? Secondly, what is the tool's validity? Is the outcome measure specific to the aspect of function it is aiming to test? Is it consistent? As part of reliability, there needs to be consideration for the sensitivity and specificity of the test. Finally, responsiveness – does it detect changes to the outcome measure over a period of time? Some outcome measures have been statistically tested to determine these aspects and therefore some have been shown to be more valid and reliable than others. These aspects are a part of the CSP core standards for physiotherapists...

> 'Taking account of the patient's problems, a published, standardised, valid, reliable

*and responsive outcome measure is used to evaluate the change in the patient's health status.'*

*(Core standards of physiotherapy practice, 2005)*

So what type of outcome measure should be used to inform my psychologically informed practice? (Table 10.1) These outcome measures can come in many formats and many can be accessed in the public domain. They include questionnaires which are simple, may be used and are included in a relevant published article as a part of that researcher's data collection. Other methods may involve gaining purchase through the copyright holder or even purchasing software systems via a commercial company.

Patient-centred care has always been at the forefront of physiotherapy. Patients' experience of their treatment can be an indicator of quality and in the last three decades there has

been a dramatic increase in the number of outcome measures that have been developed to measure this (questionnaires, rating scales and interview tools). These outcome measures which provide evidence from the patients' perspective are known as patient-reported outcome measures (PROMs). Recommendations from Lord Darzi's interim report suggested that PROMs should play a greater role in the National Health Service (NHS) and as part of the new standard NHS contract for acute services it has been a requirement from 2009 to report on PROMs for four different pathways (primary unilateral hip and knee replacements, groin hernia surgery or varicose vein surgery).There are several different types of this outcome measurement tool which can be applied to different situations.

In Table 10.2 we can see the pros and cons for each of these type of tools.

| TABLE 10.1 |
| --- |
| **Outcome Measurement Tools** |

| | |
| --- | --- |
| Disease specific instruments look specifically at the measurement of a specific disease/pathology or health problem; for example, low back pain (LBP) or chronic obstructive pulmonary disease (COPD) | 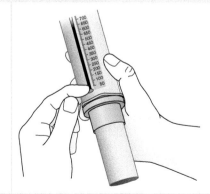 |

*Continued*

## TABLE 10.1 *cont*

### Outcome Measurement Tools

| | |
|---|---|
| Population specific instruments looking specifically at the demographics of a group; for example, the elderly, teenagers or paediatrics | 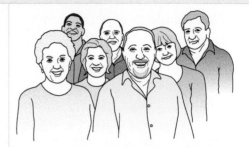 |
| Dimension specific – focuses on a particular aspect of the person's health; for example, pain, range of movement, anxiety or depression | 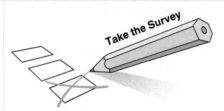 |
| Generic specific instruments – measure wide ranging aspects of a person's health; for example, Short Form 36 Health Survey is a measure of health and disability (including different aspects, such as physical functioning, bodily pain, emotional and social function, mental health) | 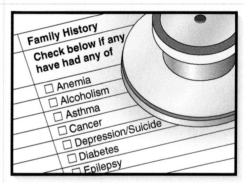 |
| Individualized – allow the patient to select the content and rate the importance of the tool; the patient generated index outcome tool allows the individual to select the five most important aspects to them that are affected by their condition and allows the individual to rate these aspects as targets for treatment | 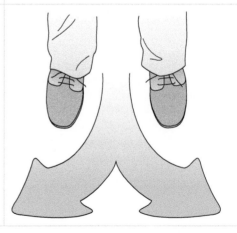 |

## TABLE 10.2
### Advantages and Disadvantages of Outcome Measures

| Instrument | Advantages | Disadvantages |
|---|---|---|
| Disease/ condition specific | Clinically relevant; very specific to a disease/ condition; clinical relevance apparent so high acceptability/compliance | Not widely applicable; limited transferability; outcomes cannot be compared with normal populations, thus limits economic evaluation |
| Population specific | Tailored to specific groups, makes them more relevant and more accessible | Not widely applicable; limited transferability; outcomes cannot be compared with normal populations, thus limits economic evaluation |
| Dimension specific | Can be more detailed than disease specific or generic; many have been widely used so data are available for comparing results | Measures of psychological wellbeing in dimension specific tools may not have been originally developed as outcome measures, but rather for diagnosis or needs assessment |
| Generic | Used across a broad range of health conditions for comparisons between treatments; can be used with healthy populations to develop normative data | Broad nature means they are less able to detect detail, therefore may be less responsive |
| Individualized | Addresses the concerns of the patient and therefore highly individualized; may have high validity | As a result of these tools having to be individually delivered they can effect feasibility |

*(Patient Reported Outcomes Measurements Group, 2010)*

## ADDITIONAL CONSIDERATIONS WHEN EVALUATING PSYCHOLOGICALLY INFORMED PHYSIOTHERAPY

When deciding on ways in which to measure outcomes in psychologically informed practice it is also important to think for whom you are providing information and how it may be used. In strained health care systems, when evaluating practice, we must consider how measurements will be used to make decisions that could affect individual patients or the funding for programmes. We will discuss these factors now to highlight some of the issues you may want to consider.

### Programme Evaluation and Commissioning

Most physiotherapists will be aware of the importance of working as closely as possible with local decision makers such as the Clinical Commissioning Groups (CCGs), local authorities, and the Health and Wellbeing Boards (HWB) (Chartered Society of Physiotherapy, 2016). Those involved in commissioning come from a variety of perspectives, both clinical and nonclinical, and need access to a range of sources to support their decision making.

Evidence-based commissioning is supported by library resources, such as Knowledge 4 Commissioning (2016). However, it has been suggested that professional background, gender and seniority can have a significant effect on the reliance on and choice of evidence used for decision making: those trained in public health being more likely to use empirical evidence; senior commissioners being more likely to use practical local evidence (Clarke et al., 2013). There may or may not be a physiotherapy expert on the panel for the CCG or the HWB and it would be wise to find out who is on your local boards and how you might be able to access them to establish their priorities. Also remember that boards will often have patients and members of the public involved so you should keep your information jargon free and avoid overuse of medical terminology.

NHS England's 'Five Year Forward View' (2014) emphasizes the importance of measuring and publishing meaningful and comparable measurements, measuring 'what matters'. The primary goal of the health service identified in the Dr Foster Ethics Committee Report (Appleby and Devlin, 2004) is improving people's health; in particular their health related quality of life (HRQoL). It was suggested that this type of PROM would help establish which treatments and delivery models are most effective and how services and clinicians are performing in comparable areas: including HRQoL data in the revalidation of clinicians, performance management of hospitals, tracking changes in clinical opinion and patient choice.

According to Garratt et al. (2002) some HRQoL measures, including the SF36 (Ware and Sherbourne, 1992), sickness effect profile (Bergner et al., 1981) and Nottingham health profile (Hunt et al., 1985) have been widely evaluated: across numerous patient populations and translated into several languages, with widely available population norms. There are also utility measures, developed for economic evaluation and targeting particular conditions, such as the EuroQol (EuroQol Group, 1990).

Although monitoring condition specific PROMs at national level is largely focused around four surgical procedures at the moment, there seems to be an appetite for expanding this approach into other sectors. The CSP recommended the use of the EuroQol-5Dimensions-5Levels (EQ-5D-5L) as a standard outcome measurement for outpatient musculoskeletal physiotherapy practice, in conjunction with appropriate and specific clinical outcome measures, and acquired an agreement for its free use in physiotherapy for a trial period (CSP, 2012).

Values based commissioning, a complementary approach to evidence based commissioning, aims to empower service users and carers to have more direct control over decisions relating to treatment, access to services and choice about care (England et al., 2013). Although this is currently focused on mental health services, it is a model that resonates with a psychologically informed physiotherapy practice in other settings where a biopsychosocial approach is used. Fulford (2011) proposed values based practice as a complementary approach to evidence based practice in order to address the growing complexity of values in contemporary health care decision making. He highlighted the increasing cultural diversity and values in society; the growth of multidisciplinary fields with a variety of professional value perspectives; and the advances in science and technology that have opened up wider ranges of choice with more complexity in decision making.

Maintaining a patient-centred approach in your practice requires a similarly appropriate measurement of outcomes, covering all aspects of that method. Although it remains important to use condition- or population-specific measures for some elements of the biopsychosocial approach (eg, symptoms and physical function) it is important to ensure that psychosocial aspects are also measured. If you are not already using them, PROM and HRQoL measures can bring some objectivity to what is essentially a subjective evaluation process in patient-centred care.

## Use of Measures at an Individual Patient Level

Nielsen et al. (2014) found that physiotherapists felt that public expectations of what physical therapy treatment should be may be a barrier to implementing a psychologically informed practice. To offset this, screening tools to identify potential predictors of poor outcome or ongoing disability may be used effectively in the clinical context as a starting point for discussion in the clinical interview, setting the scene for a more holistic approach for the patient. Rather than simply scoring a tool to identify the degree of likelihood of ongoing disability (filing the tool away in the notes), the physiotherapist can discuss the individual responses with the patient: providing opportunity for reinforcing the patient's more helpful attitudes, beliefs, or behaviours and exploring further and more specifically those that are less helpful in order to inform goals and treatment planning. This may be revisited at different stages in the rehabilitation process as a method of monitoring progress and renegotiating goals and treatment plans in a partnership with the patient.

Screening tools and outcomes in clinical practice can act as decision aids and as a method of facilitating communication among multidisciplinary teams (MDTs) to improve the discussion and detection of HRQoL problems (Greenhalgh, 2009); though it would appear that some practitioners may benefit from additional training to help them to identify, discuss and manage psychosocial aspects with their patients more effectively (Bishop and Foster, 2005; Overmeer et al., 2004; Synnott et al, 2015).

Taking time to review your caseload in relation to patient screening and outcomes will also provide you with opportunities to reflect on your own practice. Whether evaluating your own clinical effectiveness in a psychologically informed practice and identifying areas for learning and development, or reevaluating your choice of tools, you may want to revisit earlier sections of this chapter. Have you chosen tools that are valid, reliable and applicable to your population and setting? Are you using the tools in the way that they were designed and validated for use? Are you administering and scoring them appropriately? They should be sensitive enough to identify change and specific enough to ensure (so far as is possible) that the change is related to the intervention.

## Practical Issues

There are costs to using questionnaires for screening and outcome and, although they may be small per capita, they can present challenges in some settings. Costs may include a license for use, administration, equipment, training in their use, extended appointment times for completion of tools and printing. Care should be taken to avoid poor quality print versions of your questionnaires that are difficult to read and easy to misinterpret: 'someone lost the master copy!'

Not all measures are accessible in larger print, translated into different languages or adapted to different cultural groups (in a valid format) for the increasingly diverse socioeconomic and ethnic populations with whom we work. This can create a bias, excluding some sections of the population so that

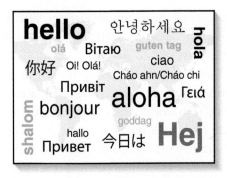

FIGURE 10.5 ■ Are we including all populations equally?

some patients may need an interpreter or other assistance in completing their questionnaires. There should be strategies in place to encourage equal opportunity for engagement and these should be regularly reviewed to ensure currency.

In psychologically informed practice there is a constant tension between keeping measures short and simple for routine clinical use (not overburdening the patient) and ensuring that they provide enough information to pick up change. There is also an ethical requirement to only gather necessary information and not information that is not subsequently used. Sometimes in practice clinicians routinely collect information out of habit, or because this is the 'done thing' in this department, without evaluating its use. You must be transparent in your intended use of any information collected.

## CASE STUDIES

To give some examples of decision making with regards to a psychologically informed practice and measurement of effectiveness, the case studies from Chapter 9 are revisited next.

## Case Study 1: the Use of Counselling Skills

If you think back to the Chapter 9, this physiotherapist was working in a respiratory outpatient clinic and treating people with chronic hyperventilation syndrome. She decided to train in counselling skills after raising her doubts over how she could discuss emotional subjects with patients. Her mentor was a physiotherapist who had previously trained in counselling so she was aware of the benefits of using counselling skills to explore emotions and suggested this type of training. The physiotherapist explored potential training opportunities surrounding counselling skills. Although an evidence based literature search was not completed in this example, the physiotherapist used the expertise of her team and more senior physiotherapists who were directed by evidence based practice.

When implementing her training in patient-centred counselling skills, the physiotherapist wanted to measure her effectiveness to inform her practice. The purpose of this measurement was to demonstrate clinical effectiveness of her reflection and to show improvements to the patient. Therefore she decided that the main effect of using counselling skills would be on the patient's psychological distress and wanted to assess this aspect before and after her treatment. She chose the Hospital Anxiety and Depression Scale (HADS) for this purpose as she had recently read about the scale's psychometric properties (Pallant and Tennant, 2007). This outcome could be tested before and after treatment to measure effectiveness at an individual patient level, to inform the physiotherapist of their effectiveness and to demonstrate improvement to patients if it was felt pertinent to do so.

If measuring outcome for a different purpose, for example to demonstrate effectiveness of this technique for all patients with chronic hyperventilation syndrome, different measurements and approaches would need to be considered in order to evaluate this in more depth. Managers and commissioners may want to see more holistic effects of using psychologically informed practice, and more measures may need to be obtained, eg, quality of life and functioning measures. There is potential to develop your practice evaluation to generate new knowledge and create a research project to inform all physiotherapists, clinicians, managers and commissioners relevant to this area. This could be measured quantitatively with a control group of participants who are not treated using psychologically informed practice to evaluate effectiveness for this population. Alternatively, it could be evaluated qualitatively to explore or generate a new theory to explain how it is experienced by the population. Obviously if the project was expanded to generate new research, full ethical and research development procedures should be adhered to.

## Case Study 2: the Use of Acceptance and Commitment Therapy

Looking at the case study of the school teacher with low back pain (LBP) 'Using Counselling and Psychological Strategies within Physiotherapy', this patient had already been seen by several physiotherapists with unsuccessful outcomes. The therapist knew that she had to take a different treatment approach in order to be effective and she wanted to be more holistic with assessment and treatment. She had recently read an article about physiotherapy that is informed by acceptance and commitment therapy for persistent LBP (Critchley et al., 2015), and decided to explore this treatment approach. After reading about the subject, looking at the evidence and further discussion with colleagues, she implemented this psychosocial strategy.

The therapist really wanted to explore how she could evaluate the intervention's effectiveness and discussed this with her senior clinicians. The EQ-5D-5L tool was suggested as a validated self-administered generic health status questionnaire that encompasses the holistic aspects of therapy (including mobility, ability to self-care, ability to undertake usual activities, pain and discomfort, and anxiety and depression). It aims to 'provide a simple generic measure of health for clinical and economic appraisal'. This can be used before and after intervention and these data can be collated to calculate quality of life adjusted years (QALY). QALY is the unit of measure that is currently used by the National Institute of Clinical Excellence (NICE) to assess the value of health outcomes. EQ-5D-5L is also one of the key measures utilized in the Department of Health in England to evaluate and benchmark some surgical pathways. This outcome measure can therefore be used at an individual level but also can be used to collate data to support the wider clinical picture of treatment and services, should this be required.

## Case Study 3: the Use of Motivational Interviewing Strategies

When the physiotherapy team identified problems with longer-term adherence to physical activity following discharge from group rehabilitation programmes for patients with osteoarthritic hips and knees they reflected on their practice together. One of them was already reading about motivational interviewing (MI) as a psychological strategy to try and encourage patients to articulate and resolve their ambivalence with regards to rehabilitation and maintenance of their physical activity. They identified that this might be an aspect the team had not been addressing. Hence individuals may not necessarily be working towards goals that were important to them and therefore may not be taking control of their own plans and solutions for the longer term. This also may have been why people did not carry on with their activities during class sessions.

The practitioner read evidence and literature on the effectiveness of MI and found some conflicting results and varying quality research; but in relation to maintaining healthy lifestyles (including physical activity adherence) and in relation to similar populations (with long-term conditions seen in primary care) he felt that there was enough evidence to implement MI as a low risk improvement to his current assessment approach. He had been reading about MI and how to implement it and had spoken to a colleague who participated in a training day and was using it in a weight management clinic.

The physiotherapy team decided to trial a new approach: they put together a small group session of three to four patients to explore their feelings about doing the exercises and physical activity in relation to their condition. The physiotherapist facilitating the group used MI techniques to enable participants to identify their ambivalence and then identify solutions. This served to engage them in self-management and long-term planning from the outset. The team also added an individual session for each patient at the conclusion of their rehabilitation to revisit their goals and planning.

In terms of evaluating their practice, this team did not feel that they should add to the patient load in terms of measurement as they already had a routine measurement and evaluation 'pack' in place. They used the following:

■ The revised short form McGill Pain Questionnaire (SFMPQ-2) as this was used throughout the orthopaedic department
■ Some functional measurements that they had collated themselves: range of motion; timed get up and go from sitting to a 5 metre point; number of sit-to-stands in 2 mins; and self-reported 'comfortable walking distance on the flat' (perceived average in the last week)
■ The EQ-5D-5L which had been used throughout the outpatient physiotherapy unit for the last few years
■ Telephone follow-up at 3 months post discharge to ask whether the patients were able to maintain their physical activity levels (by an administrator). They were asked (a) the EQ-5D-5L questions and (b) their self-reported 'comfortable walking distance on the flat' (perceived average in the last week).

In order to see whether the implementation of MI techniques and the new programme model was having any effect they decided that they would do a comparison of the EQ-5D-5L scores, at discharge and at the 3 month review, with previous groups.

## CONCLUSION

The aim of this chapter was to explore the challenges in identifying appropriate psychologically informed practice and when measuring effectiveness of psychosocial strategies among other outcome measures in clinical practice. To do this, the benefits and drawbacks of quantitative, qualitative and mixed methods have been considered to allow you to recognize how decisions could be made based on the available evidence. This can be particularly challenging in psychologically informed practice because of the range of methodologies used and the inherent problems when investigating patient-centred approaches. You may also have to weigh up the degree of risk in implementing a new strategy where there may be limited or inconclusive evidence to support you. Your decision will incorporate reflection on your own practice, your knowledge and skills in the area, the training you might be able to access before implementing it, whether formal training is required, critical reflection with peers and opportunities for support and supervision (eg, shadowing others). For example, using a cognitive behavioural approach in your physiotherapy practice is different from practicing as a cognitive behavioural therapist, which requires formal training and case experience.

Looking at different tools to measure effectiveness and the issues that would need to be considered when collecting information has also been explored. As discussed in the beginning of this chapter, it will be unlikely that you will be able to pick out psychologically informed aspects of your practice to measure specifically and in isolation. Although your psychological strategies will be applied in an effort to elicit improvement in psychological factors, as a physiotherapist you will be using it to facilitate further improvement in function. As such, your physical and psychological strategies will be integrated and difficult to assess separately. Hence most of the tools discussed are not aimed at measuring psychosocial strategies in isolation, but rather as part of a holistic approach.

Finally, clinicians need to be mindful of who the information they are collecting is for and what purpose it is to serve; if gaining information to provide proof of effectiveness for managers or commissioners, different measurements and tools may be needed than if using the information to inform patients on their clinical progress. Case studies have been used in an attempt to try and contextualize and bring together strategies and measurement tools to give examples of how decisions can be made and justified.

### References

Al-Busaidi, Z.Q., 2008. Qualitative research and its uses in health care. Sultan Qaboos Univ. Med. J. 8 (1), 11–19.

Appleby, J., Devlin, N., 2004. Measuring success in the NHS: Using patient-assessed health outcomes to manage the performance of healthcare providers. Dr Foster Ethics Committee. Accessed on 03.02.16 at: <www.drfoster.co.uk/documents/Measuring%20success.pdf>.

Bergner, M., Bobbitt, R.A., Carter, W.B., Gilson, B.S., 1981. The sickness impact profile: development and final revision of a health status measure. Med. Care 19, 787805.

Bishop, A., Foster, N.E., 2005. Physical Therapists in the United Kingdom Recognize Psychosocial Factors in Patients with Acute Low Back Pain? Spine 30 (11), 1316–1322.

Chartered Society of Physiotherapy (CSP), 2012. EQ-5D-5L Terms and Conditions. Accessed 11.02.16 at <http://www.csp.org.uk/documents/eq-5d-5l-terms-conditions>.

Chartered Society of Physiotherapy (CSP), no date. Get to grips with England's new health system – presentation, fact-sheets and resources. Accessed 11.02.16 at

<http://www.csp.org.uk/professional-union/nhs-changes/england/get-grips/presentations-factsheets>.

Clarke, A., Taylor-Phillips, S., Swan, J., et al., 2013. Evidence-based commissioning in the English NHS: who uses which sources of evidence? A survey 2010/2011. BMJ Open 3 (5), e002714. doi:10.1136/bmjopen-2013-002714.

Clay, R., 2010. More than one way to measure. Monit. Psychol. 41 (8), 52. Retrieved from: <http://www.apa.org/monitor/2010/09/trials.aspx>.

Creswell, J.W., Plano Clark, V.L., 2009. Designing and conducting mixed methods research. Sage Publications, London.

Critchley, D.J., McCracken, L.M., Talewar, R., Walker, N., Sanders, D., Godfrey, E., 2015. Physiotherapy informed by acceptance and commitment therapy for persistent low back pain. Physiotherapy 101 (1), 277.

Curry, L.A., Nebhard, I.M., Bradley, E.H., 2009. Qualitative and mixed methods provide unique contributions to outcomes research. Circulation 119, 1442–1452.

England, E., Singer, F., Perry, E., Barber, J., 2013. Guidance for implementing values-based commissioning in mental health. Joint Commissioning Panel for Mental Health. Accessed from <www.jcpmh.info> on 09.02.16.

EuroQol Group, 1990. EuroQol—a new facility for the measurement of health-related quality of life. Health Policy (New York) 16, 199208.

Fulford, K.W.M., 2011. The value of evidence and evidence of values: bringing together values-based and evidence-based practice in policy and service development in mental health. J. Eval. Clin. Pract. 17, 976–987.

Garratt, A., Schmidt, L., Mackintosh, A., Fitzpatrick, R., 2002. Quality of life measurement: bibliographic study of patient assessed health outcome measures. BMJ 324, 1417.

Greenhalgh, J., 2009. The applications of PROs in clinical practice: what are they, do they work, and why? Qual. Life Res. 18 (1), 115–123. doi:10.1007/s11136-008-9430-6; PMID: 19105048.

Halcomb, E., Hickman, L., 2015. Mixed methods research. Nurs. Stand. 29 (32), 41–47.

Hall, H., Griffiths, D., McKenna, L., 2013. From Darwin to constructivism: the evolution of grounded theory. Nurse Res. 20 (3), 17–21.

Hammond, R., 2002. An introduction to clinical effectiveness. In: Physiotherapy Pain Association Yearbook: Topical Issues in Pain 3. CNS Press, Cornwall, UK.

Harris, A.D., McGregor, J.C., Perencevich, E.N., Furuno, J.P., Zhu, J., Peterson, D.E., et al., 2006. The use and interpretation of quasi-experimental studies in medical informatics. J. Am. Med. Inform. Assoc. 13 (1), 16–23.

Hunt, S.M., McEwen, J., McKenna, S.P., 1985. Measuring health status: a new tool for clinicians and epidemiologists. J. R. Coll. Gen. Pract. 35, 1858.

Knowledge 4 Commissioning. Providing an Evidence Based NHS. <http://www.knowledge4commissioning.nhs.uk/> Accessed 11.02.16.

Lavelle, E., Vuk, J., Barber, C., 2013. Twelve tips for getting started using mixed methods in medical education research. Med. Teach. 35, 272–276.

Lewis, S.C., Warlow, C.P., 2004. How to spot bias and other potential problems in randomised controlled trials. J. Neurol. Neurosurg. Psychiatry 75, 181–187.

Lopez, K.A., Willis, D.G., 2004. Descriptive versus interpretive phenomenology: Their contributions to nursing knowledge. Qual. Health Res. 14, 726–735.

NHS England, 2014. Five Year Forward View. Accessed on 03.02.16 at <https://www.england.nhs.uk/ourwork/futurenhs/#doc>.

Nielsen, M., Keefe, F.J., Bennell, K., Jull, G.A., 2014. Physical therapist–delivered cognitive-behavioral therapy: a qualitative study of physical therapists' perceptions and experiences. Phys. Ther. 94, 197–209.

Overmeer, T., Linton, S.J., Boersma, K., 2004. Do physical therapists recognise established risk factors? Swedish physical therapists' evaluation in comparison to guidelines. Physiotherapy 90, 35–41.

Pallant, J.F., Tennant, A., 2007. An introduction to the Rasch measurement model: An example using the Hospital Anxiety and Depression Scale (HADS). Br. J. Clin. Psychol. 46, 1–18.

Patient Report Outcomes Measurements Group, 2010. Retrieved 10th January, 2016, from <http://phi.uhce.ox.ac.uk/home.php>.

Pope, C., van Royen, P., Baker, R., 2002. Qualitative methods in research on healthcare quality. Qual. Saf. Health Care 11, 148–152.

Rahman, S., Majumder, A.A., 2013. Qualitative research in medicine and healthcare: Is it subjective, unscientific or second class science? South East Asia J. Public Health 3 (1), 69–71.

Synnott, A., O'Keeffe, M., Bunzli, S., Dankaerts, W., O'Sullivan, P., O'Sullivan, K., 2015. Physiotherapists may stigmatise or feel unprepared to treat people with low back pain and psychosocial factors that influence recovery: a systematic review. J. Physiother. 61, 68–76.

Ware, J.E., Sherbourne, C.D., 1992. The MOS 36-item short-form health survey (SF36): I. conceptual framework and item selection. Med. Care 30, 47383.

Weiner, B.J., Amick, H.R., Lund, J.L., Lee, S.-Y.D., Hoff, T.J., 2011. Use of qualitative methods in published health services and management research: a 10-year review. Med. Care Res. Rev. 68 (1), 3–33.

Wisdom, J.P., Cavaleri, M.A., Onwuegbuzie, A.J., Green, C.A., 2012. Methodological reporting in qualitative, quantitative, and mixed methods health services research articles. Health Serv. Res. 47 (2), 721–745.

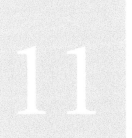

# 11

# USING PSYCHOLOGICAL INTERVENTIONS AS A STUDENT OR NEWLY QUALIFIED PHYSIOTHERAPIST – PERSONAL REFLECTIONS 1 YEAR POST QUALIFYING

KATHERINE E CROOK

## CHAPTER CONTENTS

## INTRODUCTION

A plethora of information about human psychology is available to the reader. I have been invited to write this chapter as a real-time record chronicling my first year of experience post qualifying and how psychology has informed my clinical practice. It is therefore important that the reader recognize that this is partly a reflective piece which partly draws on academic literature. It is envisaged that the chapter will be useful for future undergraduates on their journey and newly qualified graduates alike. Although the methods and principles explored and the examples discussed are based on a musculo-skeletal outpatient department setting, they are also transferable to a wide range of clinical settings. It is worth noting that implementing psychological methods in the treatment of specific client groups – paediatric, mental health, chronic pain – is outside the remit of this chapter.

The term 'psychology' is broad and often misused and a misunderstood subject, especially when embedded within another. It is useful, at this early stage, to define the term 'psychology' within the specific arena of physiotherapy and the new practitioner, with the aim of creating malleable boundaries within which to begin our discussion. As such, in this chapter psychology means any technique, verbal or nonverbal, used by a physiotherapist in order to enhance the patient's therapeutic experience and facilitate a timely recovery.

## CHAPTER AIM AND CONTENTS

The aim of this chapter is to provide the student and new graduate with an overview of psychological interventions used in the management of patients; building upon the skills learned at the undergraduate level and providing ways in which to develop as a practitioner.

This chapter will begin by identifying the importance of psychology within physiotherapy and current undergraduate teachings on the topic. It will then move on to the identification of the range of emotional states that the new graduate will encounter, the discussion of the significance of pain and how a patient deals with this and the importance of a patient's locus of control and the effect this can have on the therapist. The next part will look at touch as a nonverbal communication technique and will discuss the biopsychosocial model. The final part of the chapter will look at my personal reflections throughout my first year post qualifying and identify important psychological experiences. Finally the chapter will look at limitations

### IMPORTANT BACKGROUND INFORMATION

As of 2013 the importance of 'psychological wellbeing' had been removed from the Chartered Society of Physiotherapists (CSP) website in both the definition of physiotherapy and from the learning and development principles for CSP accreditation of qualifying programmes in physiotherapy. This differs from 2002 when the CSP stated that physiotherapists should use 'physiological approaches to promote, maintain and restore physical, psychological and social wellbeing' (CSP, 2002).

In contrast, the Health and Care Professions Council (HCPC) is clear that they require physiotherapists to incorporate psychology by being able to 'identify and take account of the physical, psychological, social and cultural needs of individuals and communities' (HCPC, 2013). The HCPC highlights that psychology can influence a person's response to the management of their health and related physiotherapy intervention and, crucially, helps to inform an understanding of health, illness and health care in the context of physiotherapy and the incorporation of this knowledge into physiotherapy practice (HCPC, 2013).

of psychology in physiotherapy practice and will give a number of real-life scenarios with questions to stimulate discussion.

## THE IMPORTANCE OF PSYCHOLOGY WITHIN PHYSIOTHERAPY AND AN OVERVIEW OF WHAT IS CURRENTLY BEING TAUGHT WITHIN UK PHYSIOTHERAPY SCHOOLS

It has been proposed that the appropriate use of psychology can help to improve patient satisfaction, empowerment, motivation and pain management (George, 2008; Green et al., 2008; Margalit et al., 2004; Middleton, 2004; Miller et al., 2009).

Recent research has highlighted that, although psychology in some form is currently taught in the UK in physiotherapy schools, the content (amount, type and delivery), depth and breadth of what is taught varies markedly both within and between schools. The authors report the 'most significant finding of this study is that of inconsistency' and the integrated nature of teaching psychology hinders the study further (Heaney et al., 2012). However, the study also found that there was an inconsistency between the importance placed on psychology and the amount of time given to the topic, calling it 'limited visibility' (Heaney et al., 2012). The study concluded that more needs to be done to standardize the course content of UK physiotherapy programmes (Heaney et al., 2012). Students focus on anatomy and physiology, reflection and development, vivas and placements, but have little time to work on (perceived) peripheral issues, including psychology. It is little wonder then that physiotherapy graduates feel ill-prepared to use psychologically informed interventions in their working day (Alexanders et al., 2014). As such, it is important early on in one's career to identify the benefits of psychology and develop this skill alongside clinical competence. It is also important that psychology is not seen as a separate entity from the positivistic world of musculoskeletal physiotherapy practice, where it can be easy to reduce patients to a collection of body parts and symptoms.

In recent years there has been a shift away from the emphasis on the traditional medical model (although this still has its place) to the biopsychosocial model of assessment and treatment of patients. This dictates that the patient's psychological status is of equal significance as that of the medical pathology. However, qualified physiotherapists report feeling ill-trained to fully carry out this type of assessment and utilize these interventions (Alexanders et al., 2014).

## THE RANGE OF EMOTIONAL STATES THE NEW GRADUATE WILL ENCOUNTER; DISCUSSION OF THE SIGNIFICANCE OF PAIN AND HOW A PATIENT DEALS WITH THIS; IMPORTANCE OF A PATIENT'S LOCUS OF CONTROL AND ITS EFFECT ON THE THERAPIST

In any clinical setting a patient's psychological status will affect directly what the therapist can or should do. The patient may feel worried, angry, unsure of why they are attending or conversely be motivated and eager to begin rehabilitation. These elements may affect the patient's psychological state. Such contributing factors all have the potential to change a person's character and behaviour: bereavement, preexisting comorbidities of physical or mental health, long-term unemployment and financial difficulties are just a few examples. All of these factors can influence the experience of pain, the main driver in seeking professional intervention. As an aside, this demonstrates the importance of objective assessment throughout the course of treatment, as this can help a patient see the progress from a factual standpoint and facilitate discharge or appropriate onward referral.

Most patients that physiotherapists treat will complain of pain in some form, among other symptoms. This can affect each person differently: person A may exhibit anger, whereas person B may exhibit anxiety or depression as a result of their pain or disability and person C may be stoic and offer very little for the therapist to 'work with' regarding their psychological state. There is no set pattern or response, nor is there a 'right' or 'wrong' reaction to illness or resultant disability. The skill of the therapist lies in identifying their patient's response and managing both their psychology and medical conditions simultaneously. The development of yellow flags has provided a more structured approach allowing the therapist to acknowledge, but not be overwhelmed by, their presence. (For more information on the 'flag system', please see Chapters 2)

In connection with this is the extent to which a patient believes their recovery is controlled by themselves or others – the extent to which the patient has an internal or external locus of control (see Figs 11.1 and 11.2)

Perhaps a more accurate reflection shows these as blurred boundaries rather than as distinct beliefs, ie, Figure 11.3.

The patient may perceive themselves to have no control over their symptoms, situation or indeed the best ways to change for the better – the most appropriate treatment. This

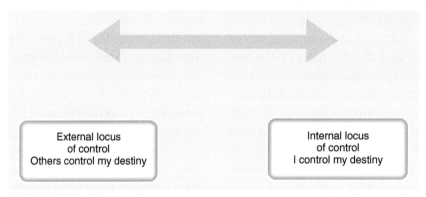

FIGURE 11.1 ▪ Simplified diagram of the concept of internal *versus* external locus of control.

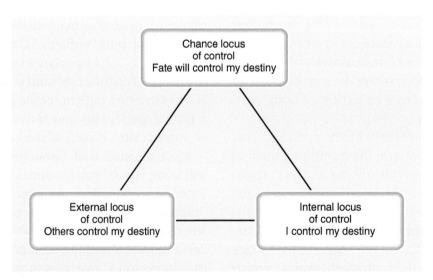

FIGURE 11.2 ▪ The inclusion of chance locus of control.

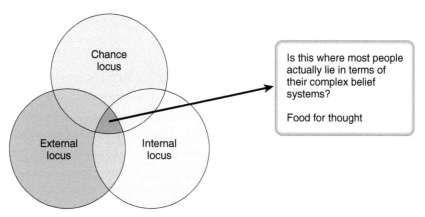

Is this where most people actually lie in terms of their complex belief systems?

Food for thought

FIGURE 11.3 ■ A more accurate reflection shows these as blurred boundaries rather than distinct beliefs.

may make a patient more aggressive and demanding, questioning every treatment modality and never quite believing in the efficacy of a treatment. The theory was first put forward in 1954 by clinical psychologist Julian B. Rotter and developed into a multi-dimensional health locus of control scale in 1978 (MHLC; Rotter, 1966; Wallston et al., 1978).

After Levenson's (1974) splitting of Rotter's internal-external construct into three dimensions – internal, powerful others, and chance – the MHLC scale was born. The MHLC scales consist of two forms, A and B that are the 'general' health locus of control scales (Wallston et al., 1978). Subsequently Wallston et al. (1994) developed form C in which they further split the powerful others dimension into two subscales: doctors and other people (Wallston et al., 1994). Finally, Wallston et al. (1999) refined the model by adding a new subscale assessing beliefs about God as a locus of control of one's health status. Chaplin et al. (2001) used factor analysis for this four-factor scale. Their findings showed that despite a desirable correlation

between the three external factors of God, powerful others, and chance, the four-factor condition which takes into account an internal control factor yields the best outcome.

Rotter's model offers an internal locus of control whereby success is believed to be based on the individual's hard work and belief that they control their own life. Alternatively those with an external locus of control attribute success, importantly for the therapist's failure, to outside influences and individuals. The external locus also contains a second element: that of chance whereby an improvement in pain or range of movement, for example, is as a result of fate or chance with no other forces at work (Keedy, 2009). Most people will be a mix of internal, external and chance and will exhibit one or a mix of loci depending on a given situation – however, in a health care setting a dominant side may surface. Consider two patients who you are treating for the same condition, one with an internal locus and one with an external locus. Patient A and B have had nonspecific lower back pain for several years, have never had any treatment and prefer instead to self-manage with the support of their general practitioner (GP). Both have sedentary lives with desk based jobs. However, what splits the two is their locus of control. Patient A has an external locus – he believes his back pain is from years of a desk job; he has never had an ergonomic assessment at work and has had no support from higher management for his back pain. His GP refers him to physiotherapy. He has never had treatment or physiotherapy before for any condition and his expectation is that the therapist will cure his pain. He does not expect to have to do anything actively and thinks that hands on treatment will solve his problem. Patient B has an external locus of control, he is aware that he has had poor posture for many years after a desk based career. He is underactive. He too has had no treatment for his back pain, but his expectations of physiotherapy are that it is unlikely to help. After six treatment sessions both patients' symptoms have resolved somewhat, but not completely improved. Patient A is angry that his back pain is still present and feels that the physiotherapist did not do enough hands on, fobbing him off with exercises and advice on posture. Patient B tried all the exercises but still feels he could have done more. It is clear from these two examples that the locus of control can have an effect on every stage of physiotherapy intervention. Patients with external, internal and chance loci present the therapist with various challenges and there are benefits and problems with their various ways of thinking. A patient with a strongly dominant internal locus of control may push themselves to work at a harder intensity too soon in their rehabilitation and may be reluctant to see their progress or have unrealistic goals. A patient with a strongly dominant external locus may want passive treatments, be noncompliant with home exercises or blame past treatments for lack of improvement in symptoms. A patient with a chance locus may be unmotivated, noncompliant with home exercises or request a discharge without treatment. Questions should be in the therapists' mind concerning: will the patient expect passive treatment; does the patient understand the importance of taking control of the situation, of completing exercises regularly? Does the patient understand that their pain may not resolve completely or take months and a change of lifestyle to resolve? Additionally have you, as the therapist, explained the treatment, its aims and goals in terms that each patient will benefit most from?

It is important for a therapist to try and identify a person's locus of control. In addition to illness cognitions, individuals maintain belief systems with regards to control over their health. The concept of Health Locus of Control (HLC) states that through a learning process, individuals will develop the belief that certain outcomes concerning their health are either a result of their own action (internals), other independent forces (externals) or chance (Levenson, 1973). Consequently many health education programmes, such as the Expert Patient Programme (EPP), emphasize responsibility and reinforcement of internal beliefs.

Research into control of chronic disease and locus of control is fascinating; for example, in ankylosing spondylitis (AS) Barlow et al. (1993) administered locus of control questionnaires to AS self-help group members analysing health locus of control beliefs along three dimensions – internality, powerful others and chance – and suggested that they could be distinguished with a sensitivity of 71.9% from nongroup members by their low reliance on powerful others, a greater satisfaction with available support and increased frequency of exercise. What is less clear is whether a person's locus of control can change over time, although there is grounded evidence that AS patients act as sophisticated problem solvers who describe the need to predict and respond to a changing disease trajectory and employ a number of informed strategies for long- and short-term exercise management (Porter, 2010). Participants here described a process of ongoing appraisal of their AS status and used approaches similar to cost–benefit analyses to make decisions about exercise behaviour.

MHLC validity and usefulness have been questioned and there are other available measures, for example the McGill pain questionnaire (Main and Waddel, 1991; Wallston, 2005).

## NONVERBAL COMMUNICATION

As mentioned earlier, the use of psychology is important in physiotherapy as it can facilitate the speedy recovery and discharge of a patient. Similarly efficient and effective communication is the basis of any therapist's training and interaction with a patient (Al-Abri and Al-Balushi, 2014). The next section of this chapter engages in nonverbal communication as a psychological technique. Nonverbal communication consists of several interconnecting components which are largely developed from social interaction. These begin in childhood and evolve as social

**BOX 11.2**

Eye contact
Facial expressions
Smiling
Appropriate body space
Body posture
Movement

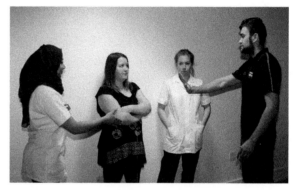

FIGURE 11.4 ■ Nonverbal communication.

situations demand. Examples of these are highlighted in Box 11.2 and Fig. 11.4.

### To Touch or Not to Touch ... That Is the Question (Apologies to Shakespeare)

Touch as a nonverbal communication technique is a key skill in a physiotherapist's role both for diagnostic assessment and treatment see Fig. 11.5. Physiotherapists are known in Western culture for massage and hands on treatment techniques. Physiotherapy carries NHS funding and accreditation. Whether it be offering soft tissue massage or the expectation that the physiotherapy treatment is only occurring once the therapist is 'hands on', demonstrates the general public's appreciation of the profession. Touch, in a clinical setting, can take on many forms. The objective assessment usually consists of touch

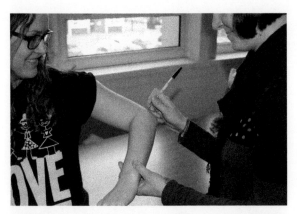

FIGURE 11.5 ■ Student physiotherapists first encounter touch during induction week at the University of Salford, United Kingdom. *(With thanks to Rachel Amelot and Rachael Kenny, Class of 2014)*

– feeling and moving body segments to assess movement and strength. Being too forceful in the objective assessment may cause excessive and needless pain, may give 'false positives' on assessment or may prevent a full assessment from taking place. This in turn can have a detrimental effect on your treatment as the patient is reluctant to be touched, tensing up when you attempt passive movements. Fundamentally the development of trust will be diminished which is essential to patient-centred care.

At the start or end of a treatment session a handshake can convey many things – power and strength, but it can also show compassion and trustworthiness. For example, understanding not to shake the hand of an elderly patient with rheumatoid arthritis will demonstrate nonverbally that you understand the patient's condition and will help to forge a trusting working relationship from the outset.

Of course there is a debate about the efficacy of hands on treatment versus no contact. Patients may believe that they are only receiving treatment once the therapist touches them; they do not understand that their treatment may consist of other factors such as education and advice or a home exercise programme to complete independently. This links into a patient's locus of control demonstrating the importance of identifying a patient locus accurately at each stage of treatment. By correctly identifying the locus it will alert the therapist to the possibility that once manual treatment is started the patient will rely solely on passive treatments to improve. If this improvement does not happen, the conclusion may be that physiotherapy 'doesn't work' for them or their condition. Additionally if the patient exhibits health behaviours, whereby they are a chronic pain patient, this perceived failure of physiotherapy will only add to their belief that the condition is what defines them. In turn this can affect employability, mental health or quality of life. Alternatively a patient may not want, require or be suitable for manual therapy. This may be as a result of skin viability issues, or pain or cultural/religious reasons; if a patient has an external locus of control they may want to be the sole generator of their improvement. In such cases no contact is indicated, indeed it could be said that it is contraindicated if we give the patient's psychological state as much influence as their physical state. As with outcome measures it is important to reassess the patient's psychological state and provide what is most appropriate for the patient at that particular time. A patient's psychological state can change and will require the therapist to identify these changes and act accordingly, for example a patient may require one session of soft tissue massage in order to initiate the recovery on the physiological/psychological/

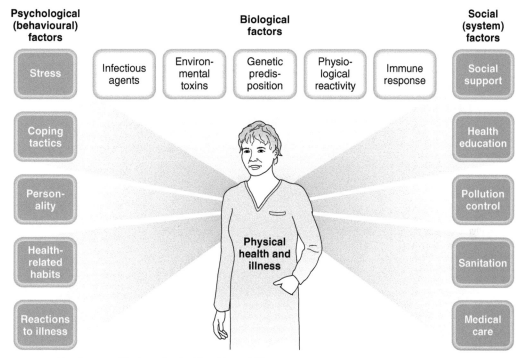

FIGURE 11.6 ■ The factors affecting physical health and illness.

placebo level, or all of the above; it is beyond the scope of this chapter to argue the ethical nature of this debate.

## DISCUSSION OF THE BIOPSYCHOSOCIAL MODEL IN MY CLINICAL PRACTICE

This part of the chapter will look at the biopsychosocial model of assessment. By way of a reminder, the following diagram illustrates the BPS approach in terms of factors affecting health and, secondly, pain.

A focus on patient-centred health care has moved us towards the BPS model which has resulted in its increasing acceptance in a clinical setting and support by the World Health Organization (WHO) (Green et al., 2008; WHO, 2002). The BPS approach argues that nonmedical factors have an equal impor-

tance in the understanding, and therefore treatment, of a patient's medical condition. The approach differs from the traditional medical paradigm as it aims to highlight and acknowledge the range of psychological and social factors which may affect a person's health. Table 11.1 illustrates some key psychological and social parameters commonly found to affect a person in clinical physiotherapy practice see Fig. 11.6 and Table 11.1. This is reflected in the WHO definition of health which states that health is not merely the absence of disease, rather that health is a state of complete physical, mental and social wellbeing (WHO, 1948). The definition has not been amended since 1948, this is therefore not a new concept.

In a careful and logical physiotherapy assessment the therapist may discover factors

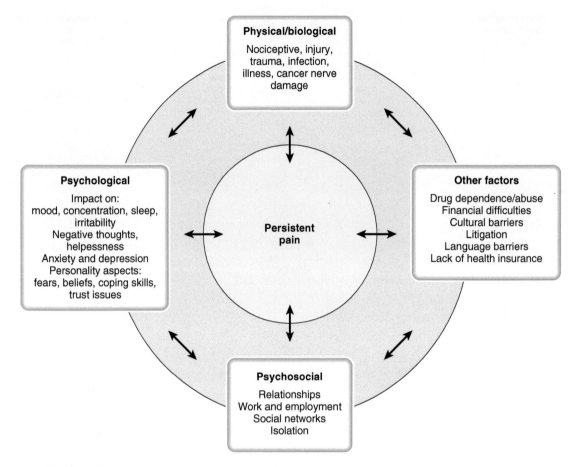

Factors affecting pain.

### TABLE 11.1

**Social and Psychological Parameters Affecting Health**

| Psychological | Social |
|---|---|
| Depression | Employment/career |
| Anxiety | Housing |
| Comorbidities | Relationship(s) |
| Fear of pain and resultant fear avoidance cycles | Bereavement and grief |
| Yellow flags | Finances |

which will disrupt a patient's progress to good health – this may be as a result of a recent bereavement, self-employment related financial concerns or the psychological effects of chronic pain. These all relate back to the concept of locus of control, mentioned previously, and can all motivate or restrict the patient's progress. Use of the BPS model can help with the assessment of a patient and ultimately with their treatment.

Within physiotherapy, the BPS model is most often used with chronic pain patients (the vast majority of NHS physiotherapists' workload) where there is no cure *per se* and the focus is on long-term management looking at helping the patient deal with and maximize their quality of life and improve their ability to cope with their pain and any resulting disabilities. Thus the focus becomes about the individual rather than the removal of the problem (pain) through medication, surgery or other forms of treatment.

Keele University in the UK has utilized the model as a part of a tool used in relation to lower back pain. The Keele STarT Back Screening Tool (SBST) is used to help therapists identify those patients who may be 'at risk' of developing chronic back pain. Calculating a score from nine questions places a patient within one of three categories – low, medium and high – with a matching treatment package most appropriate for the patient. The high risk category indicates that a biopsychosocial assessment is most appropriate with the option of treatment, such as manual therapy or acupuncture. A biopsychosocial assessment of back pain consists of asking questions about the patient's life, activity levels, mobility, thoughts about their condition and trying to improve some of these factors. For example, asking about a patient's understanding of the reasons for their pain may result in the patient explaining they were told they had 'crumbling discs' or 'something had come out'. Over time this interpretation can become cruder and quite far removed from the realities of the x-ray or scan initially used to explain the degenerative changes associated with spondylosis. By spending time, using accurate wording and written information reeducating the patient on their condition the therapist can help to alleviate worry and reduce the importance of the patient's medical symptoms. In turn this allows for psychological change in relation to stress, pain, activity and long-term management. This demonstrates that as a part of BPS assessment, (re)education is a key element of what physiotherapists can offer (Burton et al., 1996; Waddell, 1987).

Understanding a patient's attitude towards, and expectations of, physiotherapy can ensure that the patient understands the scope and limitations of physiotherapy interventions. It can provide the therapist with information about whether the patient is realistic in their expectations of what physiotherapy can achieve and what they think about their condition. For example, a patient with severe spondylosis hoping for 'a cure' or 'for the pain to stop' would need reeducation about their condition. This may also demonstrate whether a patient's coping strategies are passive (manual therapy, acupuncture) or active (exercise/movement, pacing). The therapist can then adjust their interventions accordingly.

Asking the patient if there are any activities, movements or situations they avoid or restrict because of pain can offer the therapist avenues to explore to help increase activity or areas to avoid which may be unrealistic. For example, a patient may limit their outdoor mobilizing and this could be an area to develop, ie, leaving the house three times daily rather than twice. Alternatively a patient may explain that they used to attend a gym regularly, but because of transport or confidence issues they have stopped. The therapist may be aware of local council initiatives which would suit the patient to help them get back into a gym. The focus is on increasing patient self-efficacy – the extent or strength of one's belief in one's own ability to complete tasks and reach goals (Ormrod, 2006).

Pain, reduced activity and a change in social and work status can all have an effect on a patient's mood, however there is no universal acceptable response. Anxiety and depression can be triggered or exacerbated by pain or a change in circumstances. There may be changes in diurnal patterns which can influence what the patient can undertake or it may be useful to direct the patient to their GP for appropriate medication or talking therapies to begin to deal with these feelings.

In a musculoskeletal or any other therapeutic assessment it is useful to have an arsenal of questions or topics to gain as much relevant information as possible. This will build up a picture of the patient's life and how they are currently coping with their pain, thus allowing one to see where gaps and opportunities may be to bring about change. This may be something as simple as learning that the patient has grandchildren they wish to interact with more or that they currently visit a bingo hall once a week. By identifying positive elements in this way it is easier to build on these rather than trying to implement completely new activities into a person's life. So asking if the patient may be able to manage walking to the garden path with their grandchild or increasing their visits to the bingo to twice weekly would be more manageable than twice weekly visits to a local gym or swimming pool. By harnessing the patient's current positive behaviour, change becomes more acceptable and less daunting. It is important to recognize that inclusion of the BPS as a core part of an assessment will need more investment at the undergraduate level and is still not without its difficulties.

The findings of Sanders et al. (2013) documents the recognition by physiotherapists of the need to identify and address the social and psychological obstacles to recovery that patients with low back pain experience. They go on interestingly, however, to affirm that physiotherapists often struggle to find ways to understand and address these psychosocial factors, often claiming that these problems fall outside of their immediate scope of physiotherapy practice. Sanders et al. (2013) also engage with the distinction between psychosocial factors or obstacles affecting patients' abilities to manage their back pain and their health beliefs, which may be more problematic to change. Consequently physiotherapists must both recognize patients' health beliefs and respond with appropriate clinical advice. Providing advice without first understanding a patient's beliefs could lead to reduced recovery or compliance because the patient may respond negatively to clinical recommendations that do not sufficiently connect with their experiences of living with back pain.

Examples of BPS issues that have had a bearing on treatment decisions in my recent clinical practice include the following:

1. A recently bereaved patient referred for nonspecific lower back pain. Home exercise programme, advice, education and reassurance offered on the nature of their symptoms. The patient was offered a range of treatments, including the option of self-management with an open appointment for 6 weeks. The patient chose the latter option as she felt unable to commit to a structured course of treatment involving leaving her home and being in an alien environment.

2. A patient referred after several months of ongoing back pain and symptoms resulting in lumbar spine surgery. Medically the patient was doing well and her rehabilitation was uneventful; however, as a result of the long-term nature of her condition she struggled with anxiety surrounding the success of the surgery and rehabilitation. With this patient I focussed on listening to her concerns and worries and spent time on reassurance and discussion of anatomy with exercise prescription taking on a smaller role.

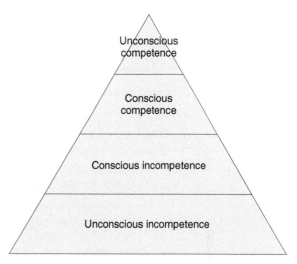

FIGURE 11.8 ■ Stages of competence.

## PERSONAL REFLECTIONS ON THE CONTINUING PROFESSIONAL DEVELOPMENT OF A NEWLY QUALIFIED PHYSIOTHERAPIST

This part of the chapter will be engaged in psychological elements through the key stages of a physiotherapist's training from preapplication through to qualifying and securing a Band 5 post. The stages demonstrate four states – 'lack'; 'awareness'; 'familiarity' and 'competence' – and will be linked to my evolving knowledge and application of psychology in my practice as well as my developing skills as a clinician. This is similar to the competence model of learning, shown in Figure 11.8, but does not correlate exactly with this because of the requirement for CPD in physiotherapy practice. It is perhaps useful to begin by explaining the four stages of competence. The origins of this theory are unclear but are represented next.

Table 11.2 takes these stages further and provides content and physiotherapy-specific examples using passive movements.

Before beginning my undergraduate physiotherapy university degree my knowledge and understanding of psychology was limited to the completion of a basic introductory course to counselling and I was therefore aware of Maslow's hierarchy of needs, open and closed questions, cognitive behavioural therapy (CBT), and the requirements of empathy and self-awareness. However, the course was brief and was meant as an introduction only. Although I had some knowledge and understanding, I lacked a great deal of the basic psychological understanding and skills relevant to physiotherapy. At the beginning of training I was not aware that psychology would form a huge part of the curriculum, I was highly focused on anatomy, physiology, vivas and doing as well as I could in all formal examinations. The first year consisted of learning muscle origins and insertions, the stages of inflammation, bony points and movement analysis – the main event was the vivas at the end of each semester. This relates to the first stage – 'lack' or unconscious

## TABLE 11.2

### Content- and Physiotherapy-Specific Examples Using Passive Movements

| Stage of Competence | Explanation of Concept | Physiotherapy-Specific Example |
|---|---|---|
| Unconscious incompetence | Person does not understand or know how to do something and does not recognize their deficit; may deny the usefulness of the skill<br><br>Person must first recognize their own incompetence, and the value of the new skill, before moving on to the next stage; how long they remain in this stage depends on the strength of their drive to learn | I don't know what passive movements are and I have no idea why or when I would use them |
| Conscious incompetence | Person does not understand or know how to do something, but does recognize the deficit and value of a new skill; making mistakes can be integral to the learning process at this stage | I know what passive movements are but I am unable to perform them at this point |
| Conscious competence | Person knows how to do something; however, demonstrating the skill or knowledge requires concentration | I can perform passive movements but I still have to think about my position, gaining consent, health and safety, dosages and so on |
| Unconscious competence | Person has had so much practice with a skill that it has become almost automatic<br><br>As a result, the skill can be performed while executing other tasks; person may now be able to teach it to others | I can perform passive movements in a variety of settings and can advise more junior staff on how to perform them |

incompetence, as I was unaware that I was missing certain skills. At this stage 'lack' should not be viewed as a negative, rather an appropriate springboard from which to learn.

However, as training progressed, there was a slight shift in emphasis not unconnected with the impending clinical placements and prospect of hands-on experience and real patients. Nonverbal communication was highlighted and discussed; subjective assessments were based around open questions to elicit as much information as possible and miss nothing; the concept of 'Yellow Flags' was introduced to help identify important information; goal setting in conjunction with the patient was promoted; internal and external loci of control was mentioned; self-efficacy and empowerment were discussed and the biopsychosocial model was introduced as the method with which it was best to work with patients. Interestingly it was only in clinical practice and after an in-service training that I understood how to begin to use the BPS model. After completing Keele University's screening tool, STarT Back, and being considered to be at high risk for persistent symptoms (currently recommended only for use with back pain), a patient is then assessed, not with the traditional biomedical model, but by using the biopsychosocial approach. This approach focuses on encouraging the patient to identify what the problem(s) is/are, what they want to start doing (or get back to doing) and working out ways in which to make these goals achievable. For example, if a patient's main problem is inactivity and they identify a love of walking the therapist must pick up on this and say this could be a goal – walking for 5 minutes every day. The focus here is on the patient – their goals, ability and their own management and understanding of the condition. It takes practice to become skilled at such assessments and this can be developed throughout a person's career through action, but also by observing others in the act.

Towards the end of training more concepts were introduced such as care of the complex patient and motivational interviewing – therapeutic alliance was touched upon as an emerging and potentially significant way of treating patients. This method is in its infancy within physiotherapy; however, it has been used widely within other spheres, namely counselling and mental health interventions. This relates to the awareness stage or conscious incompetence, where I was beginning to see that I did not have a certain skill set. I was being introduced to psychological techniques and was given the opportunity to use them in an academic setting.

On graduating and securing a position, I was more concerned with treating patients correctly, to the best of my ability in a timely manner and did not feel capable of consciously implementing psychological interventions until I felt I was able to do a 'good job'. However, once I had reached this stage I began to develop my understanding of the aforementioned concepts with real life scenarios. For example, I was able to identify Yellow Flags and crucially develop this to think how it could affect my assessment,

treatment efficacy and potential for discharge. With one reticent patient I used open questions and learned of a recent bereavement, I acknowledged this and moved on to discuss the medical complaint – thoracic pain –and realized that the bereavement was more significant; the pain could have been coming from the bereavement; the patient's physical pain may have been heightened as a result of psychological distress. In the first session I gave the patient basic movement exercises to do at home but my main focus was on allowing the patient to talk. This consisted largely of listening to the home situation, the days leading to the death of the relative and the inevitable ensuing emotions. The second treatment session focused again on listening to the patient speak about going on holiday; tellingly the pain had eased slightly but was still present intermittently. At the third and final session the patient had visibly relaxed; however, she still talked more of her deceased relative than the pain she was experiencing and reported that she was no longer concerned with the pain. In this situation the referral had come internally and the patient had already been screened for more serious pathology so I felt it appropriate to discharge on this third session with advice, education and an open appointment. It is difficult to measure what effect my management of this patient had on her medical and psychological condition. If I had not listened or allowed the patient to talk would the outcome have been the same; would the patient have had a different attitude towards physiotherapists reporting to family and friends that she felt listened to?

In short I felt that without incorporating psychological principles into my treatment, I was safe and effective to a basic standard;

however, I am now beginning to achieve better long-term patient outcomes and have become more attentive to the holistic picture, hence my effectiveness is increasing exponentially.

As I grew more in confidence with my clinical skills I was able to begin to use psychological interventions with proficiency and, most significantly, I was able to adapt and change the interventions to suit my needs. For example, I had become adept at using open questions to elicit information; however, one particular patient group – those loquacious individuals who are difficult to interrupt – required a change in intervention. This consisted of using closed questions much more readily so as to gain all relevant information and use the allocated time most effectively. As with all skills the repetitive usage of them improves your proficiency level and in the case of effectively having to stop someone from talking this can feel rude and difficult. Using eye contact for a similar effect has also been a useful tool. In this case offering the patient eye contact and allowing them to speak until they become aware of their own voice can also bring about silence, allowing for a return to relevant questioning.

This relates to the third stage – familiarity – as I was beginning to use the skills learned at the undergraduate level in a clinical setting. It is important to state that, although I may have developed conscious competence in some areas of clinical treatment, there are many elements which I have not and these continue to require development.

With continued clinical experience I did not change my approach to patients, instead I continued to learn from my patients, colleagues and senior members of staff and have developed as a clinician in all ways. My confidence in my own abilities has increased and

I am now treating more complex and challenging cases. One of my weaker areas was the management of more challenging patients; these patients would overwhelm me and I would pass them over to senior colleagues. The common theme with many of these patients was my inability to manage the patient *rather* than their condition or required treatment. Now I am able to manage these patients appropriately and to a timely discharge. My improvement in this area has occurred for a number of reasons: my own understanding of the pathways through the service, appropriate discharge, understanding the limitations of the service and, quite simply, having had more patient contact. This relates loosely to the final stage of competence, as I have developed my skills and am able to carry out my duties within my scope of practice as an autonomous practitioner. As mentioned earlier, with any occupation where continuing professional development is a key factor, I would not state I had reached unconscious competence at this early stage in my career.

However, that is not the whole story. As my clinical skills have improved and I have gained confidence in the identification of conditions and my handling and manual therapy skills, so too has my understanding of psychology. Psychology is another piece of the ever-expanding jigsaw of continuing professional development.

## PHYSIOTHERAPISTS AND PSYCHOLOGY – WHERE DO WE DRAW THE LINE?

Thus far this chapter has focussed on the importance of psychology and how physiotherapists may be able to implement it in patient contact. The, albeit limited, research suggests that it is a useful tool to develop and an area ripe for further study and discussion. However, it is worthwhile pausing and reflecting on the limitations of what we, as physiotherapists, should be doing with this tool and where our expertise ceases.

Physiotherapists often work very closely alongside a range of other health care professions – the list is long and varied dependent on the particular setting. Multidisciplinary team (MDT) working is an essential skill often noted on application forms for newly qualified posts. Indeed, multidisciplinary training, whereby health professions study a module together with a mixed cohort of health care professions, has recently been developed to aid in the communication and working as a part of a MDT once qualified. The benefits of understanding another profession's role are clear from recent research – colleagues understand the boundaries and scope of practice each other has, thus allowing for more effective communication and ultimately a smoother transition along the health care pathway for patients. For example, in an oncology discussion of cases within MDTs the planning of therapy was found to be much improved, as was the adherence to recommended preoperative assessment, pain control and adherence to medications (Taplin et al., 2016).

The reason for beginning the MDT training was as a result of a traditional hostility between professions based on protecting what each would see as 'their role; their duties'. For example, if an occupational therapist, as a part of their role, can encourage a patient to increase their physical activity around the home *and* provide them with equipment to help the patient achieve this, is the role of the physiotherapist redundant? It is important to know your limitations and identify when a patient may require professional help, the inclusion of psychology in physiotherapy interventions is not to eradicate the need or option of onward referral. Understanding our scope of practice is vital if we are to work within the CSP and HCPC professional codes of conduct.

## CLINICAL SCENARIOS

Four different scenarios with basic information about a potential patient are presented next. Answer the questions that follow each and discuss your answers with colleagues.

### Case Study 1

A 34-year-old female patient was diagnosed with fibromyalgia 7 years ago. She is attending physiotherapy as a result of a recent flare up of chronic pain. During the initial subjective assessment it becomes clear that the patient expects hands on treatment, possibly in the form of massage.
1. What do you think the patient believes are the benefits of therapeutic touch?
2. What do you believe, as her therapist, will be the benefits?
3. What are the potential pitfalls of touch?
4. What preconceptions may the client have about massage?

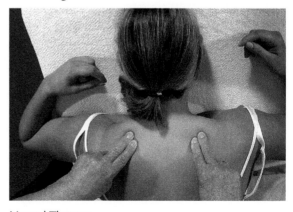

Manual Therapy.

## Case Study 2

A 67-year-old male patient with shoulder pain has been referred by his GP for increased levels of pain. The patient has not had acupuncture previously but is open to all treatment options.

1. What do you think the patient believes are the benefits of acupuncture?
2. What do you believe, as his therapist, will be the benefits?
3. How do the 'patients' lay beliefs about Western medicine *versus* traditional Chinese medicine affect the treatment outcome in this case?
4. Should lay beliefs be a factor, after all you are the professional?
5. How will you assess the importance of patient choice versus research evidence?

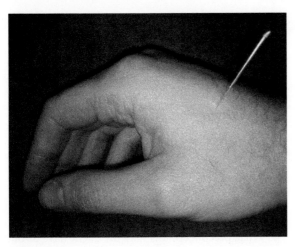

Acupuncture.

## Case Study 3

A 43-year-old female patient with a clinical diagnosis of unilateral carpal tunnel syndrome has previously found ultrasound to be beneficial (for a different condition) and asks if it would be a possibility for the present condition.

1. What do you think the patient believes are the benefits of therapeutic touch?
2. What do you believe, as her therapist, will be the benefits?
3. The department you work in is very 'anti' electrotherapy but the patient has had positive experiences with ultrasound in the past, discuss the approach you would take.
4. What are the patient benefits of using a machine to treat a person rather than hands on approaches?

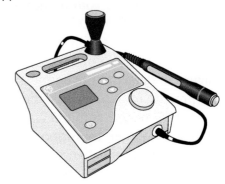

Ultrasound.

## *Case Study 4*

As part of a new initiative, your department has offered a patient education session with an excerpt marathon runner patient who has persistent shin splints. The session would consist of a discussion between the physiotherapist and excerpt patient on their condition, treatment, self-management and long-term outcomes.

1. What is/are the patient benefit(s) of this approach?
2. What is/are the drawback(s) to this type of treatment session?
3. What is/are the psychological effect(s) of such therapy?
4. No touch is involved – is this a problem?
5. This is a patient who has paid privately and is demanding a massage – discuss the approach that you would adopt with this patient.

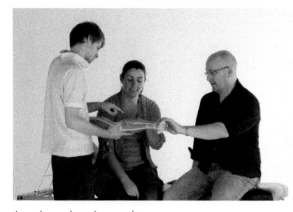

A patient education session.

## References

Al-Abri, R., Al-Balushi, A., 2014. Patient Satisfaction Survey as a Tool Towards Quality Improvement. Oman Medical Journal 29 (1), 3–7. doi:10.5001/omj.2014.02.

Alexanders, J., Anderson, A., Henderson, H. Musculoskeletal physiotherapists' use of psychological interventions: a systematic review of therapists' perceptions and practice Published Online: 11 November 2014 DOI: <http://dx .doi.org/10.1016/j.physio.2014.03.008> physiotherapy June 2015 Volume 101, Issue 2, Pages 95–102.

A qualitative and quantitative investigation of the psychology content of UK physiotherapy education.

Barlow, J.H., Macey, S.J., Struthers, G.R., 1993. Health locus of control, self-help and treatment adherence in relation to ankylosing spondylitis patients. Patient Educ. Couns. 20 (2–3), 153–166.

Burton, A.K., Wadell, G., Burtt, R., Blair, S., 1996. Patient education material in the management of low back pain in primary care. Bull. Hosp. Jt. Dis. 55, 138–141.

Chaplin, W.F., Davidson, K., Sparrow, V., Stuhr, J., van Roosmalen, E., Wallston, K.A., 2001. A structural evaluation of the expanded Multidimensional Health Locus of Control scale with a diverse sample of Caucasian/ European, Native, and Black Canadian women. J. Health Psychol. 6, 447–455.

CSP, 2002. Curriculum Framework for Qualifying Programmes in Physiotherapy. Chartered Society of Physiotherapy, London.

George, S.I., 2008. What is the effectiveness of a biopsychosocial approach to individual physiotherapy care for chronic low back pain? Internet J. Allied Health Sci. Pract. 6 (1), 1–10.

Green, A.J., Jackson, D.A., Klaber Moffett, J.A., 2008. An observational study of physiotherapists' use of cognitive-behavioural principles in the management of patients with back pain and neck pain. Physiotherapy 94 (4), 306–313.

HCPC, 2013. Standards of Proficiency Physiotherapists. Health and Care Professions Council, London.

Heaney, C., Green, A., Rostron, C., Walker, N., 2012. A qualitative and quantitative investigation of the psychology content of UK physiotherapy education. J. Phys. Ther. Educ. 26 (3)

Keedy, N.H., 2009. Health locus of control, self-efficacy, and multidisciplinary intervention for chronic back pain. Diakses pada 29 September 2014 19.38pm dari http:// ir.uiowa.edu/cgi/viewcontent.cgi?article=1571&context =etd.

Levenson, H., 1973. Multidimensional locus of control in psychiatric patients. J. Consult. Clin. Psychol. 41, 397–404.

Levenson, H., 1974. Activism and powerful others: Distinctions within the concept of internal external control. J. Pers. Assess. 38, 377–383.

Main, C.J., Waddell, G., 1991. A comparison of cognitive measures in low back pain: statistical structure and clinical validity at initial assessment. Pain 46 (3), 287–298.

Margalit, A.P.A., Glick, S.M., Benbassat, J., Cohen, A., 2004. Effect of a biopsychosocial approach on patient satisfaction and patterns of care. J. Gen. Intern. Med. 19 (5), 485–491.

Middleton, A., 2004. Chronic low back pain: patient compliance with physiotherapy advice and exercise, perceived barriers and motivation. Phys. Ther. Rev. 9 (3), 153–160.

Miller, J.S., Litva, A., Gabbay, M., 2009. Motivating patients with shoulder and back pain to self-care: can a videotape of exercise support physiotherapy? Physiotherapy 95 (1), 29–35.

Ormrod, J.E., 2006. Educational psychology: Developing learners, 5th ed. Pearson/Merrill Prentice Hall, Upper Saddle River, N.J.

Porter, S.B. (2010) Determinants of exercise behaviour in ankylosing spondyitis. PhD thesis. University of Central Lancashire UK.

Rotter, J.B., 1966. Generalized expectancies for internal versus external control of reinforcement. Psychol. Monogr. 80 (1), 1–28.

Sanders, T., Foster, N.E., Bishop, A., Ong, B.N., 2013. Biopsychosocial care and the physiotherapy encounter: physiotherapists' accounts of back pain consultations. BMC Musculoskelet. Disord. 14, 65. doi:10.1186/1471-2474-14-65.

Taplin, S.H., Weaver, S., Salas, E., Chollette, V., Edwards, H.M., Bruinoogeand, S.S., et al., 2016. Reviewing Cancer Care Team Effectiveness. J. Oncol. Pract. 12 (1).

Thomas, L., Schwenk, M.D., Dwight, L., Evans, M.D., Sally, K., Laden, M.S., et al., 2004. Treatment Outcome and Physician-Patient Communication in Primary Care Patients With Chronic, Recurrent Depression. Am. J. Psychiatry 161 (10), 1892–1901. <http://dx.doi.org/10.1176/ajp.161.10.1892>.

Waddell, G., 1987. A new clinical model for the treatment of low-back pain. Spine 12, 632–644.

Wallston, K.A., 2005. The validity of the multidimensional health locus of control scales. J. Health Psychol. 10 (5), 623–631.

Wallston, K.A., et al., 1999. Does God determine your health? The God locus of health control scale. Cognit. Ther. Res. 23, 131–142.

Wallston, K.A., Stein, M.J., Smith, C.A., 1994. Form C of the MHLC scales a condition – specific measure of locus of control. J. Pers. Assess. 63, 534–553.

Wallston, K.A., Wallston, B.S., DeVellis, R., 1978. Development of the multidimensional health locus of control (MHLC) scales. Health Educ. Monogr. 6, 160–170.

WHO, 2002. Towards a Common Language for Functioning, Disability and Health ICF. World Health Organization, Geneva. Preamble to the Constitution of the World Health Organization as adopted by the International Health Conference, New York, 19-22 June 1946; signed on 22 July 1946 by the representatives of 61 States (Official Records of the World Health Organization, no. 2, p. 100) and entered into force on 7 April 1948.

# INDEX

Page numbers followed by 'f' indicate figures, 't' indicate tables, and 'b' indicate boxes.